Immunology of
Renal Diseases

IMMUNOLOGY AND MEDICINE SERIES

Immunology of Endocrine Diseases
Editor: A. M. McGregor

Clinical Transplantation: Current Practice and Future Prospects
Editor: G. R. D. Catto

Complement in Health and Disease
Editor: K. Whaley

Immunological Aspects of Oral Diseases
Editor: L. Ivanyi

Immunoglobulins in Health and Disease
Editor: M. A. H. French

Immunology of Malignant Diseases
Editors: V. S. Byers and R. W. Baldwin

Lymphoproliferative Diseases
Editors: D. B. Jones and D. H. Wright

Phagocytes and Disease
Editors: M. S. Klempner, B. Styrt and J. Ho

Immunology of Sexually Transmitted Diseases
Editor: D. J. M. Wright

Mast Cells, Mediators and Disease
Editor: S. T. Holgate

Immunodeficiency and Disease
Editor: A. D. B. Webster

Immunology of Pregnancy and its Disorders
Editor: C. M. M. Stern

Immunotherapy of Disease
Editor: T. J. Hamblin

Immunology of Prophylactic Immunization
Editor: A. J. Zuckerman

Immunology of Eye Disease
Editor: S. Lightman

Lymphoproliferative Diseases
Editors: D. B. Jones and D. H. Wright

Immunology of Renal Diseases
Editor: C. D. Pusey

Biochemistry of Inflammation
Editors: J. T. Whicher and S. W. Evans

Immunology of ENT Disorders
Editor: G. Scadding

Immunology of Infection
Editors: J. G. P. Sissons, J. Cohen and L. K. Borysiewicz

Immunology of HIV Infection
Editor: A. G. Bird

Immunology of Gastrointestinal Diseases
Editor: T. T. MacDonald

IMMUNOLOGY

SERIES · SERIES · SERIES · SERIES AND SERIES · SERIES · SERIES · SERIES

MEDICINE

Volume 16

Immunology of Renal Diseases

Edited by
C. D. Pusey
Renal Unit, Department of Medicine
Royal Postgraduate Medical School
Hammersmith Hospital, London

Series Editor: K. Whaley

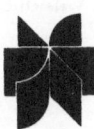

SPRINGER SCIENCE+BUSINESS MEDIA, B.V.

British Library Cataloguing in Publication Data

Immunology of renal diseases.
  1. Kidneys. Diseases
  I. Pusey, C. D.   II. Series
  616.61079

  ISBN 978-94-010-5738-7

Library of Congress Cataloging in Publication Data

Immunology of renal diseases/edited by C. D. Pusey.
      p.   cm. — (Immunology and medicine series; v. 16)
    Includes bibliographical references and index.
      ISBN 978-94-010-5738-7   ISBN 978-94-011-3902-1 (eBook)
      DOI 10.1007/978-94-011-3902-1
    1. Kidneys — Diseases — Immunological aspects. I. Pusey, C. D.
  II. Series.
      [DNLM: 1. Kidney Diseases — Immunology.   W1 IM53BI v.
  16/WJ 301 I33]
  RC903.I46   1991
  616.6'1079 — dc20
  DNLM/DLC
  for Library of Congress   91-7062
                                                                       CIP

Typeset by Technical Keying Services, Manchester.

Contents

Series Editor's Note   vii

Preface   viii

List of Contributors   ix

1   Immunogenetics of nephritis   1
A. Burns, P. Li and A. Rees

2   Introduction and regulation of autoimmune experimental glomerulonephritis   29
P. Druet

3   Molecular mechanisms of *in situ* immune complex formation in experimental membranous nephropathy   45
D. Kerjaschki

4   Immune complex handling in systemic lupus erythematosus   59
K. A. Davies and M. J. Walport

5   The membrane attack complex of complement in renal injury   81
G. M. Hänsch

6   Cell-mediated immunity in glomerulonephritis   97
S. R. Holdsworth and P. G. Tipping

7   Eicosanoids and cytokines in glomerular injury   123
J. D. Williams and M. Davies

8   Immunology of minimal-change nephropathy   161
G. Clark and D. G. Williams

9   IgA nephropathies and Henoch–Schonlein purpura   183
F. W. Ballardie

CONTENTS

10   C3 nephritic factor and membranoproliferative
     glomerulonephritis   215
       Y. C. Ng

11   Anti-glomerular basement membrane disease   229
       N. Turner and C. D. Pusey

12   Autoimmunity in systemic vasculitis   255
       D. R. W. Jayne and C. M. Lockwood

13   Immunopathogenic mechanisms of interstitial nephritis 271
       C. M. Meyers and C. J. Kelly

     Index   289

Series Editor's Note

The interface between clinical immunology and other branches of medical practice is frequently blurred and the general physician is often faced with clinical problems with an immunological basis and is expected to diagnose and manage such patients. The rapid expansion of basic and clinical immunology over the past two decades has resulted in the appearance of increasing numbers of immunology journals and it is impossible for a non-specialist to keep apace with this information overload. The *Immunology and Medicine* series is designed to present individual topics of immunology in a condensed package of information which can be readily assimilated by the busy clinician or pathologist.

K. Whaley, Glasgow
June 1991

Preface

Although it has been appreciated for many years that immune processes underlie most types of glomerulonephritis, it is the recent explosion in knowledge of cellular and molecular immunology that has prompted another book on the subject. The understanding of the mechanisms involved in renal injury requires the integration of information from *in vitro* cell-culture systems, experimental models of disease, and clinical studies. This volume draws on all of these sources in an attempt to explain current concepts of nephritis.

Increased emphasis is placed on autoimmune processes, as opposed to the deposition of circulating immune complexes, although it will be apparent that these may overlap in the area of "*in situ*" immune complex formation. Of central importance in autoimmunity is the relationship between antigen presenting cells (including B cells) expressing MHC class II molecules, autoantigenic peptides, T helper lymphocytes, and various effector cells. The mechanisms by which the immune system may lead to tissue injury are also becoming better understood, and consideration is given to the role of inflammatory cells, the complement proteins, and soluble factors such as cytokines and eicosanoids.

The way in which some of these basic processes operate in renal disease is considered in the early chapters, but much of the book is devoted to reviewing our current understanding of the immunology of the better-defined forms of nephritis. It is perhaps disappointing that this great increase in knowledge has led to so few major therapeutic advances, but as we continue to dissect out the cellular and molecular basis for these disorders, such advances must surely follow.

I would like to record my thanks to Professor Keith Peters for inspiring my interest in the immunology of nephritis, to my many colleagues for maintaining it, to all of the contributors for their excellent work, and to the publishers for their patience and encouragement.

C. D. Pusey

List of Contributors

F. W. BALLARDIE
Department of Medicine
Manchester Royal Infirmary
Oxford Road
Manchester M13 9WL
UK

A. BURNS
Renal Unit
Department of Medicine
Royal Postgraduate Medical School
Du Cane Road
London W12 0NN
UK

G. CLARK
United Medical and Dental Schools
  of Guy's and St Thomas' Hospitals
Clinical Science Laboratories
Guy's Tower
London Bridge
London SE1 9RT
UK

K. A. DAVIES
Rheumatology Unit
Department of Medicine
Royal Postgraduate Medical School
Du Cane Road
London W12 0NN
UK

M. DAVIES
Institute of Nephrology
Cardiff Royal Infirmary
Newport Road
Cardiff CF2 1SZ
UK

P. DRUET
INSERM U28
Hôpital Broussais
96 rue Didot
75674 Paris Cedex
France

G. M. HÄNSCH
Universität Heidelberg
Institut für Immunologie
Heidelberg
Germany

S. R. HOLDSWORTH
Monash University
Department of Medicine
Monash Medical Centre
Melbourne
Australia 3004

D. R. W. JAYNE
Department of Medicine
Clinical Medical School
Addenbrookes Hospital
Cambridge CB2 2QQ
UK

C. J. KELLY
Renal Electrolyte Section and the
  Immunology Graduate Group
University of Pennsylvania School
  of Medicine
700 Clinical Research Bldg.
422 Curie Blvd.
Philadelphia
Pennsylvania 19104
USA

D. KERJASCHKI
Department of Anatomical Pathology
University of Vienna
Allgemeines Krankenhaus
Spitalgasse 4
1090 Vienna
Austria

P. LI
Renal Unit
Department of Medicine
Royal Postgraduate Medical School
Du Cane Road
London W12 0NN
UK

LIST OF CONTRIBUTORS

C. M. LOCKWOOD
Department of Medicine
Clinical Medical School
Addenbrookes Hospital
Cambridge CB2 2QQ
UK

C. M. MEYERS
Renal Electrolyte Section
University of Pennsylvania School
 of Medicine
700 Clinical Research Bldg.
422 Curie Blvd.
Philadelphia
Pennsylvania 19104
US

Y. C. NG
Division of Molecular and Clinical
 Rheumatology
The Johns Hopkins University
 School of Medicine
Baltimore
Maryland 21205
USA

C. D. PUSEY
Renal Unit
Department of Medicine
Royal Postgraduate Medical School
Du Cane Road
London W12 0NN
UK

A. J. REES
Renal Unit
Department of Medicine
Royal Postgraduate Medical School
Du Cane Road
London W12 0NN
UK

P. G. TIPPING
Monash University
Department of Medicine
Monash Medical Centre
Melbourne
Australia 3004

N. TURNER
Renal Unit
Department of Medicine
Royal Postgraduate Medical School
Du Cane Road
London W12 0NN
UK

M. J. WALPORT
Rheumatology Unit
Department of Medicine
Royal Postgraduate Medical School
Du Cane Road
London W12 0NN
UK

D. G. WILLIAMS
United Medical and Dental Schools
 of Guy's and St Thomas' Hospitals
Clinical Science Laboratories
Guy's Tower
London Bridge
London SE1 9RT
UK

J. D. WILLIAMS
Institute of Nephrology
Cardiff Royal Infirmary
Newport Road
Cardiff CF2 1SZ
UK

1
Immunogenetics of Nephritis

A. BURNS, P. LI and A. REES

Since the earliest attempts to understand the pathogenesis of nephritis there has been great interest in genetic factors that may contribute to susceptibility. For example, Wells in 1812[1], noted that the siblings of a child who developed nephritis after an attack of scarlet fever were much more likely to develop nephritis than the siblings of children who did not develop nephritis after scarlatina. This observation, which has been confirmed many times, implies that constitutional factors influence susceptibility to nephritis. Experimental models have provided more detailed information. Germuth and colleagues showed that suceptibility to, and severity of, nephritis in chronic serum sickness were determined by variation in the magnitude of the antibody response[2]. Inheritance determines both the magnitude and avidity of antibody response in mice[3,4], and Devey and Stewart have shown that these differences are important in the pathogenesis of chronic serum sickness[5]. These early studies concentrated on factors which had generalized effects on antibody responses to exogenous antigens, because it was widely believed at the time that glomerulonephritis was caused by circulating immune complexes with resultant granular deposits of immunoglobulin in the glomeruli.

The realization that granular deposits could also be caused by antibodies to cell surface antigens raised the question of whether autoimmunity might be a common cause of nephritis, and not just restricted to anti-glomerular basement membrane (GBM) antibody-mediated disease. It was not long before this was shown to be the case in rodents[6] and there is now similar, though necessarily more preliminary, evidence for this in patients[7-11]. This important change in emphasis focused attention on the control of individual immune responses rather than on immune responsiveness in general.

The critical event in the development of an immune response is presentation of antigen to helper T lymphocytes, and it is this that is probably responsible for discrimination of self from foreign antigen. Antigen 'processing' is the first stage and involves antigen being internalized by antigen-presenting cells before being partially digested. Processed antigen is re-expressed on the cell

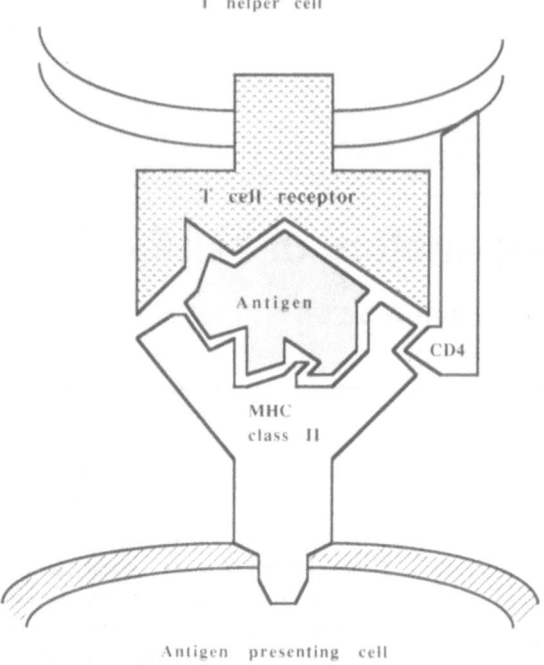

Figure 1 Diagrammatic representation of the trimolecular complex

surface bound to a major histocompatibility complex (MHC) molecule[12]. T cell receptors can only recognize antigenic peptides when bound to MHC molecules. Recent crystallographic studies of the three-dimensional structure of MHC molecules have shown that the outer domains, which are highly polymorphic, form an antigen-binding groove[13]. Single amino acid substitutions can change the three-dimensional conformation of the groove and alter the range of antigenic peptides that it can bind[14]. This is thought to be the basis of the allele-specific effects which define the 'immune response genes' that are believed to be responsible for many of the MHC associated influences on autoimmunity.

Antigen-bearing MHC molecules bind directly to T cell receptors[15] and this trimolecular complex (Figure 1) is crucial to the development of immune responses. It may initiate the destruction of autoreactive T cells during ontogeny in the thymus[16,17]; it is essential for the generation of T cell help to delayed hypersensitivity and antibody responses[18]; and it is possibly responsible for antigen-specific suppression[19]. Thus the trimolecular complex provides important opportunities for directing immune responses and for eliminating potentially harmful responses during development, a process referred to as 'moulding of T cell repertoire'.

The contribution of the MHC to susceptibility to glomerulonephritis is

2

MHC

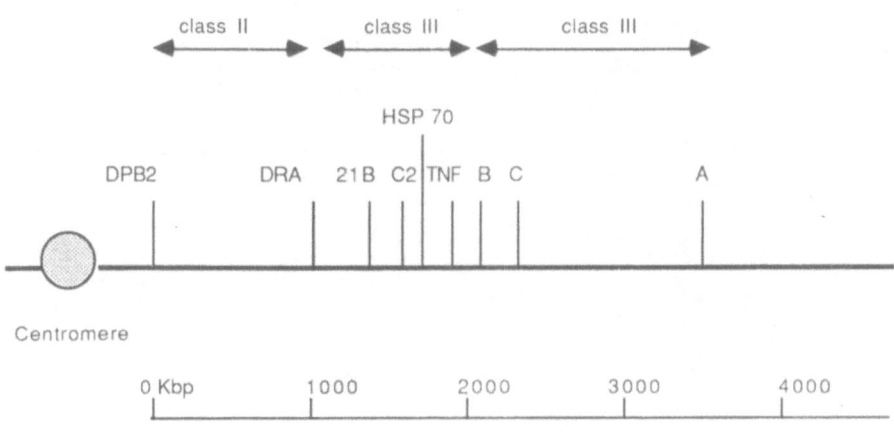

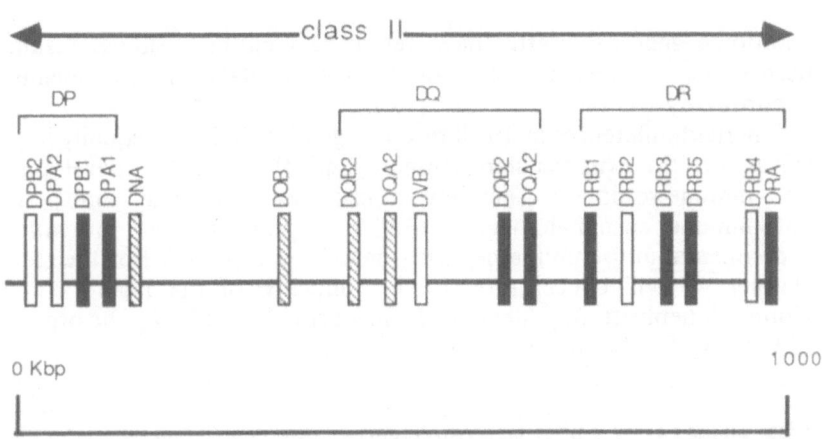

Figure 2 Physical map of the human MHC. The number of expressed genes and pseudogenes varies according to the haplotype. For the Class II region, expressed genes are depicted in black, pseudogenes in white, and undefined genes with cross-hatched markings

increasingly obvious. Druet and his colleagues (1977) used classical breeding techniques to show that the MHC played an essential role in the development of anti-GBM antibody-mediated disease in Brown Norway (BN) rats injected with mercuric chloride[20]. They bred various combinations of susceptible BN strain rats with non-susceptible Lewis rats, to show that the response was determined by the BN class II genes together with a small number of

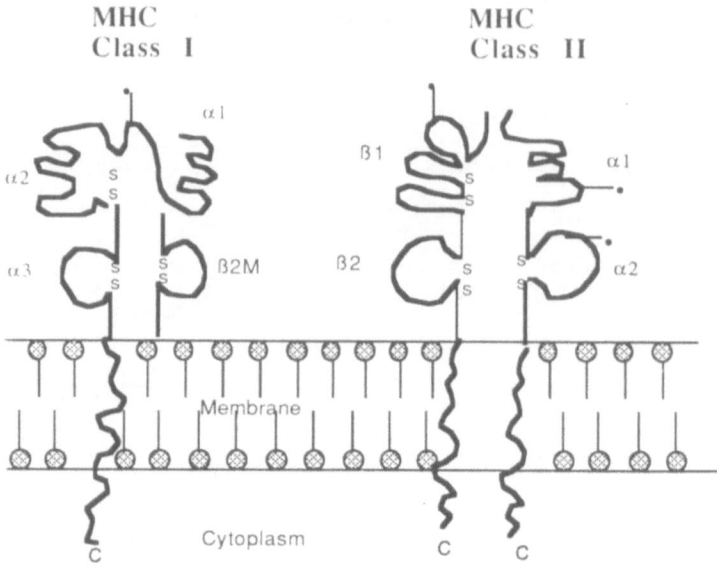

Figure 3 Class I and Class II HLA antigens are similar in structure. S–S indicates disulphide bonds between cysteine residues; C indicates carboxy-terminus; ● indicates carbohydrate side-chains

additional genes; the latter have yet to be identified. Similar results have been reported in Heymann nephritis, the experimental analogue of membranous nephropathy[6].

Inherited differences in T cell receptor genes could have equally important effects on the trimolecular complex and thus on the development of autoimmune responses. They have already been implicated in experimental autoimmune encephalomyelitis (EAE)[21-23], but to date no studies on experimental autoimmune nephritis have been reported. For the rest of the chapter we will concentrate on the influence of the HLA complex on glomerulonephritis in patients and will start by considering the organization of human MHC in detail.

THE HUMAN MAJOR HISTOCOMPATIBILITY COMPLEX

One major focus of the efforts to understand the inheritance of autoimmune nephritis has been the attempt to identify genes within the human MHC which confer susceptibility to nephritis. These studies have been based largely on finding associations between Class II serological specificities and disease. The results have been difficult to interpret and complicated further by the nomenclature that is used to describe the HLA Class II system. The advent of DNA recombinant technology, however, has greatly expanded knowledge of this system and has facilitated more accurate assignment of HLA alleles. It will ultimately simplify the hitherto very difficult nomenclature, as alleles will be assigned definitive names on the basis of their nucleotide sequence.

Several recent technical developments have facilitated more detailed studies of this region. First, restriction fragment length polymorphism (RFLP) analysis using cDNA probes to MHC genes; this can be used to assign MHC types from genomic DNA. Second, the nucleotide sequence of HLA Class II genes can now be established relatively easily, and third, analysis of DNA for the presence of particular polymorphisms can readily be accomplished by differential hybridization with sequence-specific oligonucleotide probes. These latter two techniques have become possible with the development of the *in vitro* DNA amplification technique, the polymerase chain reaction (PCR), which greatly increases the number of copies of a target DNA sequence.

The genes that encode the MHC lie on the short arm of the chromosome 6 in the distal portion of the 6p21.3 band (Figure 2)[24,25]. The complex contains three regions, designated classes II, III and I in order from the centromere. Their genetic organization has been elucidated using gene cloning and DNA sequencing. Class I and II genetic loci are highly polymorphic[26], the Class III locus less so. The products of these classes have been characterized serologically and biochemically.

The Class I region consists of HLA-A, B and C loci. Genes at these loci encode cell surface antigens which are expressed on most nucleated cells. At least 24 different HLA-A antigens, 50 HLA-B antigens and 11 HLA-C antigens have been identified serologically. Class I molecules consist of two polypeptide chains. The 44 kD heavy chain spans the plasma membrane and has an extracellular portion divided into three domains (α_1, α_2 and α_3), each of about 90 amino acids encoded by separate exons. The heavy chain is bound covalently to β_2 microglobulin (β_{2m}). The α_3 domain and β_{2m} are relatively conserved, while the α_1 and α_2 domains are highly polymorphic (Figure 3).

The three-dimensional structures of two different Class I molecules, HLA-A2 and HLA-A68, have been revealed by X-ray crystallography[13]. The α_1 and α_2 domains form a platform composed of a single beta-pleated sheet topped by alpha helices, which together form a long antigen-binding groove[15]. Differences in amino acid sequence influence the three-dimensional shape of the antigen-binding groove, and presumably the peptides that they are able to bind[14]. Antigen-bearing MHC Class I molecules bind to CD8$^+$ cells of cytotoxic or supressor phenotypes.

The MHC Class II region contains genes encoding at least three expressed Class II molecules DR, DQ, and DP (Figure 2). Each of these is a heterodimer consisting of an α and β chain (Figure 3). The α chains are encoded by single functional genes (DPα1, DQα and DRα), but the beta chains are more complicated. DP and DQ β chains are also encoded by single functional genes (DPβ1, DQβ), but the DRα chain products can combine with products of at least two beta chains (DRβi and DRβiii). Binding to the βi chain is responsible for DR specificities 1–10, whereas binding to the βiii chain is responsible for DRw52 and DRw53 specificities. Finally, there are at least eight other genes in this region which are not expressed and are referred to as pseudogenes. The products of Class II genes are heterodimers consisting of heavy (α) and light (β) chains with molecular weights 30–34 kD and 26-29 kD respectively. They form four external domains, two on each chain—α_1

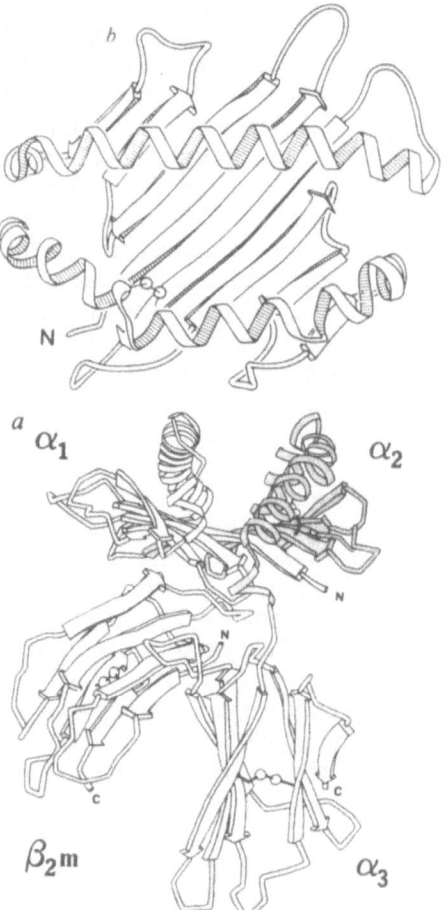

Figure 4 Structure of the HLA Class I molecule HLA-A2 as deduced by Bjorkman *et al.*[13] The upper figure shows the antigen-binding groove viewed from above, while the lower figure shows a side-on view of the molecule (reproduced with permission)

and α_2 and β_1 and β_2 respectively. The α_2 and β_2 domains lie closest to the plasma membrane and are highly conserved immunoglobulin-like molecules, while the two distal (N-terminal) domains α_1 and β_1 carry the polymorphic determinants[27].

All the expressed Class II β chain genes are polymorphic. There are at least 18 DRβ alleles, 10 DQβ alleles and 14 DPβ alleles. There is much less polymorphism of the α chain genes. Only DQα is extensively polymorphic and it has at least eight alleles. HLA-DR1 has been crystallized and shown to have a structure broadly similar to that of the Class I molecules, though the exact three-dimensional structure has yet to be elucidated. Nevertheless, a hypothetical model of the foreign antigen-binding site of Class II histocompatibility molecules has been proposed by Brown *et al.*, and is generally thought to be very accurate (Figure 4)[13].

HLA-DR molecules bind antigenic peptides, and experiments using site-directed mutagenesis have shown that single amino acid substitutions at critical positions alter their capacity to bind antigenic peptides. MHC Class II molecules are expressed principally on macrophages, B lymphocytes and activated T cells. Antigen-bearing Class II molecules bind to T cell receptors on CD4$^+$ lymphocytes of helper phenotype. It is not yet clear which domains on class II molecules perform which functions.

The Class III region is very diverse, spans 120 kb between Class I and Class II, and is less well characterized. It contains an undertermined number of apparently unrelated genes, including those encoding complement components C4, C2, and factor B, tumour necrosis factor α and β, heat-shock proteins of the HSP60 family, collagen type XI and adrenal steroid 21-hydroxylase enzymes. Other, as yet unidentified, genes are also though to be located there.

The genes for C2 and factor B lie about 400 bp apart and both are polymorphic, though much less so than Class I and II genes. Endonucleases have been used to define RFLPs of the C2 and BF genes[28]. At least five DNA polymorphisms have been defined in a 20 kb segment of DNA encompassing the C2 and BF loci. These reflect polymorphisms of the complement components and are usually detected serologically on the basis of electrophoretic mobility. C2 has three variants, C2A, C2B and C2C; C2C is the commonest with a gene frequency of 0.97, whereas C2A and C2B are much rarer. There are patients who are C2-deficient with a C2Q0 gene (Q0: quantity zero). Polymorphisms of BF have been detected by agrose gel electrophoresis. The two major variants are BFF (fast gene product) and BFS (slow gene product). There are two minor variants and up to 14 rarer variants. In caucasoids, the BFS allele is the commonest with a gene frequency of 0.7, and no factor B deficiency has been identified.

C4 is a serum glycoprotein which occurs in two forms C4A and C4B. C4A and C4B are both extensively polymorphic in man, with 13 alleles at the C4A locus and 22 at the C4B locus identified by protein electrophoresis. Null alleles are characterized by the absence of any bands, and are designated Q0, for example C4AQ0 and C4BQ0. Null alleles at either C4A or C4B are relatively common and are found in about 25% of caucasoids. Complete deficiency of C4, i.e. an individual with two null alleles at both loci, is found in less than 5% of people. C4B is more active than C4A in haemolytic assays, but although it is the subject of considerable interest there is no information about the relative activities of allelic variants.

Recombination between C2, BF, C4A and C4B loci has not been observed in man, so genes in this region display very strong linkage disequilibrium. This means that identifying the allele at a particular locus allows one to predict those that will be present at other loci and for this reason combinations of alleles at C2, BF, C4A and C4B are often referred to as complotypes[29]. Only 15 of these complotypes are observed in caucasians, the commonest being BFS, C2C, C4A3, C4B1, abbreviated SC31, which has a gene frequency of about 40%. In many cases this linkage disequilibrium extends to neighbouring HLA-B and HLA-DR loci; when this occurs they are termed extended haplotypes[30]. It is interesting that the three commonest extended haplotypes, namely B8, SC01, DR3 and B7, SC31, DR2 and B44, SC30, DR4, have all been associated with autoimmunity. This phenomenon has obvious implications when trying to interpret the reasons for associations between HLA genes and disease. It is often impossible to decide which genetic locus is more important in disease susceptibility, and indeed it may be that these alleles occurring together confer disease susceptibility.

Analysis of Data

Specific genetic loci can only be linked to a disease by studying families with more than one affected member[31]. The rarity of such affected kindred effectively precludes this approach in patients with glomerulonephritis. It follows that the involvement of the HLA complex must be inferred from the association with a particular HLA gene product. This can be ascertained from samples of patients and healthy controls, but only after certain preconditions have been satisfied. First, the population from which disease and control samples are drawn must be homogeneous, because the same disease may be associated with different HLA-molecules in different racial groups. This is illustrated in Table 1, which compares the HLA markers for nephritis in European caucasoids and Japanese. The need for study population homogeneity presents considerable difficulties when attempting to study populations such as those of the United States, where considerable racial admixture has occurred recently through immigration. The second precondition is that associations are much more likely to be found when the disease under consideration is a single entity, and when all patients are studied at the same stage of their disease. Lastly, appropriate statistical approaches must be used[32].

Table 1 Differences in significant HLA associations between European caucasiodes and Japanese

	Associated HLA antigen	
Disease	Caucasoids	Japanese
Membranous nephropathy	DR3	DR2
Minimal-change nephropathy	DR7	DR8
Mesangial IgA disease	–	DR4

Associations between HLA antigens and disease are defined in terms of their statistical significance and their strength. The various methods to determine statistical significance have been reviewed by Thompson[33]. The usual approach is to calculate the probability from contingency table and then make an appropriate correction for multiple comparisons[34]. Probability values from the first study of a particular disease are multiplied by the number of comparisons made because of the lack of a prior hypothesis. Subsequent studies to confirm a previously suspected association need no correction. Two basic measures are commonly used to define the strength of an association (Table 2). The relative risk (RR) is a simple measure of the increased risk of developing the disease conferred by a genetic marker. It does not measure the closeness of association between marker and disease,

Table 2 Measures of the strength of association between HLA antigens and disease

Test	Calculation
Relative risk (RR) (scale: >0)	$\dfrac{\text{Patients}\ (+)\ \text{marker}}{\text{Patients}\ (-)\ \text{marker}} \times \dfrac{\text{Control}\ (-)\ \text{marker}}{\text{Control}\ (+)\ \text{marker}}$
Etiological fraction (EF) (scale: 0–1)	$\dfrac{(RR-1)}{RR} \times \dfrac{\text{Patients}\ (+)}{\text{Total patients}}$
Preventive fraction (PF) (scale: 0–1)	$\dfrac{\dfrac{(1-RR)}{RR} \times \dfrac{\text{Patients}\ (+)}{\text{Total patients}}}{1 - \dfrac{\text{Patients}\ (+)}{\text{Total patients}} + \dfrac{\text{Patients}\ (+)}{\text{Total patients}}}$

and is strongly influenced by the frequency of the marker in the control sample. The closeness of associations is most easily assessed by the aetiological fraction (EF). This measure has only recently been applied to HLA data[32], but it is traditional in epidemiology where it is known as the population attributable risk. Essentially, it measures the proportion of the disease that can be attributed to the associated marker. It is independent of the frequency of marker in the control sample and can be used to compare directly the strengths of association of different markers[32]. It can also be used to estimate the degree of linkage disequilibrium between marker and susceptibility genes, provided the mode of inheritance is known[35]. The EF can only be calculated when the frequency of the marker is greater in patient samples than in controls, i.e. the RR is greater than 1. Some HLA antigens are significantly less frequent in patients than in controls and appear to confer protection. The degree of protection can be estimated by a method, analogous to the EF, which is called the preventive fraction (PF)[36]. The method for calculating it is shown in Table 2.

The difference between RR and EF is exemplified by the results of studies in membranous nephropathy. In one set of studies[37], the frequency of HLA-DR3 in patients was 75% and in controls 20%, while the frequencies of the complement allotype BfF1 were 22% and 1.7% respectively. Thus the relative risk conferred by BfF1 was greater than for DR3 (16 compared to 12) even though it was found in fewer patients. By contrast, the EF associated with BfF was considerably less than that of HLA-DR3 (0.20 compared to 0.72).

These basic measures should be used to assess the statistical and biological significance of HLA and disease associations, but can often be used to deduce more. It is comparatively simple to test various models of inheritance of disease susceptibility genes and to look for interactive effects of gene products inherited at different loci. Whether the increased frequency of the second antigen is merely a consequence of linkage disequilibrium or whether the inheritance of both antigens together is important in determining susceptibility is clearly very important. Karlin and Piazzi[38] have compared methods of analysing this kind of problem, and Porta and McHugh[39] have devised a method applicable to testing the association of two HLA antigens with a disease. The availability of such methods, and the ability to combine data from separate studies emphasizes the need for reporting complete HLA data and the need to avoid the statement 'no significant differences were observed'. This is particularly important in interpreting data from loci which are in strong linkage disequilibrium, such as those involving extended haplotypes.

ASSOCIATION WITH DISEASE

It is obvious from the preceding discussion that the interpretation of studies correlating HLA alleles with disease is complicated and fraught with uncertainty. Most of the information from patients with glomerulonephritis comes from four diseases: Goodpasture's syndrome due to anti-GBM antibodies, membranous nephropathy, mesangial IgA disease, and steroid responsive minimal change nephropathy. These will be discussed first and used to illustrate the difficulties of interpreting statistical as well as biological significance.

Anti-glomerular basement membrane disease

Human anti-GBM disease is an autoimmune disorder characterized by the presence of autoantibodies directed against a target restricted to the glomerular and a few other specialized basement membranes. It is unique amongst the nephritides in that the antibody which characterizes the disease is known to be pathogenic[40]. Anti-GBM antibodies have highly restricted specificity and are thought to react with epitopes that reside in a novel chain of type IV collagen[41,42]. Genetic factors undoubtedly play a role in susceptibility to this disease. A familial incidence has been described and the disease has been reported in four sibling pairs[43,44], including two sets of identical twins[43,45]. However, the importance of non-genetic factors is emphasized by two sets of identical twins, in our series, who are discordant for the disease[46].

The first report of an HLA association with anti-GBM disease came from the UK, when the frequency of the Class II allele HLA-DR2 was found to be greatly increased[47]. It was present in 88% of 17 patients diagnosed by immunohistology and radioimmunoassay compared to 32% of a panel of 100 controls. The strength of the association (relative risk 16) meant that the association was statistically significant despite the small numbers. The incidence of HLA-B7 was also increased in these studies, though to a lesser extent, and this was due to the high degree of linkage disequilibrium between HLA-DR2 and B7. A later study extended this series to 38 patients, 34 of whom (88%) had DR2 compared to 19% of 153 controls[48]. Currently, 75% of all 95 patients on whom we have DR types are DR2. Thus, the findings are remarkably consistent and there is little doubt that, in the UK at least, HLA-DR2, or genes in strong linkage disequilibrium with them, confer susceptibility to anti-GBM disease. Two studies elsewhere support this conclusion. Perle *et al.* in Australia reported that 7 of 8 patients with anti-GBM disease had DR2[49], and Garavoy in the United States found a lower but still significantly increased frequency of DR2, which was present in 23 of 46 patients, although no clinical details were provided[50].

The association of HLA alleles with anti-GBM disease is now recognized to be more complicated. The frequency of DR4 was consistently increased in the early studies from the UK, but never reached statistical significance. This was partly because of the small number of patients studied, but also because of limitations in the serological typing procedures used at the time. In a more recent study of 53 patients who were allogenotyped using RFLP analysis[51], the frequencies of DR2 (77% compared to 31%) and DR4 (44% compared to 37%) were increased, although DR2 remained the stronger and only significant association. DR4 was found in 8 of 13 (62%) non-DR2 patients, and overall 92% of patients possessed DR2, DR4 or both. Association of more than one DR allele with a disease is not unique, and has previously been described in diabetes (DR3 and 4) and in rheumatoid arthritis (DR1 and 4). DR alleles can also confer protection against disease, as has been described for DR2 in diabetes mellitus. This appears to be the case in anti-GBM disease, as DR1 and DRw6 are both found very infrequently (2.7% and 7.5% respectively) in our patients.

The very strong linkage disequilibrium between DR and DQ genes means that a given DR allele is almost invariably inherited together with a particular DQ allele. For example, almost all DR2 caucasoid individuals also inherit DQw6, and similarly caucasoid individuals who inherit DR4 also have either DQw7 or DQw8 (in a ratio of 30:70 in control caucasoid populations). This has considerable influence on the frequency of DQ allotypes in our patients with anti-GBM disease. HLA-DQw6, 7 and 8 were found in 79%, 34% and 25% respectively ($n = 53$), compared to control frequencies of 41%, 27% and 36% ($n = 1103$).

The obvious questions are which genes in these haplotypes are responsible for susceptibility, and why different haplotypes confer susceptibility to the same disease. These questions have been studied extensively in diabetes, in which it appears that the absence of an aspartic acid residue at position 57 of the DQβ chain is important for susceptibility[52], but that this has to be inherited in the context of particular DR alleles[53] or by implication as part of an extended haplotype. This type of analysis of DQ and DR genes in anti-GBM disease suggests that phenylalanine at position 26 of the DRβ chain may be important. It is easy to speculate that differences such as these could be involved in presentation of the autoantigen. Very soon it will be possible to test these predictions *in vitro* using purified autoantigen, mouse cells transfected with particular DR and DQ genes, and antigen-specific T cells, to assess the ability of individual Class II molecules to present autoantigen effectively.

Idiopathic membranous nephropathy

Idiopathic membranous nephropathy (IMN) is a major cause of nephrotic syndrome in adults. It is characterized by diffuse thickening of the glomerular capillary wall with granular deposition of immunoglobulins and complement visible on immunofluorescence and subepithelial electron-dense deposits

Table 3 Idiopathic membranous nephropathy: HLA-DR3 antigen frequency in caucasians

Author (year)	Ref.	Country	Patients % (n)	Controls % (n)	RR* >1	EF** 0-1
Klouda (1979)	[63]	UK	75 (32)	20 (60)	12	–
Garovoy (1980)	[110]	UK	73 (55)	21 (3184)	8.7	–
Garovoy (1980)	[110]	Spain	67 (39)	21 (3184)	7.5	0.58
Garovoy (1980)	[110]	USA	33 (33)	21 (3184)	1.9	0.16
Muller (1981)	[59]	Germany	76 (21)	23 (122)	10.7	0.70
Le Petit (1982)	[111]	France	65 (26)	20 (74)	7.42	0.57
Rashid (1983)	[62]	UK	53 (35)	27 (325)	3.05	0.35
Papiha (1987)	[73]	UK	52 (55)	23 (70)	3.64	–
Zucchelli (1987)	[108]	Italy	55 (55)	25 (65)	3.67	0.397
Roccatello (1987)	[112]	Italy	61 (18)	17 (526)	7.6	–
Vaughan (1989)	[58]	UK	65 (31)	37 (55)	2.9	0.41

* Relative risk
** Aetiological fraction

Table 4 Idiopathic membranous nephropathy: HLA-DR2 antigen frequency in Japanese

Author (year)	Ref.	Country	Patients % (n)	Controls % (n)	RR* >1	EF** 0-1
Tomura (1984)	[61]	Japan	74 (50)	30 (158)	6.5	–
Hiki (1984)	[60]	Japan	80 (50)	36 (884)	7.12	–

* Relative risk
** Aetiological fraction

evident on electron microscopy. There is little doubt that IMN is an immunologically mediated disease, although the mechanism is uncertain. Identical appearances can be produced experimentally, either by autoantibodies to glomerular epithelial cells in rats with Heyman nephritis[54] or by 'serum sickness' after injection of cationic antigens into rabbits.

Familial membranous nephropathy has been described in five pairs of brothers[55,56], two pairs being monozygotic twins[56,57]. Results from studies of the HLA complex show that heredity plays an important part in susceptibility. IMN has been repeatedly associated with certain HLA antigens, especially the Class II allele HLA-DR3. The various studies of DR3 in IMN are summarized in Table 3. In caucasoids, 55–78% of patients who develop IMN have the DR3 allele compared with 20–25% of controls. Similar studies in Japanese patients show an equally strong association between IMN and HLA-DR2 (Table 4). HLA-DR3 is very uncommon in Japanese, but even so it is not clear why IMN should be associated with different DR alleles in caucasoid and Japanese populations.

There are at least three plausible explanations: first, that both DR molecules share the properties needed to confer susceptibility to the disease; second, that the DR molecules themselves do not confer susceptibility, but are in linkage disequilibrium with the single true susceptibility gene and that the

Table 5 Idiopathic membranous nephropathy: MT (supertypic) DR antigen frequency

Author (year)	Ref.	Country	Patients % (n)	Controls % (n)	RR* >1	EF** 0–1
MT2						
I.H.W.*** (1980)		USA	92 (24)	53 (>3000)	9.7	–
Muller (1981)	[59]	Germany	6 (21)	53 (122)	5.4	–
MT1						
Tomura (1984)	[61]	Japan	86 (43)	60 (158)	4.1	–
Hiki (1984)	[60]	Japan	96 (50)	49 (103)	24.5	–

*   Relative risk
**   Aetiological fraction
*** International Histocompatibility Workshop

linkage is different in Japanese and caucasoids; and third, that the pathogenesis of MGN is different in different populations.

A recent report by Vaughan et al.[58] adds support to the second hypothesis. Using RFLP analysis of genomic DNA they confirmed the serological association between DR3 and IMN in a group of 31 patients. Only one of two subtypes of DR3 was found to be increased and, in addition, they observed a 4.5 kb DQA RFLP to occur with even greater frequency in the IMN patients than DR3. This RFLP pattern defines the DQA1 allele which is inherited exclusively with DR3 and DR5. Using data from two other published studies, Vaughan et al. made an indirect estimate of the likely frequency of this 4.5 kb DQA RFLP in the two reported groups of IMN patients and found them to be remarkably similar to their own findings. Thus, it is proposed that the DQ rather than the DR region is important in susceptibility to IMN, and that the DR3 and DR5 DQA1 allele, which is different from other DQA1 genes, is an important susceptibility factor in caucasoid IMN.

The MT system was defined by a collection of sera that react to 'public' determinants common to several DR specificities. MT1 is usually associated with DR1 and 2, MT2 with DR3, DR5, DRw6 and DRw8, and MT3 and DR4 and DR7. Not surprisingly, results using sera to define these specificities reflect inheritance of underlying DR types and provide no additional data. MT2 has been associated with IMN in the United States and Germany[59]. In Japanese populations, however, the association is with MT1[60,61] (Table 5).

HLA Class I genes have also been associated with IMN, though again this probably reflects linkage disequilibrium. Rashid[62] in a study of 34 patients found 53% had B8 compared to 25% of controls ($p < 0.001$, RR = 3.3). Others have reported significant associations with B18[63]. Both B8 and B18 are in linkage disequilibrium with DR3. Rashid[62] found that the association with B8 was statistically significant, whereas the association with DR3 was not. Even so, inspection of Tables 3 to 5 indicates that the differences in this study are likely to be due to the small number of patients, rather than to be biologically significant. Muller[59] and Le Petit[64] agree that the primary and stronger association is with DR3, and that the secondary association is with B8 by virtue of linkage disequilibrium.

Genes which code for the complement protein-factor B of the alternative pathway may also be important in the development of IMN. Dyer et al.[65] reported a very significant increase in the rare allotype BfF1 in patients with IMN compared with controls. This allele is in linkage disequilibrium with B18 and DR3.

Mesangial IgA nephropathy

Mesangial IgA nephropathy (IgAN) is probably the commonest primary glomerulonephritis in the world[66], and a significant proportion of affected patients develop end-stage renal failure[67]. Patients with IgA nephropathy have a generalized disease of cellular and humoral immunity[7,68]. An autoimmune model has been postulated for the disease recently, because IgG autoantibodies against specific determinants on mesangial cells have been found in sera from some patients[8].

The familial incidence of IgAN is well described in both caucasoid and Japanese populations, and there are reports of disease in HLA-identical siblings and in twins. A number of studies[17,69-74], though not all[75,76], have linked familial IgAN to particular alleles, but are not powerful enough to implicate the HLA system in susceptibility. The results of population studies attempting to correlate IgAN with specific HLA alleles have been even more confusing. In 1978, Berthoux and colleagues reported IgA nephropathy to be significantly associated with HLA-Bw35, but only a minority of subsequent studies have had similar findings (Tables 6 and 7). Attempts to explain these

Table 6 Mesangial IgA nephropathy: HLA-Bw35 antigen frequencies in caucasians

Author (year)	Ref.	Country	Patients % (n)	Controls % (n)	RR* >1	EF** 0-1
Berthoux (1978)	[113]	France	39 (43)†	13 (105)	4.2	0.2
Brettle (1978)	[114]	UK	18 (34)	13 (200)	1.34	0.04
Noel (1978)	[115]	France	48 (29)†	19 (112)	3.199	0.36
Nagy (1979)	[116]	Hungary	4 (24)	15 (60)	0.25	0.36
Savi (1979)	[117]	Italy	9 (23)	23 (236)	0.32	–
Macdonald (1980)	[118]	Australia	70 (17)	15	–	–
Bignon (1980)	[119]	France	14 (73)	12 (284)	1.17	0.02
Faucet (1980)	[120]	France	29 (42)	13 (356)	2.7	0.18
Mustonen (1981)	[121]	Finland	33 (33)	23 (114)	1.69	0.14
Arnaiz-Villena (1981)	[122]	Spain	33 (27)	22 (330)	1.76	0.14
Rambausek (1982)	[123]	FRG	17 (36)	14 (800)	1.23	0.04
Le Petit (1982)	[124]	France	26 (78)	13 (104)	2.22	0.14
Julian (1983)	[125]	USA	18 (28)	23	–	–
Feehally (1984)	[126]	UK	11 (46)	14 (385)	0.78	–
Hanly (1984)	[127]	Ireland	11 (56)	12 (453)	0.88	–
Waldo (1986)	[128]	USA	20 (27)	15	–	–
Berthoux (1988)	[113]	France	24 (259)†	9 (164)	3.19	0.16

* Relative risk
** Aetiological fraction
† Significant result

Table 7 Mesangial IgA nephropathy: HLA Bw35 antigen frequency in Japanese

Author (year)	Ref.	Patients % (n)	Control % (n)	RR* >1	EF** 0–1
Komori (1979)	[129]	10 (40)	14 (115)	0.68	–
Kashiwabara (1982)	[74]	29 (42)	13 (140)	2.7	0.18
Kasahara (1982)	[130]	15 (104)	16 (147)	1.0	–
Hiki (1982)	[131]	25 (103)†	14 (950)	12.1	0.13
Komori (1983)	[81]	16 (82)	16 (790)	1.01	–
Kohara (1985)	[132]	12 (41)	10 (63)	1.31	0.02
Hiki (1990)	[106]	30 (130)†	15 (472)	2.3	–

* Relative risk
** Aetiological fraction
† Significant result

Table 8 Mesangial IgA nephropathy: HLA DR4 antigen frequency in caucasians

Author (year)	Ref.	Country	Patients % (n)	Control % (n)	RR* >1	AF** 0–1
Brettle (1978)	[114]	UK	24 (17)	33 (208)	0.62	–
Mouzan-Cambon (1980)	[133]	France	0 (11)	12 (90)	–	–
Bignon (1980)	[119]	France	14 (35)	21 (56)	0.61	–
Faucet (1980)	[120]	France	49 (45)†	19 (113)	3.96	0.37
Rambausek (1982)	[123]	FRG	17 (36)	26 (248)	0.56	–
Le Petit (1982)	[124]	France	22 (49)	34 (74)	0.57	–
Berger (1984)	[67]	France	43 (30)†	13 (106)	5.02	0.34
Feehally (1984)	[126]	UK	37 (46)	32 (385)	1.01	–
Hanly (1984)	[127]	Ireland	30 (46)	33 (212)	0.88	–
Waldo (1986)	[128]	USA	40 (27)	28	–	–
Berthoux (1988)	[113]	France	25 (1985)	32 (124)	0.69	–

* Relative risk
** Aetiological fraction
† Significant result

inconsistencies on the basis of the stage of the disease or its tendency to progress to end-stage renal failure have not been convincing.

Faucet[120] reported the frequency of DR4 to be significantly increased in a group of 45 French patients, but this has not been confirmed (Table 8). The situation is quite different in Japanese, in which seven separate studies have all shown an increased prevalence of HLA-DR4, with an incidence of about 60% in patients compared with 32–44% in healthy controls (Table 9).

Two recent studies[77,78] analysed genomic DNA from caucasian patients with IgA nephropathy by RFLP techniques using probes to polymorphic DR and DQ genes. Although there was no significant difference between patients and controls using the DRB gene probe, there was a significant increase in the frequency of two RFLPs using the DQβ probe. Although, in their study Moore et al.[77] did not assign specific alleles to these RFLPs, they described two bands (2 kb and 6 kb respectively) which were significantly

Table 9 Mesangial IgA nephropathy: HLA DR4 antigen frequency in Japanese

Author (year)	Ref.	Patients % (n)	Controls % (n)	RR* >1	EF** 0–1
Kashiwabara (1982)	[74]	66 (42)‡	39 (158)	3.1	0.45
Kasahara (1982)	[130]	60 (104)‡	36 (147)	2.6	0.36
Hiki (1982)	[131]	66 (80)‡	41 (884)	2.78	0.42
Komori (1983)	[81]	55 (51)	44 (114)	1.6	0.2
Kohara (1985)	[132]	58 (41)	32 (63)	3.03	0.39
Naito (1987)	[87]	58 (70)‡	34 (100)	2.7	0.37
Hiki (1990)†	[106]	60 (130)‡	42 (472)	2.1	–

* Relative risk
** Aetiological fraction
† 80 patients included in Hiki (1982) study
‡ Significant result

more frequent in patients with IgAN (50%, $n = 78$) than in controls (15%, $n = 94$, RR $= 5.75$, $p < 0.0001$). Li et al.[78], in a study of 35 Caucasian patients, showed similar findings, using RFLPs, but, in addition used allele-specific oligotyping to assign DQ specificities to the patients. The patients had an increased prevalence of both DR4 (52%) and DR5 (31%), neither of which reached statistical significance. This contrasted with a highly significant increase in DQw7, which was probably responsible for the 6 kb band described by Moore. DQw7 was present in 71% patients ($n = 32$) compared to 28% of controls ($n = 1103$, RR6.2). This result could have been expected given the results of the DR studies, because both DR4 and DR5 are in linkage disequilibrium with DQw7. The Japanese results could also be explained by a primary association with a DQ allele, either DQw7 itself or Dw4, which is the commonest DQ allele found in linkage disequilibrium with DR4 in Japanese and differs at only four polymorphic amino acid residues from DQw7. DQw4 is found almost exclusively in Japanese populations. This means that DR4 would be a good reporter gene for a DQw7 or DQw4 in Japanese, although a poor one for DQw7 in caucasoids. This suggests that susceptibility to IgAN is more closely associated, with the DQ locus than the DR locus and identifies DQw7 and its Japanese equivalent as the susceptibility gene. In addition, it illustrates the power of comparing HLA associations between different populations.

Steroid-responsive (minimal-change) nephrotic syndrome of childhood

Minimal change-nephrotic syndrome (MCNS) is the commonest form of nephrotic syndrome in childhood but can occur at any age. There are plenty of clues to suggest that MCNS is an immunological disease, but the exact pathogenesis is unknown. There have been a large number of studies to look for MHC associations with MCNS, and these are considered in detail in Chapter 8. Thompson et al. in 1976 reported an association with HLA-B12[79]; 54% of 71 affected children inherited HLA-B12 compared with 15% of 39

Table 10 Minimal-change nephrotic syndrome: HLA Class I antigen associations

Author (year)	Ref.	Country	Patients % (n)	Controls % (n)	RR* >1	EF** 0–1
HLA B8						
Thompson (1976)	[79]	UK	42 (71)	28 (39)	1.9	0.2
Lenhard (1980)	[134]	Germany	30 (107)	18 (800)	2.0	0.15
Alfiler (1980)	[135]	Australia	36 (45)	25 (300)	1.7	0.14
O'Regan (1980)	[105]	Ireland	65 (54)	35 (253)	3.6	0.46
Mouzon-Cambon						
(1981)	[136]	France	20 (54)	12 (91)	1.9	0.09
Noss (1981)	[137]	Germany	42 (95)	20 (1000)	2.8	0.27
Meadow (1982)	[138]	UK	35 (72)	25 (458)	1.6	0.13
Ruder (1982)	[139]	Germany	26 (94)	13 (100)	2.3	0.14
Rashid (1983)	[62]	UK	71 (14)	25 (325)	7.4	–
HLA B12						
Thomson (1976)	[79]	UK	54 (71)	15 (39)	6.3	0.45
Trompeter (1980)	[80]	UK	44 (45)	25 (1036)	2.4	0.26
Lenhard (1980)	[134]	Germany	24 (107)	22 (800)	1.1	0.02
Alfile (1980)	[135]	Australia	33 (45)	30 (308)	1.2	0.04
O'Reagan (1980)	[105]	Ireland	41 (54)	37 (253)	1.3	0.08
Mouzon-Cambon						
(1981)	[136]	France	30 (54)	46 (91)	0.5	–
Noss (1981)	[137]	Germany	18 (945)	22 (1000)	0.8	–
Meadow (1981)	[138]	UK	36 (72)	31 (458)	1.3	0.07
Ruder (1982)	[139]	Germany	38 (94)	24 (100)	2.0	0.19

* Relative risk
** Aetiological fraction

controls (RR 6.3, EF 0.45). Trompeter[80] confirmed this association in a larger group of patients from the same institution, but the results were much less striking. Since then at least seven other studies of caucasoid children, from various European countries and from Australia, have failed to show a convincing association with HLA-B12 (Table 10), but have almost all demonstrated an association with the Class II antigen DR7 (Table 11). It is notable that HLA-DR7 is in linkage disequilibrium with B12, which probably accounts for the original suggestion of a B12 association. However, the association of MCNS with DR7 does not extend to other racial groups, and Japanese children suffering from MCNS appear to inherit the Class II antigen DR8 more frequently than controls (13/18 compared with 9/114 respectively, RR 10.1, EF 0.42[81]). Clearly, studies of the DQ loci will be needed in both populations before these differences can be interpreted.

Post-streptococcal glomerulonephritis

Post-streptococcal glomerulonephritis (PSGN) is an extremely common type of glomerulonephritis in many parts of the world, though no longer in Europe and the USA. It is often considered a model of immune complex-mediated glomerulonephritis. The fact that not all patients who suffer streptococcal infections develop acute glomerulonephritis would suggest that genetic

Table 11 Minimal-change nephrotic syndrome: HLA Class II antigen frequencies

Author (year)	Ref.	Country	Patients % (n)	Controls % (n)	RR* >1	EF** 0–1
HLA-DR7						
Alfiler (1980)	[135]	Australia	71 (42)	30 (121)	5.9	0.59
Mouzon-Cambon						
(1981)	[136]	France	74 (38)	30 (91)	6.3	0.62
Ruder (1982)	[139]	Germany	59 (54)	18 (100)	6.6	0.50
Nunez-Rolden						
(1982)	[140]	Spain	72 (50)	38 (179)	4.2	0.155
Komori (1983)	[81]	Japan	3.6 (28)	2.6 (114)	NS	NS
HLA-DRw8						
Komori (1983)	[81]	Japan	46 (28)	8 (114)	10.1	0.42

* Relative risk
** Aetiological fraction

susceptibility may play at least some part in this condition. A familial incidence has been reported in epidemic outbreaks[82–84], which may reflect the inheritance of susceptibility. Initial studies failed to show associations between Class I and PSGN, but Layrisse et al.[85], though unable to show any evidence of linkage to the HLA complex in 18 Venezuelan families, did show a weak association with the Class II antigen DR4 in 42 unrelated patients. Sasazuki et al.[86] have also described similar findings in the Japanese population. Patients with PSGN had a significantly increased prevalence of a Class II molecule defined by mixed lymphocyte culture and designated D"EN", which is closely related to HLA-DRw6. More recently, Naito[87] has suggested, again in a Japanese study, an association between the Class II antigen DR1 and PSGN; DR1 was found in 40% of patients ($n = 11$) compared with 12% of controls ($n = 100$) (RR = 4.9, $p < 0.02$ uncorrected; corrected p value non-significant). These results are too preliminary to draw firm conclusions, but these Class II genes, or immunoregulatory genes linked to them, may determine susceptibility to PSGN. Thus, a particular antigenic determinant of the nephritogenic streptococci may also lead to disease when presented together with particular MHC molecules.

Rapidly progressive glomerulonephritis

Rapidly progressive glomerulonephritis (RPGN) is a clinical term used to describe patients with focal necrotizing glomerulonephritis which, if left untreated, progresses to end-stage renal failure in weeks or months. Glomeruli from these patients have a common histological appearance with widespread crescent formation, but this can be due to a variety of different immunopathologies including anti-GBM disease. Nevertheless, there are a group of these patients who either have small-vessel vasculitis, Wegener's granulomatosis (WG) or microscopic polyarteritis (MPA), or apparently isolated crescentic glomerulonephritis. This last group is often referred to as having idiopathic RPGN, but there is increasing evidence that this represents a more localized form of microscopic polyarteritis. The prevailing view is that these diseases are immunologically mediated and possibly autoimmune, because of recent findings that anti-neutrophil cytoplasmic antibodies (ANCA) are closely correlated with vasculitis and idiopathic RPGN[10].

Early studies to look for immunogenetic factors associated with RPGN were flawed by the heterogeneity of disease leading to crescentic nephritis. Nevertheless, Muller et al.[88], in 1984, reported that idiopathic RPGN was associated with HLA-DR2, MT3 and the complement allotype BfF, especially when inherited together as an extended haplotype. None of his patients was said to have had evidence of systemic disease, which is surprising in view of the high incidence of systemic symptoms in most series of RPGN. This was the case in 45 patients presenting with RPGN, studied by Elkon et al.[89], in whom the overall frequency of DR2 was not increased. However, it became clear that when the patients were segregated by the clinical diagnosis of Wegener's granulomatosis or microscopic polyarteritis, the patients with WG had a significantly increased frequency of DR2 (65%, $n = 17$) compared with normal controls (21%, $n = 113$, $\chi^2 = 12.1$). There was no significant HLA-DR association with MP. It is too early to draw any conclusions from these studies, and further work will not be worthwhile until the problem of heterogeneity has been resolved. New laboratory techniques such as ANCA detection will undoubtedly facilitate more meaningful searches for immunogenetic influences on the development of RPGN.

Systemic lupus erythematosus

Systemic lupus erythematosus (SLE) is the prototype of a non-organ-specific autoimmune disease, with immune complexes deposited in pathological lesions, and antibody-mediated damage occurring in both lymphoid and non-lymphoid tissues. The occurrence of familial cases suggests a role for genetic factors which predispose to SLE. As many as 5% of patients with SLE have a relative with the same disease and 57% of monozygotic twins are concordant for SLE. The occurrence of SLE in dizygotic twins is similar to that of other first-degree relatives. Thus, both genetic and environmental factors play a role in susceptibility to SLE.

Clinically detectable evidence of renal involvement in SLE is seen in about 50% of patients, although electron microscopic abnormalities are ubiquitous even when renal function and sediment are entirely normal. Thus, when considering the immunogenetics of lupus nephritis, one must necessarily consider the genetic aspects of SLE in general and the wide variety of autoimmune systems involved.

Some patients developing lupus nephritis progress inexorably to end-stage renal failure, while others suffer exacerbations and remissions. The diversity of the pathological and clinical features of this condition may reflect disease heterogeneity, which makes study of immunogenetics in this condition difficult. The strongest disease susceptibility genes identified in humans are those responsible for deficiencies of the proteins of the classical pathway of complement, encoded both within (C2 and C4) and without (C1q) the MHC. Inherited complete deficiencies of these proteins account for only a tiny minority of patients suffering from SLE, although the prevalence of SLE in patients with hereditary deficiencies of classical pathway components of complement is 68–88%. Recognition of these facts has stimulated detailed studies of complement proteins to look for partial deficiencies.

C4 and C2 are encoded within the MHC and it has been suggested that the association of SLE with deficiency of these components occurs as a result of genetic linkage with other immune response genes, perhaps located within the Class II region. This seems unlikely to be the explanation, as patients with complete deficiencies of these proteins have a variety of MHC haplotypes[90]. Many workers have looked for evidence of partial complement deficiency in patients with SLE, and Glass et al. have found an association between heterozygous C2 deficiency and SLE[91]. The C4A and C4B proteins exhibit extensive polymorphism as discussed earlier, and a number of groups have shown a markedly raised prevalence of C4AQ0 genes in patients with lupus[92–96]. However, the majority of these C4AQ0 alleles were on DR3-bearing haplotypes[93,95,96] and the relative contributions of each of these alleles to disease susceptibility is difficult to assess, although Bachelor et al.[97] have found an increased prevalence of the C4AQ0 allele in DR3 negative lupus patients. Indeed, the C4AQ0 allele appears to occur more commonly in lupus patients from other racial groups, compared with non-lupus individuals of similar descent.

Initial studies of Class II antigens demonstrated a raised prevalence of HLA-DR2 and HLA-DR3 in caucasian SLE patients, but subsequent studies have only confirmed the DR3 association. Woodrow, however, combining the data from eight publication reports, found that the presence of DR2 and DR3 was associated with an increased risk of developing SLE of 2 and 2.4 respectively[98]. The DR2 association has also been seen in a study of SLE in southern Chinese (RR = 2.64)[99]. The haplotype HLA-A1, B8, DR3 is particularly associated with SLE, as indeed it is with many other autoimmune conditions including Graves' disease, Addison's disease, type I diabetes mellitus and coeliac disease. One current hypothesis is that these Class II molecules are particularly favourable restriction elements for the presentation of antigen to T lymphocytes in lupus as well as in these other autoimmune conditions.

The recent discovery that the genes for tumour necrosis factor are encoded within the MHC has led to the search for polymorphisms of these genes. Jacob and McDevitt have found reduced TNF-α production in the offspring of lupus-susceptible (NZW) mice crossed with non-susceptible mice (NZB), and reported that regular injections of TNF-α reduced the severity of nephritis and prolonged survival in these mice[100]. Recently, they have described analogous observations in patients with SLE[101]. These observations imply that inherited variation in TNF expression may be another disease-susceptibility gene for SLE.

It does not appear that distinct allotypic variants of antibodies, T cell receptors or autoantigens are involved in disease susceptibility, although there is some evidence in mice for selective use of certain V gene families in the formation of autoantibodies. These can, however, also be found in non-lupus-prone mice[102]. There is, as yet, no evidence to support a role for genetic variation in antibody repertoire as a disease-susceptibility factor in humans. Stenezky *et al.* related Gm allotyopes to clinical features in 90 Hungarian patients with SLE, and found that patients homozygous for Gm 3;5,13 were at special risk of developing SLE-related nephropathy[103]. The association of Gm with renal disease may be related to the fact that anti-DNA antibodies in Gm 3;5,13 homozygotes bind to anionic sites on glomerular basement membranes, thus initiating tissue injury.

Much of the work on genetic influences on the development of SLE has been done using animal models. Disease can be transmitted by bone marrow transplantation from certain susceptible strains of mice to non-susceptible irradiated individuals. Interbreeding of different susceptible strains of mice, and breeding of susceptible with non-susceptible strains, has demonstrated that several genes are likely to be involved; both dominant and recessive genes have been implicated. In addition, these experiments point to the existence of disease-protective genes which inhibit disease development. The onset of SLE, in susceptible mice, can be accelerated or delayed by viral and bacterial infection. One such virus, the lactate dehydrogenase (LDH) virus, which inhibits disease development, has been shown to use Class II MHC molecules as a receptor and may thereby enter and inhibit the activities of antigen-presenting cells[104].

Although the cause of SLE in humans is likely to be multifactorial, genetic factors certainly exist. Taken alone these are relatively weak, but they may act in consort to determine disease susceptibility, or may represent linkage to another true susceptibility gene.

HLA alleles and the severity of disease

Thus far, this chapter has been concerned only with the effects of HLA alleles on susceptibility to nephritis. There is also evidence that the HLA complex influences the severity of nephritis, its tendency to relapse, or the likelihood of progression to end-stage renal failure. Often, this evidence refers to associations with particular haplotypes rather than individual alleles, and there are even fewer precedents from experimental studies to guide interpretation of such associations. Nevertheless, the existence of extended haplotypes, including the genes for complement, TNF and heat shock proteins within the Class III region, is tantalizing. There are no reports, to date, of the influence of HLA haplotypes on the intensity of inflammation, but DR2 has been reported to be associated with a reduced capacity for TNF secretion *in vitro*[101].

The severity of anti-GBM disease has been reported to be influenced by whether HLA-B7 is inherited together with DR2[48]. In a study of 38 patients, Rees *et al.* reported that those with B7 had significantly higher serum creatinine concentrations at presentation and a worse outlook, even though anti-GBM antibody titres were similar in both groups. Analysis of these data showed that these effects could not be explained merely by the strength of the known linkage disequilibrium between B7 and DR2, which suggests that B7-bearing haplotypes have independent effects on the severity of the disease.

Broadly similar data have been reported in minimal-change nephrotic syndrome in children. Trompeter[79], in his original study, suggested that HLA-B12-positive children with MCGN were more likely to have relapsed 3 years following standard doses of cyclophosphamide therapy than those who had not inherited this antigen. On the other hand, O'Regan et al.[105], in a study of 54 Irish children suffering MCGN, demonstrated an increased frequency of both B8 and B12 Class I antigens (RR = 3.5 and 1.3 respectively), but found that those with HLA B8 represented 72% (13/18) of those in remission after 3 years compared with 66% (10/15) of those in relapse. Thus, the strongest disease associations are with Class II genes, but extended haplotypes may influence the severity of disease or its response to therapy.

Hiki et al., in a study to clarify the relationship between the long-term prognosis of IgAN and the DR4 antigen, confirmed the B35 and DR4 associations with disease in Japanese but concluded that DR4 plays no role in the long-term prognosis of IgAN. The frequency of B35 seemed to be increased in patients with stable disease (35.7%) compared with those with progressive disease (20%), but this difference was not statistically significant[106].

Although there are no definite associations between HLA antigens and mesangio-capillary nephritis, a report from Welch et al. suggests that, despite treatment with steroids, patients with the extended haplotype HLA-B8 DR3 are significantly more likely to develop renal failure than patients with other haplotypes[107].

The data are much less certain for membranous nephropathy. Zucchelli has suggested that patients with the HLA-B8 DR3 haplotype have a worse prognosis than others[108], whereas Short et al.[109] reported that patients with HLA-B18 DR3 BfF1 did worse than patients with other DR3-bearing haplotypes. These directly contradictory results suggest that HLA haplotypes have little influence on the severity of IMN, at least in comparison to other factors.

CONCLUDING REMARKS

There has been a tendency to regard immunogenetic studies of nephritis as little more than 'stamp collecting', of little help in understanding pathogenesis and none in providing a basis for new therapies. Undoubtedly, there has been considerable truth in this view, largely because the diseases and immunological attributes (usually the HLA complex) were insufficiently understood. This situation is changing very fast, particularly because of the rapid accumulation in knowledge of the HLA system made possible by the techniques of molecular biology. These methods have been used to define the organization of the MHC genes and to define the structure of MHC molecules. Analogous studies on other elements of the immune response, such as T cell receptors and the immunoglobulins, are rapidly defining inherited restrictions in response, and by implication inherited predispositions to immunologically mediated disease.

References

1. Wells, W. C. (1812). Observation on the dropsy which succeeds scarlet fever. *Trans. Soc. Improve. Med. Chir. Know.*, **13**, 167–186.
2. Germuth, F. G. and Rodriguez, E. L. (1973). *The Immunopathology of the Renal Glomerulus.* (Boston: Little Brown).
3. Biozzi, G., Mouton, G., Sant'Anna, O. A., Passos, H. C., Gennari, M. and Reis, M. H. (1980). Genetics of immunoresponsiveness to natural antigens in the mouse. *Curr. Top. Microbiol. Immunol.*, **85**, 31–98.
4. Steward, M. R., Reinhardt, M. C. and Staines, N. A. (1979). The genetic control of antibody affinity. Evidence from breeding studies with mice selectively bred for either high or low affinity antibody production. *Immunology*, **37**, 697–702.
5. Devey, M. E. and Steward, M. W. (1980). The induction of chronic antigen-antibody complex disease in selectively bred mice producing either high or low affinity antibody to protein antigens. *Immunology*, **41**, 303–311.
6. Steinglen, B., Thoenes, G. H. and Gunther, E. (1978). Genetic control of susceptibility to autologous immune complex glomerulonephritis in inbred rat strains. *Clin. Exp. Immunol.*, **33**, 88–94.
7. Hale, G. M., McIntosch, S., Hiki, Y., Clarkson, A. R. and Woodroffe, A. J. (1986). Evidence for IgA specific B cell hyperactivity in patients with IgA nephropathy. *Kidney Int.*, **29**, 718–724.
8. Ballardie, F. W., Brenchley, P. E. C., Williams, S. and O'Donoghue, D. J. (1988). Autoimmunity in IgA nephropathy. *Lancet*, **2**, 588–592.
9. Niles, J., Collins, B., Baird, L., Erikson, M., Bradford, D., Pan, G., Hsuing, C. K., Schneeberger, E. and Bhan, A. (1987). Antibodies reactive with renal glycoprotein and with deposits in membranous nephritis. *Kidney Int.*, **31**, 338.
10. Falk, R. J. and Jennette, J. C. (1988). Anti-neutrophil cytoplasmic autoantibodies with specificity for myeloperoxidase in patients with systemic vasculitis and idiopathic necrotizing and crescentic glomerulonephritis. *N. Engl. J. Med.*, **318**, 1651–1657.
11. Clayman, M. D., Michaud, L., Brentjens, J., Andres, G. A., Kefalides, N. A. and Neilson, E. G. (1986). Isolation of the target antigen of human anti-tubular basement membrane antibody-associated interstitial nephritis. *J. Clin. Invest.*, **77**, 1143–1147.
12. Moller, G. (1987). Antigenic requirements for activation of MHC restricted responses. *Immunol. Rev.*, **98**, 1–187.
13. Bjorkman, P. J., Saper, M. A., Samraoui, B., Bennett, W. S., Strominger, J. L. and Wiley, D. C. (1987). Structure of the human class I histocompatibility antigen, HLA-A2. *Nature*, **329**, 506–512.
14. Bjorkman, P. J., Saper, M. A., Samraoui, B., Bennett, W. S., Strominger, J. L. and Wiley, D. C. (1987). The foreign antigen binding site and T cell recognition regions of class I histocompatibility antigens. *Nature*, **329**, 512–518.
15. Cairns, J. S., Curlsinger, C. A., Dahl, C. A., Freeman, S., Allen, B. J. and Bach, F. H. (1985). Sequence polymorphism of HLA DRβ1 alleles relating to T-cell-recognised determinants. *Nature*, **317**, 166–168.
16. Von Bohmer, H., Teh, H. S. and Kisieiow, P. (1989). The thymus selects the useful, neglects the useless and destroys the harmful. *Immunol. Today*, **10**, 57–61.
17. Nossal, G. J. V. (1989). Immunologic tolerance: collaboration between antigen and lymphokines. *Science*, **245**, 147–153.
18. Schwartz, R. H. (1986). Immune response (Ir) genes of the murine major histocompatibility complex. *Adv. Immunol.*, **38**, 31–201.
19. Wraith, D., McDevitt, H. O., Steinman, L. and Acha-Orbea, H. (1989). T Cell recognition as the target for immune intervention in autoimmune disease. *Cell*, **57**, 707–715.
20. Druet, E., Sapin, C., Gunther, E., Feingold, N. and Druet, P. (1977). Mercuric chloride-induced anti-glomerular basement membrane antibodies in the rat: genetic control. *Eur. J. Immunol.*, **7**, 348–351.
21. Acha-Orbea, H., Mitchell, D. J., Timmerman, L. and Wraith, D. C. (1988). Limited heterogeneity of T cell receptors from lymphocytes mediating autoimmune encephalomyelitis allows specific immune intervention. *Cell*, **54**, 263–273.
22. Urban, J. L., Kuman, V., Kono, D. H., Gomez, C., Horvath, S. J., Clayton, J., Ando, D. G., Sercarz, E. and Hooc, L. (1988). Restricted use of T cell receptor V genes in murine

autoimmune encephalomyelitis raises possibilities for antibody therapy. *Cell*, **54**, 577–592.

23. Burns, F. R., Li, X., Shen, N., Offner, H., Chou, Y. K., Vandenbark, K. and Heber-Katz, E. (1989). Both rat and mouse T cell receptors specific for the encephalogenic determinants of myelin basic protein use similar Va and Vb chain genes. *J. Exp. Med.*, **169**, 27–39.

24. Trowsdale, J. (1988). Molecular genetics of the MHC. *Immunology., Supp. 1*, 21–23.

25. Campbell, R. D. and Bentley, D. R. (1985). Structure and genetics of C2 and factor B genes. *Immunol. Rev.*, **87**, 19–37.

26. Dupont, B. (1988). *Histocompatibility Testing 1987*. (New York: Springer-Verlag).

27. Kaufman, J. F. and Strominger, J. L. (1982). HLA-DR light chain has a polymorphic N-terminal region and a conserved Ig-like C-terminal region. *Nature*, **297**, 694–697.

28. Cross, S. J., Edwards, J. H., Bentley, D. R. and Campbell, R. D. (1985). DNA polymorphism of the C2 and factor B genes. *Immunogenetics*, **21**, 39–48.

29. Alper, C. A., Raum, D., Karp, S., Awdeh, Z. L. and Yunis, E. J. (1983). Serum complement 'Supergenes' of the major histocompatibility complex in man (complotypes). *Vox. Sang.*, **45**, 62–67.

30. Awdeh, Z. L., Raum, D., Yunis, E. J. and Alper, C. A. (1983). Extended HLA/complement allele haplotypes: evidence for T/t like complex in man. *Proc. Natl. Acad. Sci USA*, **80**, 259–263.

31. Connealy, P. M. and Rivas, M. L. (1980). Linkage analysis in man. *Adv. Hum. Genet.*, **10**, 209–266.

32. Thomson, G., Motro, U. and Selvin, S. (1983). Statistical aspects of measuring the strength of associations between HLA antigens and disease. *Tissue Antigens*, **21**, 320–328.

33. Thompson, G. (1981). A review of theoretical aspects of HLA and disease. *Theoret. Pop. Biol.*, **20**, 168–208.

34. Svejgaard, A., Platz, P. and Ryder, L. P. (1983). HLA and disease 1982 — a survey. *Immunol. Rev.*, **70**, 193–218.

35. Bengtsson, B. O. and Thomson, G. (1981). Measuring the strength of associations between HLA antigens and disease. *Tissue Antigens*, **18**, 315–322.

36. Green, A. (1982). The epidemiologic approach to studies of association between HLA and disease. II. Estimation of absolute risks etiologic and preventive fraction. *Tissue Antigens*, **19**, 259–268.

37. Barron, K. S., Person, D. A., Brewer, E. J. Jr., Beale, M. G. and Robson, A. M. (1981). Pulse methylprednisolone therapy in diffuse proliferative lupus nephritis. Glomerulonephritis in systemic lupus erythematosus (clinical conference). *Am. J. Nephrol.*, **1**, 53–67.

38. Karlin, S. and Piazza, A. (1981). Statistical methods for assessing linkage disequilibrium at the HLA-A,B,C,loci. *Ann. Hum. Genet.*, **45**, 79–94.

39. Porta, J. and McHugh, R. (1980). Detection of HLA haplotype associations with disease. *Tissue Antigens*, **15**, 337–345.

40. Lerner, R. A., Glassock, R. J. and Dixon, F. J. (1967). The role of anti-glomerular basement membrane antibody in the pathogenesis of human glomerulonephritis. *J. Exp. Med.*, **126**, 989–1004.

41. Butkowski, R. J., Langeveld, J. P. M., Wieslander, J., Hamilton, J. and Hudson, B. G. (1987). Localization of the Goodpasture epitope to a novel chain of basement membrane collagen. *J. Biol. Chem.*, **262**, 7874–7877.

42. Wieslander, J., Kataja, M. and Hudson, BG. (1987). Characterization of the human Goodpasture antigen. *Clin. Exp. Immunol.*, **69**, 332–340.

43. d'Apice, A. J., Kincaid Smith, P., Becker, G. H., Loughhead, M. G., Freeman, J. W. and Sands, J. M. (1978). Goodpasture's syndrome in identical twins. *Ann. Intern. Med.*, **88**, 61–62.

44. Gossain, V. V., Gerstein, A. R. and Janes, A. W. (1972). Goodpasture's syndrome: a familial occurrence. *Ann. Rev. Respir. Dis.*, **105**, 621–624.

45. Simonsen, H., Brun, C., Thomsen, O. F., Larsen, S. and Ladefoged, J. (1982). Goodpasture's syndrome in twins. *Acta Med. Scand.*, **212**, 425–428.

46. Almkuist, R. D., Buckalew, V. M. Jr., Hirszel, P., Maher, J. F., James, P. M. and Wilson, C. B. (1981). Recurrence of anti-glomerular basement membrane antibody mediated glomerulonephritis in an isograft. *Clin. Immunol. Immunopathol.*, **18**, 54–60.

47. Rees, A. J., Peters, D. K., Compston, D. A. and Batchelor, J. R. (1978). Strong association between HLA-DRW2 and antibody-mediated Goodpasture's syndrome. *Lancet*, **1**, 966–968.

48. Rees, A. J., Peters, D. K., Amos, N., Welsh, K. I. and Batchelor, J. R. (1984). The influence of HLA-linked genes on the severity of anti-GBM antibody-mediated nephritis. *Kidney Int.*, **26**, 445–450.

49. Perl, S. I., Pussell, B. A., Charlesworth, J. A., Macdonald, G. J. and Wolnizer, M. (1981). Goodpasture's (anti-GBM) disease and HLA-DRw2 (letter). N. Engl. J. Med., 305, 463–464.
50. Garovoy, M. R. (1982). Immunogenetic associations in nephrotic states, Contemp. Issues Nephrol., 9, 259–282.
51. Burns, A., Li, P., So, A., Pusey, C. D. and Rees, A. J. (1991). Analysis of HLA class II genes in patients with Goodpashire's syndrome: a possible role for the DRB5 gene in susceptibility. (submitted)
52. Todd, J. A., Bell, J. I. and McDevitt, H. O. (1987). HLA-DQb gene contributes to susceptibility and resistance to insulin-dependent diabetes mellitus. Nature, 329, 599–604.
53. Sheehy, M. J., Scharf, S. J., Rowe, J. R., Neme de Gimenez, M. H., Meske, L. M., Erlich, H. A. and Nepom, B. S. (1989). J. Clin. Invest., 83, 830–835.
54. Kerjaschki, S. and Farquhar, M. G. (1983). Immunocytochemical localisation of Hayman nephritis antigen (GP330) in glomerular epithelial cells from normal Lewis rats. J. Exp. Med., 157, 667–686.
55. Sato, K., Oguchi, H., Hora, K., Furukawa, T., Furuta, S., Shigematsu, H. and Yoshizawa, S. (1987). Idiopathic membranous nephropathy in two brothers. Nephron, 46, 174–178.
56. Short, C. D., Feehally, J., Gokal, R. and Mallick, N. P. (1984). Familial membranous nephropathy. Br. Med. J. (Clin. Res.), 289, 1500.
57. Vangelista, A., Tazzari, R. and Bonomini, V. (1988). Idiopathic membranous nephropathy in 2 twin brothers (letter). Nephron, 50, 79–80.
58. Vaughan, R. W., Demaine, A. G. and Welsh, K. I. (1989). A DQA1 allele is strongly associated with idiopathic membranous nephropathy. Tissue Antigens, 34, 261–269.
59. Muller, G. A., Muller, C. A., Liebau, G., Kompf, J., Ising, H. and Wernet, P. (1981). Strong association of idiopathic membranous nephropathy (IMN) with HLA-DR3 and MT-2 withough involvement of HLA-b18 and no association to BfF1. Tissue Antigens, 17, 332–337.
60. Hiki, Y., Kobayashi, Y., Itoh, I. and Kashiwagi, N. (1984). Strong association of HLA-DR2 and MT1 with idiopathic membranous nephropathy in Japan. Kidney Int., 25, 953–957.
61. Tomura, S., Kashiwabara, H., Tuchida, H., Shishido, H., Sakurai, S., Tsuji, K. and Takeuchi, J. (1984). Strong association of idiopathic membranous nephropathy with HLA-DR2 and MT1 in Japanese. Nephron, 36, 242–245.
62. Rashid, H. U., Papiha, S. S., Agroyannis, B., Morley, A. R., Ward, M. K. and Kerr, D. N. (1983). The associations of HLA and other genetic markers with glomerulonephritis. Hum. Genet., 63, 38–44.
63. Klouda, P. T., Manos, J., Acheson, E. J., Dyer, P. A., Goldby, F. S., Harris, R., Lawler, W., Mallick, N. P. and Williams, G. (1979). Strong association between idiopathic membranous nephropathy and HLA-DRW3. Lancet, 2, 770–771.
64. Laurent, B., Berthoux, F. C., Le Petit, J. C., Genin, G., Laurent, P., Broutin, F., Touraine, F. and Touraine, J. L. (1983). Immunogenetics and immunopathology of human membranous glomerulonephritis. Proc. Eur. Dial. Transplant. Assoc., 19, 629–634.
65. Dyer, P. A., Klouda, P. T., Harris, R. and Mallick, N. P. (1980). Properdin factor B alleles in patients with idiopathic membranous nephropathy. Tissue Antigens, 15, 505–507.
66. D'Amico, G. (1987). The commonest glomerulonephritis in the world: IgA nephropathy. Q.J. Med., 245, 709–729.
67. Berger, J. (1984). IgA mesangial nephropathy. 1968–1983. Contrib. Nephrol., 40, 4–6.
68. Lai, K. N., Lai, F. M., Chui, S. H., Chan, Y. M., Tsao, G., Leung, K. N. and Lam, C. (1987). Studies of lymphocyte subpopulations and immunoglobulin production in IgA nephropathy. Clin. Nephrol., 28, 281–287.
69. Tolkoff Rubin, N. E., Cosmi, A. B., Fuller, T., Rubin, R. H. and Colvin, R. B. (1980). IgA nephropathy in HLA identical siblings. Transplantation, 29, 505–506.
70. Sabatier, J. C., Genin, C., Assenat, H., Colon, S., Ducret, F. and Berthoux, F. C. (1979). mesangial IgA glomerulonephritis in HLA identical brothers. Clin. Nephrol., 11, 35–38.
71. Katz, A., Karanicolas, S. and Falk, J. A. (1980). Family study in IgA nephritis: possible role of HLA antigens. Transplantation, 29, 505–506.
72. Montoliu, J., Darnell, A., Toras, A., Guadalupe, E., Valles, M. and Revert, L. (1980). Familial IgA nephropathy. Report of two cases and brief review of the literature. Arch. Intern. Med., 140, 1374–1375.
73. Papiha, S. S., Pareek, S. K., Rodger, R. S., Morley, A. R., Wilkinson, R., Roberts, D. F. and Kerr, D. N. (1987). HLA-A,B,DR and Bf allotypes in patients with idiopathic

membranous nephropathy (IMN). *Kidney Int.*, **31**, 130–134.

74. Kashiwabara, H., Shishido, H., Tomura, S., Tuchida, H. and Miyajima, T. Strong association between IgAQ nephropathy and HLA-DR4 antigen. *Kidney Int.*, **22**, 377–382.

75. Julian, B. A., Quiggins, P. A., Thompson, J. S., Woodford, S. Y., Gleason, K. and Wyatt, R. J. (1985). Familial IgA nephropathy. Evidence of an inherited mechanism of disease. *N. Engl. J. Med.*, **312**, 202–208.

76. Scolari, F., Savoldi, S., Scaini, P., Amoroso, A., Prati, E. and Maiorca, R. (1989). Familial occurrence of primary glomerulonephritis: experience in an Italian centre. *Nephrol. Dial. Transplant.*, **4**, 441–442 (Abstract).

77. Moore, R. H., Hitman, G. A., Lucas, E., Richards, N., Venning, M., Papiha, S., Awad, J., Cunningham, J and Marsh, F. P. (1989). Genetic susceptibility to autoimmunity in primary IgA nephropathy. *Nephrol. Dial. Transplant.*, **4**, 428–429 (Abstract).

78. Li, P., Burns, A., So, A., Pusey, C. D. and Rees, A. J. (1991). The DQw7 allele at the HLA-DQB locus is associated with susceptibility to IgA nephropathy in Caucasians. *Kidney Int.*, (in press).

79. Thomson, P. D., Barratt, T. M., Stokes, C. R. and Turner, M. W. (1976). HLA antigens and atopic features in steroid-responsive childhood nephrotic syndrome. *Lancet*, **2**, 765–768.

80. Trompeter, R. S., Barrett, T. M., Kay, R., Turner, M. W. and Soothill, J. F. (1980). HLA atopy and cyclophosphamide in steroid responsive childhood nephrotic syndrome. *Kidney Int.*, **17**, 113–117.

81. Komori, K., Nose, Y., Inouye, H., Tsuji, K., Nomoto, Y., Tomino, Y., Sakai, H., Iwagaki, H., Itoh, H. and Hasegawa, O. (1983). Immunogenetical study in patients with chronic glomerulonephritis. *Tokai J. Exp. Clin. Med.*, **8**, 135–148.

82. Dodge, W. F., Spargo, B. F. and Travis, L. B. (1967). Occurrence of acute glomerulonephritis in sibling contacts of children with sporadic acute glomerulonephritis. *Paediatrics*, **140**, 1028–1030.

83. Rodriguez Iturbe, B., Rubio, L. and Garcia, R. (1981). Attack rates of post streptococcal glomerulonephritis in families. A perspective study. *Lancet*, **1**, 401–403.

84. Anthony, B. F., Kaplan, E. L., Wannamaker, L. W., Briese, F. W. and Chapman, S. S. (1969). Attack rates of acute nephritis after type 49 streptococcal infection of the skin and of the respiratory tract. *J. Clin. Invest.*, **48**, 1697–1704.

85. Layrisse, Z., Rodriguez Iturbe, B., Garcia Ramirez, R., Rodriguez, A. and Tiwari, J. (1983). Family studies of the HLA system in acute post-streptococcal glomerulonephritis. *Hum. Immunol.*, **7**, 177–185.

86. Sasazuki, T., Hayase, R., Iwanoto, I. and Tsuchida, H. (1979). HLA and acute post-streptococcal glomerulonephritis. *N. Engl. J. Med.*, **301**, 1184–1185.

87. Naito, S., Kohara, M. and Arakawa, K. (1987). Association of class II antigens of HLA with primary glomerulopathis. *Nephron*, **45**, 111–114.

88. Muller, G. A., Gebhardt, M., Kompf, J., Baldwin, W. M., Ziegenhagen, D. and Bohle, A. (1984). Association between rapidly progressive glomerulonephritis and the properdin factor BfF and different HLA-D region products. *Kidney Int.*, **25**, 115–118.

89. Elkon, K. B., Sutherland, D. C., Rees, A. J., Hughes, G. R. and Batchelor, J. R. (1983). HLA antigen frequencies in systemic vasculites: Increase in HLA-DR2 in Wegener's granulomatosis. *Arthritis Rheum.*, **26**, 98–101.

90. Meyer, O., Hauptmann, G., Trappeiner, G., Ochs, H. D. and Mascart-Lemone, F. (1985). Genetic deficiency of C4, C2, or C1q and lupus syndromes: associations with anti-Ro (SS-A) antibodies. *Clin. Exp. Immunol.*, **62**, 678–684.

91. Glass, D., Raum, D., Gibson, D., Stillman, J. S. and Schur, P. H. (1976). Inherited deficiency of the second component of complement: rheumatic disease association. *J. Clin. Invest.*, **58**, 853–861.

92. Fielder, A. H., Walport, M. J. and Bachelor, J. R. (1983). Family study of the MHC in patients with SLE: importance of nullalleles in C4A and C4B in determining disease susceptibility. *Br. Med. J.*, **286**, 425–428.

93. Christiansen, F. T., McCluskey, J., Dawkins, R. L., Kay, P. H., Uko, G. and Zilko, P. J. (1983). Complement allotyping in SLE: association with C4A null. *Aust. N.Z. J. Med.*, **13**, 483–488.

94. Reveille, J. D., Arnett, F. C., Wilson, R. W., Bias, W. B. and McLean, R. H. (1985). Null alleles of the fourth component of complement and HLA haplotypes in familial systemic lupus erythematosis. *Immunogenetics*, **21**, 299–311.

95. Howard, P. F., Hochberg, M. C., Bias, W. B., Arnett, F. C. and McLean, R. H. (1986). Relationship between C4 null genes, HLA-D region antigens, and genetic susceptibility to systemic lupus erythematosis in Caucasian and Black Americans. *Am. J. Med.*, **81**, 187–193.

96. Kemp, M. E., Atkinson, P. J., Skanes, V. M., Levine, R. P. and Chaplin, D. D. (1987). Deletion of C4A genes in patients with systemic lupus erythematosis. *Arthritis Rheum.*, **30**, 1015–1022.

97. Bachelor, J. R., Fielder, A. H. L. and Walport, M. J. (1987). Family study of the major histocompatibility complex in HLA-DR3 negative patients with systemic lupus erythematosis. *Clin. Exp. Immunol.*, **70**, 364–371.

98. Woodrow, J. C. (1988). Immunogenetics of systemic lupus erythematosis. *J. Rheumatol.*, **15**, 197–199.

99. Hawkins, B. R., Wong, K. L., Chan, K. H., Dunckley, H. and Serjeantson, S. W. (1987). Strong association between the major histocompatibility complex and systemic lupus erythematosus in Southern Chinese. *J. Rheumatol.*, **14**, 1128–1131.

100. Jacob, C. O. and McDevitt, H. O. (1988). Tumor necrosis factor-a in murine autoimmune lupus nephritis. *Nature*, **331**, 356–358.

101. Jacob, C. O., Fronek, Z., Lewis, G. D., Koo, M., Hansen, J. A. and McDevitt, H. O. (1990). Heritable major histocompatibility complex class II-associated differences in production of tumor necrosis factor a: Relevance to genetic predisposition to systemic lupus erythematosis. *Proc. Natl. Acad. Sci. USA*, **87**, 1233–1237.

102. Bona, C. A. (1988). V genes encoding autoantibodies: molecular and phenotyping characteristics. *Ann. Rev. Immunol.*, **6**, 327–358.

103. Stenszky, V., Kozma, L., Szegedi, G. and Fario, N. R. (1986). Interplay of immunoglobulin G heavy chain markers (GM) and HLA in predisposing to systemic lupus erythematosus. *J. Immunogenet.*, **13**, 11–17.

104. Inada, T. and Mims, C. A. (1984). Mouse Ia molecules are receptors for lactate dehydrogenase virus. *Nature*, **309**, 59–61.

105. O'Regan, D., O'Callaghan, U., Dundon, S. and Reen, D. J. (1980). HLA antigens and steroid responsive nephrotic syndrome in childhood. *Tissue Antigens*, **16**, 147–151.

106. Hiki, Y., Kobayashi, Y., Ookubo, M. and Kashiwagi, N. (1990). The role of HLA-DR4 in long-term prognosis of IgA nephropathy. *Nephron*, **54**, 264–265.

107. Welch, T. R., Beischel, L., Balakrishnan, K., Quinlan, M. and West, C. D. (1986). Major-histocompatibility-complex extended haplotypes in membranoproliferative glomerulonephritis. *N. Engl. J. Med.*, **314**, 1476–1481.

108. Zucchelli, P., Ponticelli, C., Cagnoli, L., Aroldi, A. and Tabacchi, P. (1987). Genetic factors in the outcome of idiopathic membranous nephropathy (letter). *Nephrol. Dial. Transplant.*, **1**, 265–266.

109. Short, C. D., Dyer, P. A., Cairns, S. A., Manost, J., Waltons, C., Harris, R. and Mallick, N. P. (1983). A major histocompatibility system haplotype associated with poor prognosis in idiopathic membranous nephropathy. *Dis. Markers*, **1**, 189–196.

110. Garvoy, M. R. (1980). Idiopathic membranous glomerulonephritis (IMGN): An HLA associated disease. In Terasaki, P. I. (ed.) *Histocompatibility Workshop 1980, Los Angeles*, pp. 129. (University of California Press)

111. Le Petit, J. C., Laurent, B. and Berthoux, F. C. (1982). HLA-DR3 and idiopathic membranous nephritis (IMN) association. *Tissue Antigens*, **20**, 227–228.

112. Roccatello, D., Coppo, R., Amoroso, A., Curtoni, E. S., Martina, E. S., Basolo, B., Amore, A., Rollino, C. and Picciotto, G. (1987). Failure to relate mononuclear phagocyte system function to HLA-A,B,C,DR,DQ antigens in membranous nephropathy. *Am. J. Kidney Dis.*, **31**, 130–134.

113. Berthoux, F. C., Alamartine, E., Pommier, G. and Le Petit, J. C. (1988). HLA and IgA nephritis revisited 10 years later: HLA B35 antigen as a prognostic factor. *N. Engl. J. Med.*, **319**, 1609–1610.

114. Brettle, R., Peters, D. K. and Batchelor, J. R. (1978). Mesangial IgA Glomerulonephritis and HLA antigens. *N. Engl. J. Med.*, **299**, 200–201.

115. Noel, L. H., Descamps, B., Jungers, P., Bach, J. F., Busson, M., Suet, C., Hors, J. and Dausset, J. (1978). HLA antigens in three types of glomerulonephritis. *Clin. Immunol. Immunopathol.*, **10**, 19–23.

116. Nagy, J., Hamorl, A., Ambrus, M. and Nernadi, E. (1979). More on IgA glomerulonephritis

and HLA antigens. *N. Engl. J. Med.*, **300**, 92.

117. Savi, M., Neri, T. M., Silvestri, M. G., Allegri, L. and Migone, L. (1979). HLA antigens and IgA mesangial glomerulonephritis. *Clin. Nephrol.*, **12**, 45–46.

118. Macdonald, I. M., Dumble, L. J. and Kincaid Smith, P. S. (1980). HLA Bw35, circulating immune complexes and IgA deposits in mesangial proliferative glomerulonephritis. *Aust. N.Z. J. Med.*, **10**, 480–481.

119. Bignon, J. D., Houssin, A., Soulillou, J., Denis, J., Guimbretiere, J. and Guenel, J. (1980). HLA antigens and Berger's disease. *Tissue Antigens*, **16**, 108–111.

120. Faucet, R., Le Pogamp, P., Genetet, B., Chevet, D., Gueguen, M., Simon, P., Ramee, M. P. and Cartier, F. (1980). HLA-DR4 antigen and IgA nephropathy. *Tissue Antigens*, **16**, 405–410.

121. Moutonen, J., Pasternack, A., Helin, H., Rilva, A., Penttinen, K., Wager, O. and Harmoinen, A. (1981). Circulating immune complexes, the concentration of serum IgA and the distribution of HLA antigens in IgA nephropathy. *Nephron*, **29**, 170–175.

122. Arnaiz-Villena, A., Gonzalo, A., Mampaso, F., Teruel, J. L. and Ortunno, J. (1981). HLA and IgA nephropathy in Spanish population. *Tissue Antigens*, **17**, 549–550.

123. Rambausek, M., Seelig, H. P., Andressy, K., Waldherr, R., Lenhard, V. and Ritz, E. (1982). Clinical and serological features of mesangial IgA glomerulonephritis. *Proc. EDTA*, **19**, 663–668.

124. Le Petit, J. C., Cazes, M. H., Berthoux, J. C., Van Loghem, E., Goguen, J., Seger, J., Chapuis-Cellier, C., Marcellin, M., De Lange, G., Garovoy, M. R., Serre, J. L., Brizard, C. P. and Carpenter, C. B. (1982). Genetic investigation in mesangial IgA nephropathy. *Tissue Antigens*, **19**, 108–114.

125. Julian, B. A., Wyatt, R. J., McMorrow, R. G. and Galla, J. H. (1983). Serum complement proteins in IgA nephropathy. *Clin. Nephrol.*, **20**, 251–258.

126. Feehally, J., Dyer, P. A., Davidson, J. A., Harris, R. and Mallick, N. P. (1984). Immunogentics of IgA nephropathy: experience in a UK centre. *Dis. Markers.*, **2**, 493–500.

127. Hanly, P., Garrett, P., Spencer, S. and O'Dwyer, W. F. (1984). HLA -A, -B and -DR antigens in IgA nephropathy. *Tissue Antigens*, **23**, 270–273.

128. Waldo, B. F., Beischel, L. and West, C. D. (1986). IgA synthesis by lymphocytes from patients with IgA nephropathy and their relatives. *Kidney Int.*, **29**, 1229–1233.

129. Komori, K., Nose, Y., Inouye, H., Tsuji, K., Nomoto, Y. and Sakai, H. (1979). Study of HLA system in IgA nephropathy. *Tissue Antigens*, **14**, 32–36.

130. Kasahara, M., Hamada, K., Okuyama, T., Ishikawa, N., Ogasawara, K., Ikeda, H., Takenouchi, T., Wakisaka, A., Aizawa, M., Kataoka, Y., Miyamoto, R., Kohara, M., Naito, S., Kashiwagi, N. and Hiki, Y. (1982). Role of HLA in IgA nephropathy. *Clin. Immunol. Immunopathol.*, **25**, 189–195.

131. Hiki, Y., Kobayashi, Y., Tateno, S., Sada, M. and Kashiwagi, N. (1982). Strong association of HLA-DR4 with benign IgA nephropathy. *Nephron*, **32**, 222–226.

132. Kohara, M., Naito, S., Arakawa, K., Miyata, J., Chihara, J., Taguchi, T. and Takebayashi, S. (1985). The strong association of HLA-DR4 with spherical mesangial dense deposits in IgA nephropathy. *J. Clin. Lab. Immunol.*, **18**, 157–160.

133. Mouzon-Cambon, A., Ohayon, E., Bouissou, F. and Barthe, P. (1980). HLA-DR typing in children with glomerular diseases. *Lancet*, **2**, 868.

134. Lenhard, V., Dippel, J., Muller Wiefel, D. E., Schroder, D., Seidl, S. and Scharer, K. (1980). HLA antigens in children with idiopathic nephrotic syndrome. *Proc. EDTA*, **17**, 673–677.

135. Alfiler, C. A., Roy, L. P., Doran, T., Sheldon, A. and Bashir, H. (1980). HLA-DRw7 and steroid responsive-nephrotic syndrome of childhood. *Clin. Nephrol.*, **14**, 71–74.

136. Mouzon-Cambon, A., Bouissou, F., Dutau, G., Barthe, P., Parra, M. T., Sevin, A. and Ohayon, E. (1981). HLA DR-7 in children with idiopathic nephrotic syndrome. Correlation with atopy. *Tissue Antigens*, **17**, 518–524.

137. Noss, G., Bachmann, H. J. and Obling, H. (1981). Association of minimal change nephrotic syndrome (MCNS) with HLA-B8 and B13. *Clin. Nephrol.*, **15**, 172–174.

138. Meadow, S. R., Sarsfield, J. K., Scott, D. G. and Rajah, S. M. (1981). Steroid responsive nephrotic syndrome and allergy: Immunological studies. *Arch. Dis. Child.*, **56**, 517–524.

139. Ruder, H., Scharer, K., Lenhard, V., Wingen, A. M. and Oplez, G. (1982). HLA phenotypes and idiopathic nephrotic syndrome in children. *Proc. EDTA*, **19**, 602–606.

140. Nunez-Roldan, A., Villechenous, E., Fernandez-Andrade, C. and Martin-Govanentes, J. (1982). Increased HLA-DR7 and decreased DR2 in steroid responsive nephrotic syndrome. *N. Engl. J. Med.*, **306**, 366–367.

2
Induction and Regulation of Autoimmune Experimental Glomerulonephritis

P. DRUET

An autoimmune glomerulonephritis (AIGN) results from autoantibodies and/or from effector autoreactive T cells that recognize glomerular autoantigens. Experimental autoimmune diseases may be classified according to different criteria, for example: (1) autoimmune diseases that apparently occur spontaneously, as opposed to those which are intentionally induced; or (2) organ-specific diseases, as opposed to systemic diseases. These classifications apply to AIGN as shown in Table 1. We will consider the mechanisms of induction and regulation of glomerular-specific autoimmunity, and of AIGN occurring in the context of systemic autoimmunity.

GLOMERULAR-SPECIFIC AUTOIMMUNITY

Anti-glomerular basement membrane anti-(GBM-) mediated glomerulonephritis

Anti-GBM-mediated glomerulonephritis (GN) was one of the first autoimmune diseases to be studied. Susceptibility greatly depends upon the species tested and, within a species, upon the strain used[1]. Sheep immunized with heterologous or homologous GBM develop a severe autoimmune crescentic GN responsible for renal failure and death. This model has been extensively studied by Steblay et al.[2] but, owing to the species involved, the mechanisms at play could not be dissected.

More recently several models have become available in the rat. Susceptibility to the induction of anti-GBM-mediated AIGN greatly depends upon the strain. Brown Norway (BN) rats produce auto-anti-GBM antibodies following immunization with collagenase-digested bovine GBM, but they do not

Table 1 Experimental models of autoimmune glomerulonephritis

Condition	Spontaneous	Induced
Glomerular-specific	Membranous GN	Anti-GBM nephritis
		Heymann's nephritis
In the context of systemic autoimmunity	Lupus nephritis	Lipopolysaccharide-induced
		Parasitic infections
		Allogeneic reactions
		Toxin-induced

develop either proteinuria or crescentic GN. The genetic control of autoantibody production has been studied in that situation and was shown to depend upon genes, one of which is linked to the major histocompatibility complex (MHC)[3].

Sado et al.[4] observed that WKY/NCry rats immunized with homologous or isologous GBM and complete Freund's adjuvant (CFA) produced anti-GBM antibodies which were deposited along the GBM. These rats also exhibited significant proteinuria and a focal proliferative glomerulonephritis.

Pusey et al.[5] have studied the anti-GBM antibody response of various strains of rats to homologous or isologous collagenase-digested GBM. They found circulating autoantibodies in BN rats immunized with isologous or homologous GBM, even in the absence of CFA. The magnitude of the response was higher in rats immunized with the homologous antigen and CFA and these rats developed albuminuria. A proportion of them exhibited a mild focal proliferative GN with segmental lesions; pulmonary lesions were also apparent in some animals. The other strains (PVG/c, DA, LEW, WAG) also produced autoantibodies following immunization with homologous GBM and CFA. PVG/c and DA rats produced higher amounts of antibody and kidney-bound antibodies were only found in those two strains, although there was no apparent renal injury. Finally, the autoantibody response in BN rats was sustained for 12 months before levels fell. The precise mechanisms responsible for induction and regulation of autoimmunity, as well as the autoantigen(s) involved, remain to be investigated.

It is interesting to note that BN rats are highly prone to anti-GBM antibody production when compared with other strains of rats. Such antibodies were observed following immunization with GBM antigen but also (see below) in the context of T cell-dependent polyclonal activation of B cells following drug or toxin exposure, or in the chronic graft-versus-host reaction (GVHR). This suggests a low level of tolerance to GBM antigens in that strain. A similar lack of tolerance may explain the preferential occurrence of anti-GBM nephritis in DR2-positive patients[6]. Whether the autoantigen has to be modified (by collagenase in the experimental situation or by environmental agents in humans) for the immune response to occur remains to be shown. However, this is unlikely to occur in the chronic GVHR model.

In all these models it has been considered that the autoimmune disorder observed was antibody-mediated. Several arguments support this view. However, it could not be excluded that cell-mediated responses were also involved. Evidence has been obtained from heterologous nephrotoxic nephritis that T cells are also important as effector cells[7]. An experimental model of autoimmune GN has been developed in chickens immunized with heterologous GBM. These animals develop a classical AIGN with antibodies deposited along the GBM[8]. Advantage has been taken of the fact that bursectomy inhibits antibody production to demonstrate that bursectomised chickens immunized with heterologous GBM also develop AIGN. This happens without anti-GBM antibody production. Only mononuclear cells were found in the glomeruli, and the disease has been transferred with mononuclear cells from immunized animals[9]. It is likely that GBM-specific T cells are responsible for this form of AIGN. This demonstrates that autoimmune anti-GBM-mediated GN, at least in this species, can be a consequence of both antibody and cell-mediated immune responses.

Heymann's nephritis

This autoimmune membranous glomerulonephritis is obtained following immunization of susceptible strains of rats (LEW or PVG/c) with a rat renal tubular antigen and CFA. The crude antigenic fraction (FX1A) that was initially used[10] contains the nephritogenic antigen, a 330 kD glycoprotein (gp 330), expressed on both the brush border of proximal convoluted tubules and on the epithelial cells of the glomerular capillary wall[11-13]. The gp 330 antigen is concentrated in the coated pits and is irregularly distributed at the cell surface. Heymann's nephritis is due to the fixation of circulating autoantibodies to this irregularly distributed autoantigen[14,15]. The accumulation of antibodies gives rise to 'in situ' immune complex formation, responsible for the typical granular IgG deposits observed by immunofluorescence. Besides anti-gp 330 antibodies, other antigen–antibody systems may participate in the pathogenesis of the disease, for example gp 90 (dipeptidyl peptidase IV) or even basement membrane components and their corresponding antibodies[16,17].

The mechanisms responsible for induction and regulation of Heymann's nephritis have been studied, although less extensively than the target antigen. The antibody response to FX1A plus CFA is T cell-dependent[18]. It requires the presence of antigen-specific CD4+ T cells (helper/inducer). Neonatal thymectomy, or adult thymectomy associated with irradiation and reconstitution with bone marrow B cells, abrogates the antibody response and therefore prevents the occurrence of autoimmune nephritis[18]. The disease may be induced in T cell depleted adult animals following reconstitution with normal syngeneic CD4+ T cells[18]. De Heer et al.[19] have also shown that the immune response, as assessed by the detection of autoreactive B cells, is limited to the lymph nodes draining the site of immunization; CD4+ T cells are likely to be present at this site. These experiments show that, in susceptible strains, autoreactive T and B cells are present and can be triggered following proper immunization. They also show that tolerance is broken only locally.

The cellular basis of down-regulation of autoimmunity has been approached in two different situations. In rats with active Heymann's nephritis the amount of autoantibodies produced by B cells in the draining lymph nodes decreases after the tenth week and the level of circulating autoantibodies decreases later. These observations indicate that the autoimmune response is down-regulated. De Heer *et al.*[20] have shown that CD8 + T cells appear in the spleen of rats with active Heymann's nephritis from week 12. When such T cells were transferred into syngeneic recipients, which were subsequently challenged with FX1A and CFA, the antibody response was inhibited by 80%. This is in agreement with the fact that splenectomy is associated with increased renal IgG deposits[21]. Interestingly, when CD4 + T cells collected from the spleens of such animals were transferred, the immune response in subsequently immunized recipients was increased[20]. These experiments show clearly that autoreactive B cells and CD4 + helper T cells are found in the draining lymph nodes. Antigen specific CD4 + helper T cells and CD8 + suppressor/cytotoxic T cells are found in the spleen; they may respectively enhance or down-regulate autoimmunity. The fact that adult thymectomy enhances autoantibody production has been considered as the consequence of depletion of short-lived suppressor T cells.

Other studies have shown that tolerance may be induced in susceptible LEW and PVG/c rats following immunization with high doses of antigen plus incomplete Freund's adjuvant (IFA)[18,19,22]. Tolerance can be transferred to syngeneic recipients by lymph node cells from tolerized animals. Splenic CD8 + T cells from such animals also transferred resistance into subsequently challenged recipients, while CD8 − T cells induced an enhancement of autoimmunity[18,19]. The role of CD8 + T cells in the resistance of BN or DA rats has not been studied. It is known that resistance in BN rats may be overcome following immunization with the appropriate adjuvant[23,24]. It would be interesting to test the effect of *in vivo* CD8 + T cell depletion in resistant strains.

These studies taken together show clearly that T lymphocyte subsets play an important role in the regulation of Heymann's nephritis. Both CD4 + helper T cells and CD8 + suppressor/cytotoxic T cells are involved. The former are preferentially triggered following immunization with CFA and the latter following immunization with IFA. Furthermore, CD8 + T cells are involved in the down-regulation of the active disease. Although the role of CD8 + T cells in autoimmunity has recently been questioned[25], it seems clear that they play a role in Heymann's nephritis. The development of gp 330-specific T cell clones would be of value in better understanding the cellular basis of this important autoimmune disorder.

AUTOIMMUNE GLOMERULONEPHRITIS IN THE CONTEXT OF POLYCLONAL ACTIVATION

In the situations described above, T and B cell clones, specific for a given antigen such as gp 330, are selectively triggered. In other situations, numerous T and/or B cell clones are triggered, leading to 'polyclonal activation'[26]. An autoimmune glomerulonephritis is observed if a fraction of the stimulated clones is kidney-specific. The kidney may thus be affected in this context as well as other organs.

Autoimmune glomerulonephritis induced by bacterial products

Lipopolysaccharide (LPS) is of bacterial origin. It is composed of two polysaccharidic structures and of the lipid A region. The latter probably combines with a receptor on B lymphocytes and is responsible for B cell polyclonal activation[27]. Bacterial LPS is able to trigger 10–50% of all resting B cells, which then differentiate into antibody-producing cells of any immunological specificity[28]. Anti-DNA antibodies and rheumatoid factors, as well as antibodies to exogenous antigens or haptens, are produced. Total serum immunoglobulin levels (mainly IgM) increase. Other non-bacterial agents are also able to activate B cells polyclonally[26].

Injection of these B cell mitogens into mice induces glomerular immuno-globulin deposits[29]. IgM and IgG deposits in the mesangial areas and in the capillary loops are particularly prominent following chronic injections of LPS[30]. Only slight glomerular lesions are seen at the light-microscope level. About 40% of the immunoglobulins eluted from the kidneys of these mice are DNA specific[29]. Since DNA is released following LPS injections[31], anti-DNA antibodies may combine with DNA, forming circulating immune complexes that could then become deposited in the kidney. Alternatively, DNA may bind to the collagen part of the GBM with subsequent fixation of circulating antibodies to this 'planted' antigen[32].

Since only 40% of the kidney-bound Ig was DNA specific, this suggested that other antibodies should be involved. Rheumatoid factor is produced[30] and could combine with the deposited anti-DNA antibodies, but many other systems could also be involved. For example, anti-phosphoryl choline antibodies with the T15 idiotype are produced as a consequence of polyclonal activation in this model, and anti-idiotypic antibodies (anti-T15) are also produced for the same reason. Both such antibodies have been detected in the kidney[33]. It appears therefore that following B cell polyclonal activation many antigen–antibody systems may be involved.

LPS has been used in several strains of mice. As expected, strains lacking the LPS receptor[34] do not respond, while autoimmune disease in lupus-prone mice is enhanced following LPS injections[34].

Autoimmune glomerulonephritis induced by parasites

Parasitic infections are known to be associated with glomerulonephritis in humans[26,35], although the mechanisms at play are not well understood. On the one hand, evidence has been obtained that the immune response against the parasite itself could be important. On the other hand, an hyperimmuno-globulinaemia is a common feature of parasitic infections, suggesting a role for polyclonal activation. A B cell mitogen has been recovered from Plasmodia[36]. Animals infected with Schistosome[37] or Trypanosome[38,39] also develop a glomerulonephritis. Various autoantibodies such as anti-DNA antibodies, rheumatoid factor antibodies, and more recently anti-laminin antibodies, have been demonstrated in these situations. This again strongly suggests that the parasite acts, at least in part, by inducing a polyclonal activation of B cells.

Autoimmune glomerulonephritis induced by allogeneic reactions

Two different allogeneic reactions, the graft-versus-host reaction (GVHR) and the transplantation tolerance model (TTM), will be considered.

Graft-versus-host reaction

A GVHR is observed when parental T cells from a given mouse or rat strain (X) are transferred into a semi-allogeneic (X × Y) F1 hybrid[40]. An acute, lethal GVHR is observed when both parents differ at Class I and Class II MHC antigens, while a chronic GVHR is induced when they differ only at Class II antigens.

The acute GVHR is due to the development of parental (X) alloreactive T cells that recognize Y Class II or Class I antigens in the F1 hybrid. Anti-Class II T cells provide help for the proliferation of cytotoxic anti-Class I T cells that will destroy the F1 hybrid cells, leading to bone-marrow aplasia, atrophy of the lymphoid organs, severe skin and gastrointestinal lesions, and finally death.

A chronic GVHR may occur in three situations[40,41]. First, no cytotoxic T cells develop in Class I compatible situations; only anti-allo Class II T cells are present, which polyclonally stimulate F1 B cells through their allo Class II antigen. The role of autoantigens in the induction of this B cell stimulation is considered to be very important, and only those antigens with repetitive determinants are likely to be involved[40]. Various autoantibodies (anti-DNA, anti-GBM, anti-erythrocyte, rheumatoid factor, ...) are produced, leading to a lupus-like syndrome including an autoimmune glomerulonephritis with granular IgG deposits along the glomerular capillary walls[42]. Anti-DNA antibodies have been eluted from the glomeruli. Second, a chronic GVHR may also be observed in some strain combinations in spite of an incompatibility at Class I and Class II antigens. Depletion of donor parental CD8 + T cells using monoclonal antibodies will leave the inoculum with only CD4 + T cells, among which the allo anti-Class II T cell clones will expand. Finally, in other strain combinations incompatible at both Class I and Class II antigens, parental T cells are deficient in CD8 + cytotoxic anti-allo Class I T cells. This again will allow the development of anti-allo Class II T cells that will polyclonally stimulate F1 B cells.

Transplantation tolerance model

Mice from a given strain (Y) become tolerant to the X alloantigens following injection at birth of spleen cells from (X × Y) F1 hybrids[42-44]. Such mice do not reject skin grafts from X parents and do not generate cytotoxic T cells against the X alloantigens. The F1 cells transferred at birth persist in the recipient for a long period and these tolerant mice are therefore chimaeric[44]. However, allo-anti-Class II T cells from the host escape tolerance and are able to stimulate B cells from the F1 hybrid donor[45]. Autoantibodies (anti-DNA, anti-erythrocyte, rheumatoid factor, anti-laminin) are thus produced by F1 B cells. Some of these are found deposited in the glomeruli of the host, and are responsible for an immune complex GN involving extramembranous deposits. The specificity of kidney-bound antibodies has been only partly characterized, and has been shown to contain rheumatoid factor activity. It is interesting that the autoantibodies produced have the IgG1 isotype and that total serum IgE level increases[46]. This suggests a role for TH2 cells. CD4+ T cells, at least in mice, are now divided into two different subsets: TH1 which produce γ-interferon (IFN) and IL2, and TH2 which produce IL4 and IL5. IL4 is the cytokine responsible for IgE and IgG1 production[47]. A role for TH2 cells and for IL4 production has recently been demonstrated quite convincingly. An increase in Class II antigen expression was documented on B cells from the F1 donor, and parental T cells were able to increase Ia expression on normal F1 B cells[48]. This effect, known to depend upon IL4, was inhibited following incubation with an anti-IL4 monoclonal antibody. Finally, the hypothesis that IL4 plays a major role was confirmed following treatment of mice with monoclonal anti-IL4 antibody. The increase in IgE and IgG1 production was completely abrogated. Interestingly, other isotypes (IgG2a, IgG3) were produced, suggesting that TH1 cells were now involved and implying control of TH1 cells by TH2 cells (M. Goldman et al., personal communication).

Drug-induced autoimmune glomerulonephritis

Many drugs are known to induce autoimmune glomerulonephritides in humans[49]. Hypothetical mechanisms have been suggested for a long time, but have not yet been confirmed. Drugs could act as haptens fixed on glomerular antigens; alternatively, they could release or modify autoantigens. It is of interest that drugs such as gold salts or D-penicillamine may also induce several other, non-renal, autoimmune disorders[49]. This is an indication that at least some drugs could lead to disregulation of the immune system.

Experimental models have recently been devised. Extensive studies have been performed using the BN rat as an experimental animal and $HgCl_2$ as the inducing agent[50]. Other studies using D-penicillamine and gold salts have confirmed that this strain is prone to develop drug-induced AIGN and that the mechanisms are probably quite similar to those responsible for the chronic GVHR[51,52].

$HgCl_2$-induced autoimmunity in BN rats

Induction phase

Non-toxic amounts of $HgCl_2$ (100 µg/100 g body weight injected thrice weekly for 2 months) induce autoimmune manifestations in BN rats[50] from the second week that peak during the third and fourth weeks. These include lymphoproliferation, mainly due to an increase in the number of CD4+ T cells and B cells in the spleen and lymph nodes[53]. Total serum Ig levels increase, mainly owing to an increase in IgE, IgG1 and IgG2b isotypes[53]. A number of autoantibodies are produced that recognize GBM components, (mainly laminin but also collagen IV and fibronectin)[54,55], nuclear antigens, several other autoantigens including IgG, collagen II and thyroglobulin[56]. Antibodies against non-self antigens (TNP, sheep red blood cells) are also produced[57], and the amount of circulating natural polyreactive antibodies is increased[58]. A biphasic autoimmune glomerulonephritis is observed with IgG deposited along the GBM in a linear pattern during the first phase, from day 8[59]. Later (from the third week) a typical membranous glomerulonephritis is superadded[60]. The mechanism of formation of subepithelial deposits is still unknown; however, Ig eluted from kidneys with predominantly granular deposits binds in a linear pattern when incubated on normal kidney cryostat sections[60]. Several non-exclusive hypotheses may be proposed to explain the formation of granular deposits, including deposition of circulating GBM–anti-GBM immune complexes or rearrangement of linear IgG deposits due to the deposition of anti-idiotypic antibodies. It is also possible, as suggested by Aten et al.[61], that anti-laminin antibodies react against glomerular epithelial cells. Other autoimmune abnormalities (Sjögren's syndrome, dermatitis) have been reported[62].

These data suggest that $HgCl_2$ induces in BN rats a polyclonal activation of B cells. It was indeed confirmed that T cells from $HgCl_2$-injected rats were able to collaborate in vitro with normal B cells for antibody production[57]. In vivo experiments showed that T cells were required for this polyclonal activation to occur[63]. Further experiments showed that T cells from $HgCl_2$-injected BN rats were able to recognize either B cells from other $HgCl_2$-injected rats or normal syngeneic B cells, and that this interaction was blocked by an anti-class II monoclonal antibody[64]. These self-reactive T cells were frequent (about 1/5000 at the acme of the disease)[65]. Finally, T cells from rats exposed to $HgCl_2$ transferred autoimmunity to normal syngeneic recipients, provided that the recipients were previously depleted of CD8 + T cells using an anti-CD8 monoclonal antibody[66]. These experiments suggest that $HgCl_2$ elicits the emergence of self-reactive, anti-class II, CD4 + T cells. Although recent data unequivocally demonstrate that self-reactive T cells are clonally deleted in the thymus[67,68], there are other experiments which show that some $TCR\alpha\beta +$, double negative (CD4− CD8−), T cells may escape thymic deletion and, under certain circumstances, may become CD4 + and self-reactive[69]. The exact mechanism of action of mercury remains to be elucidated. Our experiments also suggest that when autoreactive T cells from $HgCl_2$-injected rats are transferred into normal recipients, they initiate the appearance of CD8 + T cells which may prevent their expansion[66]. The nature of these cells (cytotoxic?, anti-idiotypic?) is not yet known. Since such cells apparently do not appear in $HgCl_2$-injected rats, this indicates that mercury also acts by inhibiting such cells. That $HgCl_2$ induces a defect at the T suppressor level has been shown previously in PVG/c rats[70].

The similarities between the chronic GVHR and $HgCl_2$-induced autoimmunity are striking. In both situations anti-class II T cells are produced and a defect at the CD8 + T cells level seems to be required. In order to confirm these similarities we tested the effect of normal BN T cells transferred into (LEW × BN) F1 hybrids. The F1 hybrids produced anti-laminin and anti-nuclear autoantibodies, total serum IgE levels increased, and rats developed an autoimmune glomerulonephritis characterized by linear IgG deposits along the glomerular capillary walls[52]. More interestingly, using monoclonal anti-laminin antibodies and rabbit anti-idiotypic antibodies obtained in the $HgCl_2$-induced model, we demonstrated that anti-laminin antibodies share a cross-reactive idiotype, and that this cross-reactive idiotype is also present on circulating IgG and kidney-bound antibodies in the chronic GVHR[71]. All these data strongly support the notion that these autoimmune diseases are due to anti-Ia T cells which activate the same B cell clones.

Another feature of this model is that susceptibility is genetically controlled[72,73]. Several strains of rats with the RT1-1 or -u haplotype at the MHC are resistant (BN rats bear the RT1-n haplotype). Segregants between resistant (LEW) and BN rats were tested as well as congenic rats. This allowed us to demonstrate that both MHC- and non-MHC-linked genes are involved, with about three genes being implicated in the control of susceptibility.

Regulation phase

About 50% of the rats die during the third and fourth weeks. The remaining rats recover and all the autoimmune abnormalities progressively disappear[54,60]. After 2 months, IgE levels return to normal values and most autoantibodies are no longer detected. At least two non-exclusive mechanisms have been proposed. Several arguments strongly favour a role for Ts cells: (1) rats injected with very low doses of $HgCl_2$ do not develop autoimmunity and become resistant to further challenge with higher doses[74]; (2) injection of spleen cells from convalescent $HgCl_2$-treated BN rats to naive syngeneic recipients attenuates the severity of $HgCl_2$-induced disease[75]; (3) while the number of CD8+ T cells in the blood is decreased during the induction phase, it increases significantly during the regulation phase[76]. However, treatment with an anti-CD8 monoclonal antibody does not affect significantly either the induction or the regulation phase[77]. These observations are compatible with an initial defect in Ts cells, but they also show that CD8+ T cells are not by themselves responsible for the regulation phase.

Anti-idiotypic antibodies have been proposed as another mechanism to explain the regulation phase. Chalopin et al.[78] have obtained indirect evidence that auto-anti-idiotypic antibodies are produced. Serum from $HgCl_2$-injected rats is able to enhance an anti-GBM plaque-forming cell assay, as would be expected. However, from an anti-idiotypic antibody, other factors (such as GBM–anti-GBM immune complexes) could explain this effect. Recently, a monoclonal auto-anti-idiotypic antibody has been obtained from a BN rat injected with $HgCl_2$[98]. This antibody recognizes monoclonal anti-laminin antibodies produced in the mercury model. This demonstrates that such antibodies are synthesized during the disease, but their regulatory and/or pathogenic effect is unknown.

Other mechanisms may also play a role. For example, different cytokines may be produced during the two phases of the disease, including IL4 during the former phase and γ-IFN during the latter. It has been shown that these cytokines may down-regulate TH1 and TH2 cells respectively[47].

HgCl₂-induced autoimmunity in other strains of rat and other species

HgCl$_2$-induced autoimmunity in other strains of rat and other species

As already mentioned, susceptibility depends upon the strain of rat tested[79]. As far as induction or regulation mechanisms are concerned, data are only available in PVG/c rats, in which T suppressor function is defective[70]. New Zealand rabbits injected with HgCl$_2$ exhibit an AIGN quite similar to that seen in BN rats[80]. Among the various strains of mice tested, those with the H-2^S haplotype (B10 S, A.SW) are particularly susceptible to the induction of autoimmunity[81,82]. These mice produce anti-S3 autoantibodies similar to those found in scleroderma patients[83], and these antibodies have been recovered from kidney eluates. Susceptibility is genetically controlled. As in BN rats, total serum IgE levels increase and recent results have demonstrated that IL4 plays a major role[84]. Treatment of B10 S mice with an anti-IL4 monoclonal antibody abrogates the increase in total serum IgE levels and the production of autoantibodies with the IgG1 isotype[99].

Other drug-induced autoimmune glomerulonephritides

Several models of AIGN have been described using D-penicillamine (D-pen), gold salts, or other drugs, but the mechanisms of induction were not studied. Recently, several experiments have been performed which suggest analogies between HgCl$_2$- and gold- or D-pen-[84,85] induced autoimmunity. Autoimmune glomerulonephritis has been described following D-pen[84,85] or gold exposure[51] in BN rats. Most abnormalities encountered in HgCl$_2$-induced autoimmunity were also observed in these two models. The severity of the disease was, however, less than in HgCl$_2$-induced AIGN. The cross-reactive idiotype that has been described in the mercury model[86], and in chronic GVHR, has also been found in D-pen and gold models[71]. In addition, anti-Class II T cells have also been observed[51,85]. Finally, Lewis rats do not develop AIGN after D-pen[84] or gold treatment[100]. These data strongly support a common mechanism for these three models of drug-induced autoimmunity, and show that the BN rat strain is the most appropriate in which to test the potential of drugs to induce systemic autoimmunity. Susceptible mice also develop autoimmunity following gold or D-pen exposure[81].

MURINE LUPUS NEPHRITIS

Numerous reviews have considered this topic[87,88], and the spontaneous autoimmune disease observed in female (NZB × NZW) F1 hybrids, MRL lpr/lpr or male B × SB mice will not be described here. The mechanisms leading to the 'in situ' formation and/or to the deposition of immune complexes responsible for the AIGN observed in these diseases have also been discussed in these reviews.

Concerning the mechanisms of induction of these diseases, there is general agreement on the following. (1) The major abnormality is a generalized polyclonal B cell activation[87], which does not rule out a role for autoantigens in causing a switch to IgG or IgA production (reviewed in ref. 89). (2) T cells are required for this polyclonal activation to occur[88]. (3) Genetic and non-genetic factors play a major role in inducing or accelerating autoimmunity[88].

More recent studies have been concerned with the molecular genetics of B and T cell antigen receptors[88]. It appears from these studies that the Ig germ line genes are probably normal, and that the gene segments expressed in autoantibodies[90] and in antibodies to exogenous antigens are similar. Furthermore, no reduced or increased somatic mutation in Ig genes could be defined. Concerning the T cell antigen receptor (TcR), it seems that there is no special TcR associated with autoimmunity, in spite of the unusual nature of the NZW TcR β chain[91,92], and that the repertoire is similar to that of normal mice. Self-reactive T cells are normally deleted in the thymus, and this procedure does not seem to be affected in (NZB × NZW) F1 mice. Potentially self-reactive T cells have also been shown to be normally deleted in MRL lpr/lpr mice[90].

Finally, a role for TcR $\alpha:\beta+$, double-negative, T cells has recently been proposed[88]. Such T cells exist at a very low percentage (5%) in normal BALB/c mice and may become CD4+ and anti-self Ia reactive following stimulation with Con A[69,73]. The lymphoproliferation observed in MRL lpr/lpr mice is mainly composed of double-negative T cells, and these cells contribute to (NZB × NZW) F1 mice to the helper activity for anti-DNA production. It is therefore possible that TcR $\alpha:\beta+$, CD4− CD8−, T cells represent potentially autoreactive T cells that escaped clonal elimination in the thymus and that may become autoreactive in different situations. It is interesting in this connection that CD4+ anti-Ia T cells have been obtained from MRL lpr/lpr[94] and from (NZB × NZW) F1 mice[95]. The role of double-negative T cells, their relationship with anti-Ia T cells, and their role in autoimmunity require further studies.

CONCLUSION

Although they do not always represent the exact counterpart of human AIGN, experimental models have allowed advances in our understanding of glomerular autoimmunity. We need much more information in many areas. (1) It is crucial to define better the autoantigens involved. Except for the autoantigen responsible for anti-GBM-mediated AIGN[96], very little is known in the human situation. It will be also of great interest to define the role of autoantigens in situations associated with polyclonal activation of B cells[89]. (2) It is clear from experimental models[23,72,73], and from the human situation[6,97], that MHC antigens are crucial for T cell activation. Much more will be learnt in the future from restriction fragment length polymorphism analysis and from studies at the gene level. (3) Although it has now been demonstrated that autoreactive T cells are deleted in the thymus in well-defined situations[67,68], it is nevertheless obvious that this deletion process is not absolute. Autoreactive T cells may be induced in several experimental models of AIGN. It will be of major importance to obtain T cell lines or clones to characterize the T cell receptor, and to elucidate the regulatory circuits which prevent activation of autoreactive T cells. In this respect, there is evidence that suppressor T cells[18,20], the idiotypic network[78], and/or cytokines[46] may be of major importance in several models of AIGN.

Our understanding of human AIGN has greatly improved during the last few years owing to a better understanding of experimental models and to major advances in basic immunology. Further research in these areas should contribute to the elucidation of the mechanisms of glomerular autoimmunity in the human situation.

References

1. Wilson, C. B. and Dixon, F. J. (1986). The renal response to immunological injury. In Brenner, B. M. and Rector, F. C. (eds.) *The Kidney*, pp. 800. (Philadelphia: W. B. Saunders)
2. Steblay, R. W. (1962). Glomerulonephritis induced in sheep by injections of heterologous glomerular basement membrane and Freund's complete adjuvant. *J. Exp. Med.*, 116, 253–272
3. Stuffers-Heimann, M., Günther, E. and Van Es, L. A. (1979). Induction of autoimmunity to antigens of the glomerular basement membrane in inbred Brown-Norway rats. *Immunology*, 36, 759–767.
4. Sado, Y., Okigaki, T., Takamiya, H. and Seno, S. (1984). Experimental autoimmune glomerulonephritis with pulmonary haemorrhage in rats. The dose-effect relationship of the nephritogenic antigen from bovine glomerular basement membrane. *J. Clin. Lab. Immunol.*, 15, 199–205
5. Pusey, C. D., Holland, M. J., Cashman, S. J., Sinico, R. A., Lloveras, J. J., Evans, D. J. and Lockwood, C. M. (1991). Autoimmunity to glomerular basement membrane induced by homologous and isologous in Brown Norway rats. *Nephrol. Dial. Transplant.* (in press)
6. Rees, A. J., Peters, D. K., Compston, D. A. S. and Batchelor, J. R. (1978). Strong association between HLA DRw2 and antibody mediated Goodpasture's syndrome. *Lancet*, 1, 966–968
7. Tipping, P. G., Neale, T. J. and Holdsworth, S. R. (1985). T lymphocyte participation in antibody-induced experimental glomerulonephritis. *Kidney Int.*, 27, 530–537
8. Bolton, W. K., Chandra, M., Tyson, T. M., Kirkpatrick, P. R., Sadovnic, M. J. and Sturgill, B. C. (1988). Transfer of experimental glomerulonephritis in chickens by mononuclear cells. *Kidney Int.*, 34, 598–610
9. Bolton, W. K., Tucker, F. L. and Sturgill, B. C. (1984). A new avian model of experimental glomerulonephritis consistent with mediation by cellular immunity. *J. Clin. Invest.*, 73, 1263–1276
10. Heymann, W., Hackel, D. B., Harwood, S., Wilson, S. G. F. and Hunter, J. L. P. (1959). Production of nephrotic syndrome in rats by Freund's adjuvants and rat kidney suspensions. *Proc. Soc. Exp. Biol. Med.*, 100, 660–664
11. Kerjaschki, D. and Farquhar, M. G. (1982). The pathogenic antigen of Heymann nephritis is a membrane glycoprotein of the renal proximal tubular brush border. *Proc. Natl Acad. Sci.*, 79, 5557–5561
12. Kerjaschki, D. and Farquhar, M. G. (1983). Immunocytochemical localization of the Heymann nephritis antigen (gp 330) in glomerular epithelial cells of normal Lewis rats. *J. Exp. Med.*, 157, 667–686
13. Chatelet, F., Brianti, E., Ronco, P., Roland, J. and Verroust, P. (1986). Ultrastructural localization by monoclonal antibodies of brush border antigens expressed by glomeruli. I. Renal distribution. *Am. J. Pathol.*, 122, 500–511
14. Couser, W. G., Steinmuller, D. R., Stilmant, M. M., Salant, D. J. and Lowenstein, L. M. (1978). Experimental glomerulonephritis in the isolated perfused rat kidney. *J. Clin. Invest.*, 62, 1275–1287
15. Van Damme, B. J. C., Fleuren, G. J., Bakker, W. W., Vernier, R. L. and Hoedemaeker, Ph. J. (1978). Experimental glomerulonephritis in the rat induced by antibodies against tubular antigens. V. Fixed glomerular antigens in the pathogenesis of heterologous immune complex glomerulonephritis. *Lab. Invest.*, 38, 502–510
16. Verroust, P., Ronco, P. and Chatelet, F. (1987). Antigenic targets in membranous glomerulonephritis. *Springer Semin. Immunopathol.*, 9, 341–358
17. Hogendoorn, P. C. W., Bruijn, J. A., Van Der Broek, L. J. C. M., De Heer, E., Foidart, J. M., Hoedemqaeker, Ph. J. and Fleuren, G. J. (1988). Antibodies to purified renal tubular

epithelial antigens contain activity against laminin, fibronectin and type IV collagen. *Lab. Invest.*, **58**, 278–286

18. Cheng, I. K. P., Dorsch, S. E. and Hall, B. M. (1988). The regulation of autoantibody production in Heymann's nephritis by T lymphocyte subsets. *Lab. Invest.*, **59**, 780–788

19. De Heer, E., Daha, M. R. and Van Es, L. A. (1985). The autoimmune response in active Heymann's nephritis in Lewis rats is regulated by T lymphocyte subsets. *Cell Immunol.*, **92**, 254–264

20. De Heer, E., Daha, M. R., Burger, J. and Van Es, L. A. (1986). Re-establishment of self tolerance by suppressor T-cells after active Heymann's nephritis. *Cell Immunol.*, **98**, 28–33

21. Abrass, C. (1986). Evaluation of sequential glomerular eluates from rats with Heymann nephritis. *J. Immunol.*, **137**, 530–535

22 Litwin, A., Bash, J. A., Adams, L. E., Donovan, R. J. and Hess, E. V. (1979). Immunoregulation of Heymann's nephritis. I. Induction of suppressor cells. *J. Immunol.*, **122**, 1029–1034

23. Stenglein, B., Thoenes, G. H. and Günther, E. (1978). Genetic control of susceptibility to autologous immune complex glomerulonephritis in inbred rat strains. *Clin. Exp. Immunol.*, **33**, 88–94

24. Zanetti, M., Bellon, B., Verroust, P. and Druet, P. (1980). A search for circulating immune complexes like-material during the course of autoimmune complex glomerulonephritis in Lewis and Brown-Norway rats. *Clin. Exp. Immunol.*, **41**, 189–195

25. Möller, G. (1988). Do suppressor T cells exist? *Scand. J. Immunol.*, **27**, 247–250

26. Goldman, M., Baran, D. and Druet, P. (1988). Polyclonal activation and experimental nephropathies. *Kidney Int.*, **34**, 141–150

27. Skidmore, B. J., Chiller, J. M., Morrison, D. C. and Weigle, W. O. (1975). Immunological properties of bacterial lipopolysaccharide (LPS): Correlation between the mitogenic, adjuvant and immunogenic properties. *J. Immunol.*, **114**, 770–775

28. Anderson, J., Coutinho, A. and Melchers, F. (1977). Frequencies of mitogen-reactive B cells in the mouse. I. Distribution in different lymphoid organs from different inbred strains of mice at different ages. *J. Exp. Med.*, **145**, 1511–1519

29 Izui, S., Lambert, P. H., Fournie, G. J., Turler, H. and Miescher, P. A. (1977). Features of systemic lupus erythematosus in mice injected with bacterial lipopolysaccharides. Identification of circulating DNA and renal localization of DNA–anti-DNA complexes. *J. Exp. Med.*, **145**, 1115–1130

30 Ramos-Niembro, F., Fournie, G. and Lambert, P. H. (1982). Induction of circulating immune complexes and their renal localization after acute or chronic polyclonal B cell activation in mice. *Kidney Int.*, **21**, S29–S38

31. Fournie, G. J., Lambert, P. H. and Miescher, P. A. (1984). Release of DNA in circulating blood and induction of anti-DNA antibodies after injection of bacterial lipopolysaccharides. *J. Exp. Med.*, **140**, 1189–1206

32. Izui, S., Lambert, P. H. and Miescher, P. A. (1976). In vitro demonstration of a particular affinity of glomerular basement membrane and collagen for DNA. A possible basis for a local formation of DNA-anti-DNA complexes in systemic lupus erythematosus. *J. Exp. Med.*, **144**, 428–443

33. Goldman, M., Rose, L. M., Hochmann, A. and Lambert, P. H. (1982). Deposition of idiotype-anti-idiotype immune complexes in renal glomeruli after polyclonal B cell activation. *J. Exp. Med.*, **155**, 1385–1399

34. Hang, L. M., Slack, J. H., Amundson, C., Izui, S., Theofilopoulos, A. N. and Dixon, F. J. (1983). Induction of murine autoimmune disease by chronic polyclonal B cell activation. *J. Exp. Med.*, **157**, 874–883

35. Levy, M. (1986). Infections and glomerular diseases. *Clin. Immunol. Allergy*, **6**, 255–286

36. Greenwood, B. M. and Vick, R. M. (1975). Evidence for a malaria mitogen in human malaria. *Nature*, **257**, 592–594

37. Houba, V. (1979). Experimental renal disease due to schistosomiasis. *Kidney Int.*, **16**, 30–43

38. Rose, L. M., Goldman, M. and Lambert, P. H. (1982). Simultaneous induction of an idiotype, of corresponding anti-idiotypic antibodies and of immune complexes during African trypanosomiasis in mice. *J. Immunol.*, **128**, 79–85

39. Bruijn, J. A., Oemar, B. S., Ehrich, J. H. H., Foidart, J. M. and Fleuren, G. J. (1987). Anti-basement membrane glomerulopathy in experimental trypanosomiasis. *J. Immunol.*, **139**, 2482–2488

40. Gleichmann, E., Pals, S. T., Rolink, A. G., Radaszkiewicz, T. and Gleichmann, H. (1984). Graft-versus-host reactions: Clues to the etiopathology of a spectrum of immunological diseases. *Immunol. Today*, **5**, 324–332

41. Via, C. S. and Shearer, G. M. (1988). T-cell interactions in autoimmunity: insights from a murine model of graft-versus-host disease. *Immunol. Today*, **9**, 207-213

42. Goldman, M., Feng, H. M., Engers, H., Hochmann, A., Louis, J. and Lambert, P. H. (1983). Autoimmunity and immune complex disease after neonatal induction of transplantation tolerance in mice. *J. Immunol.*, **131**, 251-258

43. Tateno, M., Kondo, N., Itoh, T. and Yoshiki, T. (1985). Autoimmune disease and malignant lymphoma associated with host-versus-graft disease in mice. *Clin. Exp. Immunol.*, **62**, 535–544

44. Luzuy, S., Merino, J., Engers, H., Izui, S. and Lambert, P. H. (1986). Autoimmunity after induction of neonatal tolerance to alloantigens: Role of B cell chimerism and F1 donor B cell activation. *J. Immunol.*, **136**, 4420–4426

45. Abramowicz, D., Goldman, M., Bruyns, C., Lambert, P. H., Thoua, Y. and Toussaint, C. (1987). Autoimmune disease after neonatal injection of semi-allogeneic spleen cells in mice; involvement of donor B and T cells and characterization of glomerular deposits. *Clin. Exp. Immunol.*, **70**, 61–67

46. Goldman, M., Abramowicz, D., Lambert, P., Vandervorst, P., Bruyns, C. and Toussaint, C. (1988). Hyperactivity of donor B cells after neonatal induction of lymphoid chimerism in mice. *Clin. Exp. Immunol.*, **72**, 79–83

47. Mosmann, T. R. and Coffman, R. L. (1989). Heterogeneity of cytokine secretion patterns and functions of helper T cells. *Adv. Immunol.*, **46**, 111–147

48. Abramowicz, D., Doutrelepont, J. M., Lambert, P., Van Der Vorst, P., Bruyns, C. and Goldman, M. (1990). Increased expression of Ia antigens on B cells after neonatal induction of lymphoid chimerism in mice: role of Interleukin-4. *Eur. J. Immunol.*, **20**, 469–476

49. Fillastre, J. P., Druet, P. and Mery, J. PH. (1988). Drug-induced glomeruloneophritis. In Cameron, J. S. and Glassock, R. J. (eds). *The Nephrotic Syndrome*, pp. 697. (New York: Marcel Dekker)

50. Pelletier, L., Hirsch, F., Rossert, J., Druet, E. and Druet, P. (1987). Experimental mercury-induced glomerulonephritis. *Springer Semin. Immunopathol.*, **9**, 359–369

51. Tournade, H., Pelletier, L., Glotz, D. and Druet, P. (1989). Toxiques et auto-immunité. *Médecine/Sciences*, **5**, 303–310

52. Tournade, H., Pelletier, L., Pasquier, R., Vial, M. C., Mandet, C. and Druet, P. (1990). Graft-versus-host reactions in the rat mimick toxin-induced autoimmunity. *Clin. Exp. Immunol.*, **81**, 334–338

53. Pelletier, L., Pasquier, R., Guettier, C., Vial, M. C., Mandet, C., Nochy, D., Bazin, H. and Druet, P. (1988). HgCl$_2$ induces T and B cell to proliferate and differentiate in BN rats. *Clin. Exp. Immunol.*, **71**, 336–342

54. Bellon, B.,, Capron, M., Druet, E., Verroust, P., Vial, M. C., Sapin, C., Girard, J. F., Foidart, J. M., Mahieu, P. and Druet, P. (1982). Mercuric chloride induced auto-immune disease in Brown Norway rats: sequential search for antibasement membrane antibodies and circulating immune complexes. *Eur. J. Clin. Invest.*, **12**, 127–133

55. Fukatsu, A., Brentjens, J. R., Killen, P. D., Kleinman, K. D., Martin, G. R. and Andres, G. A. (1987). Studies on the formation of glomerular immune deposits in Brown Norway rats injected with mercuric chloride. *Clin. Immunol. Immunopathol.*, **45**, 35–47

56. Pusey, C. D., Bowman, C., Morgan, A., Weetman, A. P., Hartley, B. and Lockwood, C. M. (1990). Kinetics and pathogenicity of autoantibodies induced by mercuric chloride in the Brown Norway rat. *Clin. Exp. Immunol.*, **81**, 76–82

57. Hirsch, F., Couderc, J., Sapin, C., Fournie, G. and Druet, P. (1982). Polyclonal effect of HgCl$_2$ in the rat, its possible role in an experimental auto-immune disease. *Eur. J. Immunol.*, **12**, 620–625

58. Hirsch, F., Kuhn, J., Ventura, M., Vial, M. C., Fournie, G. and Druet, P. (1986). Autoimmunity induced by HgCl$_2$ in Brown Norway rats. I. Production of monoclonal antibodies. *J. Immunol.*, **136**, 3272–3276

59. Sapin, C., Druet, E. and Druet, P. (1977). Induction of anti-glomerular basement membrane antibodies in the Brown Norway rat by mercuric chloride. *Clin. Exp. Immunol.*, **28**, 173–179

60. Druet, P., Druet, E., Potdevin, F. and Sapin, C. (1978). Immune type glomerulonephritis induced by HgCl$_2$ in the Brown-Norway rat. *Ann. Immunol.*, **129C**, 777–792

61. Aten, J., Bruijn, J. A., Veringa, A., De Heer, E. and Weening, J. J. (1988). Anti-laminin autoantibodies and mercury-induced membranous glomerulopathy. *Kidney Int.*, **33**, 309

62. Aten, J., Bosman, L. B., Rozing, J., Stijnen, T., Hoedemaeker, P. J. and Weening, J. (1988). Mercuric chloride autoimmunity in the Brown Norway rat. *Am. J. Pathol.*, **133**, 127–138

63. Pelletier, L., Pasquier, R., Vial, M. C., Mandet, C., Moutier, R., Salomon, J. C. and Druet, P. (1987). Mercury-induced autoimmune glomerulonephritis: Requirement for T-cells. *Nephrol. Dial. Transplant.*, **1**, 211–218

64. Pelletier, L., Paquier, R., Hirsch, F., Sapin, C. and Druet, P. (1986). Autoreactive T cells in mercury-induced autoimmune disease: In vitro demonstration. *J. Immunol.*, **137**, 2548–2553

65. Rossert, J., Pelletier, L., Pasquier, R. and Druet, P. (1988). Autoreactive T cells in mercury-induced autoimmunity. Demonstration by limiting dilution analysis. *Eur. J. Immunol.*, **18**, 1761–1766

66. Pelletier, L., Pasquier, R., Rossert, J., Vial, M. C., Mandet, C. and Druet, P. (1988). Autoreactive T cells in mercury-induced autoimmunity. Ability to induce the autoimmune disease. *J. Immunol.*, **140**, 750–754

67. Kappler, J. W., Roehm, N., and Marrack, P. (1987). T cell tolerance by clonal elimination in the thymus. *Cell*, **49**, 273–280

68. Kisielow, P., Bluthmann, H., Staerz, U. D., Steinmetz, M. and Von Boehmer, H. (1988). Tolerance in T-cell-receptor transgenic mice involves deletion of nonmature $CD4^+8^+$ thymocytes. *Nature*, **333**, 742–746

69. deTalance, A., Regnier, D., Spinella, S., Morisset, J. and Seman, M. (1986). Origin of autoreactive T helper cells. I. Characterization of Thy-1^+, $Lyt^-/L3T4^-$ precursors in the spleen of normal mice. *J. Immunol.*, **137**, 1101–1108

70. Weening, J. J., Fleuren, G. J. and Hoedemaeker, P. J. (1981). Immunoregulation and antinuclear antibodies in mercury-induced glomerulopathy in the rat. *Clin. Exp. Immunol.*, **45**, 64–71

71. Guéry, J. C., Tournade, H., Pelletier, L., Druet, E. and Druet, P. (1989). Rat anti-glomerular basement membrane antibodies in toxin-induced autoimmunity and in chronic graft-versus-host reaction share recurrent idiotypes. *Eur. J. Immunol.*, **20**, 101–105

72. Druet, E., Sapin, C., Gunther, E., Feingold, N. and Druet, P. (1977). Mercuric chloride induced anti-glomerular basement membrane antibodies in the rat. Genetic control. *Eur. J. Immunol.*, **7**, 348–351

73. Sapin, C., Hirsch, F., Delaporte, J. P., Bazin, H. and Druet, P. (1984). Polyclonal IgE increase after $HgCl_2$ injections in BN and LEW rats. A genetic analysis. *Immunogenetics*, **20**, 227–236

74. Pusey, C. D., Bowman, C., Peters, D. K. and Lockwood, C. M. (1983). Effects of cyclophosphamide on autoantibody synthesis in the Brown Norway rat. *Clin. Exp. Immunol.*, **54**, 697–704

75. Bowman, C., Mason, D. W., Pusey, C. D. and Lockwood, C. M. (1984). Autoregulation of antibody synthesis in mercuric chloride nephritis in the Brown Norway rat. I. A role for T suppressor cells. *Eur. J. Immunol.*, **14**, 464–470

76. Bowman, C., Green, C., Borysiewicz, L. and Lockwood, M. (1987). Circulating T-cell populations during mercuric chloride-induced nephritis in the Brown Norway rat. *Immunology*, **61**, 515–520

77. Pelletier, L., Rossert, J., Pasquier, R., Vial, M. C. and Druet, P. (1990). Role of $CD8^+$ T cells in mercury-induced autoimmunity or immunosuppression in the rat. *Scand. J. Immunol.*, **31**, 65–74

78. Chalopin, J. M. and Lockwood, C. M. (1984). Autoregulation of autoantibody synthesis in mercuric chloride nephritis in the Brown Norway rat. II. Presence of antigen-augmentable plaque-forming cells in the spleen is associated with humoral factors behaving as auto-anti-idiotypic antibodies. *Eur. J. Immunol.*, **14**, 470–475

79. Druet, E., Sapin, C., Fournie, G., Mandet, C., Gunther, E. and Druet, P. (1982). Genetic control of susceptibility to mercury-induced immune nephritis in various strains of rat. *Clin. Immunol. Immunopathol.*, **25**, 203–212

80. Roman-Franco, A. A., Turiello, M., Albini, B., Ossi, E., Milgrom, F. and Andres, G. A. (1978). Anti-basement membrane antibodies and antigen-antibody complexes in rabbits injected with mercuric chloride. *Clin. Immunol. Immunopathol.*, **9**, 464–481

81. Robinson, C. J. G., Balazs, T. and Egorov, I. K. (1986). Mercuric chloride-, gold sodium

thiomalate-, and D-penicillamine-induced antinuclear antibodies in mice. *Toxicol. Appl. Pharmacol.*, **86**, 159–169

82. Pietsch, P., Vohr, H. W., Degitz, K. and Gleichmann, E. (1989). Immunological alterations inducible by mercury compounds. II. HgCl₂ and gold sodium thiomalate enhance serum IgE and IgG concentrations in susceptible mouse strains. *Int. Arch. Allergy Appl. Immunol.*, **90**, 47–53

83. Reuter, R., Tessars, G., Vohr, H. W., Gleichmann, E. and Lührmann, R. (1989). Mercuric chloride induces autoantibodies against U3 small ribonuclear protein in susceptible mice. *Proc. Natl Acad. Sci.*, **86**, 237–241

84. Donker, Ab. J., Venuto, R. C., Vladutio, A. O., Brentjens, J. R. and Andres, G. A. (1984). Effects of prolonged administration of D-penicillamine or captopril in various strains of rats. *Clin. Immunol. Immunopathol.*, **30**, 142–155

85. Tournade, H., Pelletier, L., Pasquier, R., Vial, M. C., Mandet, C. and Druet, P. (1989). D-Penicillamine-induced autoimmunity in Brown Norway rats: similarities with HgCl₂-induced autoimmunity. *J. Immunol.* (In press)

86. Guéry, J. C., Druet, E., Glotz, D., Hirsch, F., Mandet, C., De Heer, E. and Druet, P. (1990). Specificity and cross-reactive idiotypes of anti-glomerular basement membrane autoantibodies in HgCl₂-induced autoimmune glomerulonephritis. *Eur. J. Immunol.* (In press)

87. Theofilopoulos, A. N. and Dixon, F. J. (1985). Murine models of systemic lupus erythematosus. *Adv. Immunol.*, **37**, 269–390

88. Theofilopoulos, A. N., Kofler, R., Singer, P. A. and Dixon, F. J. (1989). Molecular genetics of murine lupus models. *Adv. Immunol.*, **46**, 61–109

89. Dziarski, R. (1988). Autoimmunity: Polyclonal activation or antigen induction? *Immunol. Today*, **9**, 340–342

90. Theofilopoulos, A. N., Kofler, R., Noonan, D., Singer, P. and Dixon, F. J. (1986). Molecular aspects of murine systemic lupus erythematosus. *Springer Semin. Immunopathol.*, **9**, 121–142

91. Kotzin, B. L. and Palmer, E. (1987). The contribution of NZW genes to lupus-like disease in (NZB × NZW) F₁ mice. *J. Exp. Med.*, **165**, 1237–1251

92. Kotzin, B. L., Barr, V. L. and Palmer, E. (1985). A large deletion within the T-cell receptor beta-chain gene complex in New Zealand white mice. *Science*, **229**, 167–171

93. Morisset, J., Trannoy, E., deTalance, A., Spinella, S., Debrep, P., Godet, P. and Seman, M. (1988). Genetics and strain distribution of concanavalin-A reactive Ly-2⁻, L3T4⁻ peripheral precursors of autoreactive T cells. *Eur. J. Immunol.*, **18**, 387–394

94. Rosenberg, Y. J., Steinberg, A. D. and Santoro, T. J. (1983). The basis of autoimmunity in mrl-lpr/lpr mice: A role for self Ia-reactive T cells. *Immunol. Today*, **5**, 64–67

95. Ando, D. G., Sercarz, E. E. and Hahn, B. V. (1987). Mechanisms of T and B cell collaboration in the in vitro production of anti-DNA antibodies in the NZB/NZW F1 murine SLE model. *J. Immunol.*, **87**, 3185–3190

96. Wieslander, J., Kataja, M. and Hudson, B. G. (1987). Characterisation of the human Goodpasture antigen. *Clin. Exp. Immunol.*, **69**, 332–340

97. Klouda, P. T., Manos, J., Acheson, E. J., Dyer, P. A., Goldby, F. S., Harris, R., Lawler, W., Mallick, N. P. and Williams, G. (1979). Strong association between idiopathic membranous nephropathy and HLA-DRw3. *Lancet*, **2**, 770–771

98. Guery, J. C. and Druet, P. (1990). A spontaneous hybridoma producing autoanti-idiotypic antibodies that recognize a Vₖ-associated idiotype in mercury-induced autoimmunity. *Eur. J. Immunol.*, **20**, 1027–1031

99. Ochel, M., Vohr, H.-W., Pfeiffer, C. and Gleichmann, E. (1991). Il-4 required for the IgE and IgG1 increase and IgG1 autoantibody formation in mice treated with mercuric chloride. *J. Immunol.*, (in press)

100. Tournade, H., Guery, J. C., Pasquier, R., Nochy, D., Hinglais, N., Guilbert, B., Druet, P. and Pelletier, L. (1991). Experimenal gold-induced autoimmunity. *Nephrol. Dial. Transplant.*, (in press)

3
Molecular Mechanisms of *In Situ* Immune Complex Formation in Experimental Membranous Nephropathy

D. KERJASCHKI

INTRODUCTION

Membranous glomerulopathy (MGN) is characterized by the deposition of granular immune complexes in the glomerular basement membrane (GBM) that corresponds to subepithelial dense immune deposits in the lamina rara externa seen by electron microscopy[1]. The progression of this disease to renal insufficiency is not influenced in a significant number of cases, despite aggressive immunosuppressive therapies[2-4]. Therefore, a specific therapy for MGN is needed which can be only conceived when its pathogenic mechanisms are understood. This requires: (1) the identification of molecule(s) which serve as the antigen(s) in the initial immune complexes; (2) the precise analysis of the mechanisms of stablization and growth of the nascent antibody–antigen complexes to permanent subepithelial immune deposits; and (3) clarification of the secondary mechanisms which trigger complex pathophysiological reactions in the glomerulus.

The current status of knowledge about the pathogenesis of MGN was recently extensively reviewed[5-8], and some aspects of the secondary mechanisms are reviewed in Chapter 5 of this volume. In this chapter, several recent aspects of the pathogenic process of experimental MGN are summarized, some of which could eventually offer clues to how to interfere specifically with the formation of the immune deposits in human MGN.

Heymann nephritis: a model of human membranous nephropathy

Because human material for experimental work on MGN is very limited, many researchers have resorted to an experimental MGN-like disease in rats, that resembles its human counterpart in great detail. This disease model was developed by Heymann et al.[9,10] and is therefore commonly referred to as 'Heymann nephritis' (HN).

The immune deposits in HN can be induced either by active immunization of rats with the nephritogenic antigen ('active HN'), or by passive transfer, for example by intravenous injection of heterologous antibodies raised against pathogenic antigen preparations ('passive HN')[11,12]. These variants of HN differ primarily in the speed with which the immune deposits develop. Thus, passive HN has proved very useful for the analysis of the early events in the formation of immune deposits, mainly because they appear within minutes after the intravenous injection of heterologous nephritogenic antibodies[13]. By contrast, in active HN the formation of immune deposits takes several weeks, because they depend on the development of a specific endogenous immune response to the nephritogenic antigen preparation used for active immunization. There are several lines of evidence that active and passive HN are caused by similar molecular mechanisms[14,15]; for example, IgG eluted from glomeruli of rats with active HN readily induces passive HN when injected intravenously into normal rats.

Other experimental glomerular diseases in which subepithelial immune deposits occur frequently involve the 'implantation' of artificial antigens into the GBM (for example, strongly cationic molecules) which are then complexed and stabilized by cross-linking by a specific antibody[16-18]. Several general observations on the formation of immune deposits have derived from such models, although they are considered rather artificial and often resemble human MGN only in a few aspects, especially because highly cationic molecules which bind to the negative charges of the GBM presumably do not occur in human MGN. Consequently, HN is generally considered a more relevant model system for human MGN, which involves only endogenous proteins as antigens.

The origin of immune deposits in HN: circulating immune complexes and *in situ* formation

In their classic work, Dixon[19], and Germuth and colleagues[20], postulated that granular subepithelial immune deposits in the GBM (for example in chronic serum sickness) derive from direct deposition of soluble pre-formed immune complexes from the circulation. In HN, the observation that antibodies to a tubular antigen (as described later in detail) are deposited in the GBM and cause glomerular damage was explained in a similar way. It was assumed that immune complexes containing the pathogenic antigen(s) and the corresponding specific antibodies were pre-formed in the circulation and trapped in the GBM[21,22]. There are several reports about the presence of circulating antigen–antibody complexes in HN[23-26], but their direct nephritogenic role has not been convincingly demonstrated.

Alternatively, an 'in situ' mechanism for the formation of glomerular immune deposits in HN was proposed by Van Damme et al.[27] and Couser and associates[28,29]. This hypothesis is largely based on experiments in which nephritogenic antibodies, such as anti-Fx1A IgG in a blood-free salt solution, formed typical glomerular immune deposits when perfused through isolated kidney[28], thus avoiding formation of circulating immune complexes.

The *in situ* hypothesis of the formation of immune deposits in HN predicts that the HN-antigen(s) are present in the glomerulus. Thus, proof of this concept requires the identification of the nephritogenic antigen(s), and the development of monospecific antibodies which can subsequently be used for precise localization of the pathogenic antigen(s) by immunohistochemistry.

THE NEPHRITOGENIC ANTIGEN OF HN

The search for the nephritogenic antigen

HN was originally induced by immunization of rats with homogenates of autologous[9] and heterologous[22] kidney cortex. A more refined antigen preparation was subsequently developed by fractionation of homogenates of cortex (designated 'Fx1A'[21]) and is still widely used for the induction of HN. Initial biochemical approaches relied on the preparation of subfractions of Fx1A, and on testing of their ability to induce HN. These experiments yielded a highly nephritogenic large lipoprotein complex, designated RTα5[21], which was believed to be a single antigenic component. In a different approach, the nephritogenic principle was recovered in pronase digests of kidney cortex extracts[30]. More recently, a nephritogenic fraction (designated gp600), which is composed of several microvillar proteins, was recovered in the high-molecular-weight fractions obtained by gel chromatography[31]. In retrospect, these attempts used a crude cortex homogenate as the starting material for purification of the pathogenic molecule(s), in which proteolysis and aggregation of proteins were not adequately controlled. As a consequence, these previously defined 'antigens' were not purified proteins by today's biochemical standard but variable mixtures of molecules[32].

These problems were largely avoided by the use of purified fractions of brush border microvilli of proximal tubules as the source of the nephritogenic antigen. This approach is valid because the pathogenic antigen(s) was previously localized in high concentration in the brush border region of proximal tubuli[33] by indirect immunofluorescence, using sera of HN rats or IgG eluted from diseased glomeruli. In these preparations, the nephritogenic proteins were traced down to the membrane protein fraction of microvilli, and further to a lens culinaris lectin-binding subfraction of glycoproteins derived therefrom[34]. Collectively, these data indicated that the nephritogenic antigen of HN was a membrane glycoprotein of large size.

Identification of gp330 as the nephritogenic HN antigen

When IgG was eluted from isolated glomeruli of rats with HN and used for immunoprecipitation with ^{125}I-labelled, detergent-solubilized membrane proteins of isolated tubular microvilli, a single molecule was specifically precipitated[35]. This membrane glycoprotein obviously contained a rather large extracellular domain, and showed an apparent molecular weight of 330 kD. It was therefore designated as 'gp330'[35].

In order to prove its nephritogenic potential, gp330 was purified by several methods such as gel- and lectin-affinity chromatography, preparative SDS-PAGE, and affinity purification with monoclonal antibodies. When rats were then immunized with the isolated molecule, subepithelial granular immune deposits were observed in glomeruli, identical to those in HN[35]. Moreover, the animals also developed albuminuria, which, however, was less impressive than that elicited by immunization with crude antigen preparations. When, in control experiments, rats were immunized against a preparation of microvillar proteins which were depleted selectively of gp330 by gel chromatography, immune deposits were not observed.

Collectively, these data provide evidence that purified gp330 shows most, if not all, of the properties expected of the pathogenic antigen of active (and passive) HN. Several laboratories have independently confirmed these findings[36-44]. The identification and purification of the nephritogenic antigen also raised the possibility of producing monoclonal and affinity-purified polyclonal antibodies.

The localization of the nephritogenic antigen of HN

Several attempts have been made to define the distribution of the nephritogenic antigen(s) of HN by the use of currently available probes. Thus, rat anti-Fx1A serum, or heterologous rabbit anti-Fx1A IgG, or eluates from Heymann-nephritic glomeruli, have been used for immunofluorescence and immunoperoxidase studies at the light- and electron-microscopic level. Using immunofluorescence, an antigen was found in the glomerulus in a granular pattern[14,27,28,45], but at the ultrastructural level the results diverged substantially. The antigen was variously localized to the glomerular basement membrane, to the surface of all types of glomerular cells, and to the cell membrane at the base of the glomerular epithelial cells[14,27,28,45]. The reason for these discrepancies is probably the low titre and multispecificity of the antibody preparations used, and also limitations in the resolution of the diaminobenzidine reaction for immunoperoxidase[46].

Localization of gp330 in normal glomeruli

The precise localization of gp330, especially by immunoelectron microscopy, using monoclonal and affinity-purified polyclonal antibodies, has revealed important information which would not have been accessible by any other technique. The results obtained have helped to explain why immune deposits are formed in the glomerulus in HN, and have revealed the specific association of gp330 with clathrin-coated pits.

By the use of specific monoclonal or affinity-purified IgG[47], we have localized gp330 in a granular distribution in glomeruli of Lewis rats (a strain which is highly susceptible to the induction of active HN), and Sprague–Dawley rats (a low-responder strain), in a pattern which closely resembles that seen previously with anti-Fx1A antibodies[45].

The precise localization of gp330 in glomeruli was unravelled by immunoelectron microscopy, using indirect immunoperoxidase and immunogold techniques[47]. Gp330 was localized exclusively to the glomerular epithelial cells. There it was observed in the endoplasmic reticulum, in the Golgi apparatus (i.e. biosynthetic compartments of the cells), and occasionally in multivesicular bodies (considered a pre-lysosomal or lysosomal compartment). Unexpectedly, on the surface of glomerular epithelial cells, gp330 was restricted to the clathrin-coated pits of the cell membrane. The most interesting finding of these experiments was that gp330 was located in clathrin-coated pits on the base of the foot processes, where they contact the GBM[47].

From these morphological and supporting biochemical data[47], we have concluded that gp330 is a biosynthetic product of glomerular epithelial cells, and that it is concentrated in clathrin-coated pits which are known to play a key role in receptor-mediated endocytosis in several other cell systems[48]. Similar confirmatory results have been reported by several other investigators[40,49].

Screening of other tissues for the presence of gp330 by immunohistochemistry and biochemical methods has subsequently indicated that gp330 is a member of a larger family of structurally related, but not identical, membrane glycoproteins which are present in several organs[50,51]. The currently identified related molecules include the enzyme maltase (gp300)[52], and a 280 kD protein, antibodies to which are highly teratogenic in rats[53,54].

Physiological function of gp330

Because of its location in clathrin-coated pits, which is typical of all receptor molecules studied so far[48], we have speculated either that gp330 may be a receptor for which the ligands are not yet known, or alternatively that gp330 could be a ligand itself or a constituitive molecule of coated pits[55]. In a recent report, a potential ligand for which gp330 could serve as receptor was found in serum[56] by ligand blotting which was, however, performed under strongly denaturing conditions for both gp330 and its putative ligand. Molecular cloning of the gp330 gene, sequencing, and comparison of DNA-derived amino acid sequences with data banks are expected to clarify this issue.

THE FORMATION OF IMMUNE DEPOSITS IN HN

Gp330 immune complexes form in coated pits of podocytes

When rabbit anti-gp330 IgG was intravenously injected into rats, it was detected by immunofluorescence in a fine granular pattern in capillary loops after 15 minutes[13]. Injected rabbit IgG was found by immunoelectron microscopy at this time point exclusively within the coated pits on the 'soles' of the podocytes, i.e. precisely the same location in which the gp300 antigen is found. These complexes grew with time and became rather large after several days, but they remained permanently associated with clathrin-coated membrane areas of the podocytes, as shown by serial sectioning[13].

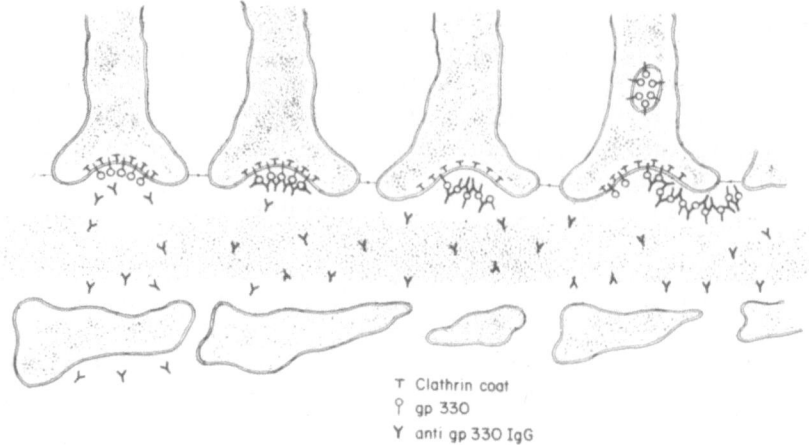

T Clathrin coat
♀ gp 330
Y anti gp 330 IgG

Figure 1 Schematic drawing of the early events in the *in situ* formation of immune deposits in passive HN. (1) Circulating anti-gp330 IgG (Y) penetrates the GBM and approaches gp330 (♀), a resident membrane glycoprotein of clathrin-coated pits located at the base of the epithelial foot processes. (2) Anti-gp330 IgG binds to its antigen gp330, presumably at specific 'pathogenic epitopes', in the coated pits, forming an initial immune complex. (3) This initial immune complex becomes attached to the GBM as early as 15 minutes after injection of the antibody, and is shed partially, but remains in contact with a coated pit. (4) The immune deposit grows in size by repeated cycles of *in situ* immune-complex formation and shedding into the lamina rara externa, until it eventually encroaches on the area of the slit diaphragm. The same result could be obtained if the immune deposit was fixed to one site of the GBM and the foot process subsequently moved over the immune deposit until positioned under the slit diaphragm. The continued growth of the immune deposit appears to require *de novo* synthesis by the foot processes of new molecules of gp330 which, like other membrane glycoproteins, are assumed to be delivered via vesicles that eventually fuse with the cell membrane at the base of the foot processes

In keeping with the in-situ complex hypothesis, these findings indicate that immune complexes are initially formed in clathrin-coated pits of the podocyte cell membranes, and that they remain in contact with these membrane domains for at least several days, presumably because newly synthesized gp330 antigen is presented by these organelles for repeated cycles of immune complex formation (Figure 1)[13].

Redistribution of gp330 on cell surfaces by anti-gp330 IgG

Several experimental data indicate that immune complexes which involve membrane proteins on the surfaces of epithelial cells redistribute and form patches and caps, similar to those found in lymphocytes[57]. These aggregated antibody–antigen complexes are then either shed from the surface or endocytosed by the cells. Patching, capping and shedding of immune complexes on the surfaces of glomerular epithelial cells *in vitro* were observed when anti-renal microvillar IgG was added to the culture medium[58], and were suppressed by chlorpromazine[59], which is known to prevent capping in lymphocytes[57]. Moreover, chlorpromazine also prevented the formation of immune deposits in passive HN[59]. While several membrane proteins of cultured glomerular epithelial cells form shedding complexes, gp330-containing complexes appear to be primarily endocytosed (G. Camussi, personal communication). These data indicate that in HN redistribution and presumably also shedding and/or endocytosis of immune complexes from the glomerular epithelial cell surface are involved in the formation of immune deposits.

Gp330 immune complexes are rapidly immobilized to the GBM

Since clathrin-coated pits are membrane domains which are specialized for receptor-mediated endocytosis[60], the intriguing question arises of why the gp330 immune complexes are not removed from the podocyte surface by these organelles.

When rats were injected with anti-gp330 IgG 15 minutes before sacrifice, and their GBMs were purified by extraction with detergents and high-salt buffers, immune complexes containing both gp330 and injected anti-gp330 IgG remained firmly associated with the lamina rara externa, as shown by immunogold double-labelling[13]. With time, the immobilized immune complexes became large immune deposits, but they were still firmly attached to the GBM[57]. Attachment appears to occur via the gp330 antigen rather than via the IgG molecules, because alkaline or acid extraction of isolated GBMs removes the IgG from the complexes but does not detach gp330. Although the precise chemistry of this interaction is unknown, we have speculated that it could be covalent, because it is not influenced by high concentrations of salts, non-denaturing detergents and various chaotropes[13]. We do not know, at present, whether a specific ligand in the lamina rara externa is needed for the interaction with gp330, or whether it is indiscriminate.

Cross-linking of immune complexes

The ability to form large cross-linked immune complexes is an important determinant for their stability and persistence in the GBM. This was demonstrated by the use of defined cationic antigens which were 'implanted' into the GBM, followed by injection of specific antibodies[60-62]. When passive HN was induced by monovalent Fab-fragments of anti-Fx1A IgG[58], or by Fab–anti gp330 IgG (unpublished observation), immune complexes in the GBM appeared only transiently. A similar phenomenon was observed when monoclonal anti-gp330 IgG was injected intravenously[63]. The simplest interpretation of these results is that in HN the formation of antibody–antigen aggregates by multiple cross-linking by bivalent IgG contributes to the stability of immune deposits.

Gp330 epitope specificity of pathogenic anti-gp330 IgG

In passive HN, several pieces of evidence indicate that the formation of stable immune deposits requires initially the binding of anti-gp330 antibody to specific epitopes of gp330. Direct experimental evidence for such 'pathogenic epitopes' of gp330 derives from the expression of fragments of the gp330 gene in λgt11 vectors in the form of β-galactosidase fusion proteins. When fusion protein-specific antibodies are raised in rabbits and are injected into rats, some form immune deposits, while others do not (unpublished observations). These experiments raise the possibility that eventually the amino acid sequence of a 'pathogenic epitope' could be determined.

Role of microvillar proteins other than gp330

Since immunization with purified gp330 induces less proteinuria than in Fx1A-induced HN, it was suspected that antigens other than gp330 could participate in functional damage to the glomerular capillary wall[39,40,64-67]. It was observed that intravenous injection of antibodies to a membrane protein of kidney microvilli, with a molecular weight of 90–116 kD, formed transient immune deposits in the GBM of normal rats[67] in the absence of gp330-containing immune complexes. Stable immune deposits were induced by these antibodies only when the rats were pre-sensitized against the heterologous injected antibody beforehand, or when an autologous phase in the host animal developed several days after injection. The 90–116 kD molecule was found also in Fx1A, and was identified as the enzyme dipeptidyl-peptidase IV (DPP IV)[68,69]. Since rats injected with anti-DPP IV antibody developed transient proteinuria which coincided with the presence of DPP IV immune complexes in the GBM[69], it appears that this system may contribute to functional damage of the glomerulus. Recently, it has been shown that anti-Fx1A antibodies prepared from a strain of rat which is genetically deficient in DPP IV induce typical passive HN in normal rats, thus indicating that DPP IV is not essential for the induction of the passive disease[70]. This is in contrast to experience in the mouse, where DPP IV appears to be the major antigen in an HN-like disease[67]. Other additional, less well-defined, antibody–antigen systems may contribute to the development of glomerular damage and proteinuria, particularly in active HN when induced by 'crude' antigens such as Fx1A[71,72].

CONCLUSIONS AND PERSPECTIVES

Factors contributing to the formation of immune deposits in HN

Obviously the formation of immune deposits is a multifactorial process. Collectively, the data summarized above indicate that a pathogenic antibody has to be specific for certain domains on the gp330 molecule. This could be associated with the firm and rapid attachment of immune complexes to the GBM, which prevents their endocytosis by glomerular epithelial cells. Furthermore, cross-linking of the antigen by divalent antibodies causes redistribution and shedding of the complexes.

It is possible that this type of immobilization and redistribution is a general prerequisite for the formation of persistent and growing immune deposits for membrane antigens other than gp330, and presumably for other glomerular diseases than MGN.

What can be learnt from HN for human MGN?

Attempts have been made to apply the observations on HN to human MGN. While several investigators have found anti-brush border antibodies in patients[73-75], the general agreement currently is that in most patients the antigens involved in MGN are different from those in HN[76-78]. This view is supported by the finding that a gp330-related molecule is present in the proximal tubules of human kidneys, but not in glomeruli[79,80], although this does not disprove that similar mechanisms are responsible for the formation of immune deposits, probably involving different antigens[81]. It should also be kept in mind that at a molecular level MGN could be a syndrome, rather than a homogenous disease, with regard to the nephritogenic antigens involved.

It will be an exciting challenge to analyse the pathogenesis of human MGN, relying on the experience with HN, because manipulation of several steps in the pathogenesis, such as specific interception of pathogenic antibodies or inhibition of the immobilization of immune complexes in the GBM, could provide the possibility for specific interference with the formation of immune deposits.

References

1. Ehrenreich, T. and Churg, J. (1968). Pathology of membranous nephropathy. *Pathol. Annu.*, **3**, 145–186
2. Cameron, J. D. (1982). Membranous nephropathy: The treatment dilemma. *Am. J. Kidney Dis.*, **1**, 371–375
3. Ponticelli, C. (1986). Prognosis and treatment of membranous nephropathy. *Kidney Int.*, **29**, 927–940
4. Couser, W. G. (1985). Glomerular diseases. In Wynngaarden, J. B. and Smith, L. R. (eds), *Cecil's Textbook of Medicine*, 17th edn., Chapter 62, pp. 568–589.
5. Couser, W. (1985). Mechanisms of glomerular injury in immune-complex disease. *Kidney Int.*, **28**, 569–583
6. Andres, G., Brentjens, J. R., Caldwell, P. R. B., Camussi, G. and Matsuo, S. (1987). Formation of immune deposits and disease. *Lab. Invest.*, **55**, 510–520
7. Brentjens, J. R. and Andres, G. A. (1989). Interaction of antibodies with renal surface antigens. *Kidney Int.*, **35**, 954–968
8. Verroust, P. (1989). Nephrology Forum: Membranous Nephropathy. *Kidney Int.* (In press)
9. Heymann, W., Hackel, D. B., Harwood, S., Wilson, S. G. F. and Hunter, J. L. P. (1959). Production of nephrotic syndrome in rats by Freund's adjuvants and rat kidney suspensions. *Proc. Soc. Exp. Biol. Med.*, **100**, 660–664
10. Heymann, W., Knutec, E. P., Wilson, S. G. F., Hunter, J. L. P., Hackel, D. B., Okuda, R. and Cuppage, L. (1965). Experimental autoimmune renal disease in rats. *Ann. N.Y. Acad. Sci.*, **124**, 310–326
11. Barabas, A. Z. and Lannigan, R. (1974). Induction of an autologous immune-complex glomerulonephritis in the rat by intravenous injection of heterologous anti-rat kidney antibody. I. Production of chronic progressive immune-complex glomerulonephritis. *Br. J. Exp. Pathol.*, **55**, 47–55
12. Sugisaki, T. J., Klassen, J., Andres, G. A., Milgrom, F. J. and McCluskey, R. T. (1973). Passive transfer of Heymann's nephritis with serum. *Kidney Int.*, **3**, 66–73
13. Kerjaschki, D., Miettinnen, A. and Farquhar, M. G. (1987). Initial events in the formation of immune deposits in passive Heymann nephritis. *J. Exp. Med.*, **166**, 109–128
14. Neale, T. J., Couser, W. G., Salant, D. J., Lowenstein, L. M. and Wilson, C. B. (1982). Specific uptake of Heymann's nephritic kidney eluate by rat kidney. *Lab. Invest.*, **46**, 450–453
15. Madaio, M. P., Salant, D. J., Cohen, A. J., Adler, S. and Couser, W. G. (1983). Comparative

study of in situ immune deposit formation in active and passive Heymann nephritis. *Kidney Int.*, **23**, 498–505

16. Oite, T. M., Batsford, S. R., Mihatsch, M., Takamiya, H. and Vogt, A. (1982). Quantitative studies of the in situ immune complex glomerulonephritis in the rat induced by planted cationized antigen. *J. Exp. Med.*, **155**, 460–474

17. Border, W. A., Ward, H. J., Kamis, E. S. and Cohen, A. H. (1982). Induction of membranous nephropathy in rabbits by administration of an exogenous cationic antigen: Demonstration of a pathogenic role for electrical charge. *J. Clin. Invest.*, **69**, 451–461

18. Adler, S. G., Wang, H., Ward, H. J., Cohen, A. H. and Border, W. A. (1983). Electrical charge: Its role in the pathogenesis and prevention of experimental membranous nephropathy in the rabbit. *J. Clin. Invest.*, **71**, 487–499

19. Dixon, F. J., Feldman, J. D. and Vazquez, J. J. (1961). Experimental glomerulonephritis. The pathogenesis of a laboratory model resembling the spectrum of human glomerulonephritis. *J. Exp. Med.*, **113**, 899–937

20. Germuth, F. G. and Rodriguez, E. (1973). Immunopathology of the renal glomerulus. In: *Immune Complex Deposition and Anti-basement Membrane Disease.* (Boston: Little Brown)

21. Edgington, T. S., Glassock, R. J. and Dixon, F. J. (1968). Autologous immune complex nephritis induced with renal tubular antigen: I. Identification and isolation of the pathogenic antigen. *J. Exp. Med.*, **127**, 555–572

22. Edgington, T. S., Glassock, R. J. and Dixon, F. J. (1967). Autologous immune complex pathogenesis of experimental allergic glomerulonephritis. *Science*, **155**, 1432–1434

23. Abrass, C. K., Border, W. A. and Glassock, R. J. (1980). Circulating immune complexes in rat with autologous immune complex nephritis. *Lab. Invest.*, **42**, 1–7

24. Naruse, T., Fukasawa, T., Umegae, S., Oite, S. and Miyakawa, Y. (1978). Experimental membranous glomerulonephritis in rats: Correlation of ultrastructural changes with the serum level of autologous antibody against tubular antigen. *Lab. Invest.*, **39**, 120–134

25. Fleuren, G. J., Grond, J. and Hoedemaeker, Ph. J. (1980). The pathogenic role of free-circulating antibody in autologous immune complex glomerulonephritis. *Clin. Exp. Immunol.*, **41**, 205–217

26. Couser, W. G. (1981). What are circulating immune complexes doing in glomerulonephritis? *New Engl. J. Med.*, **300**, 1230–1232

27. Van Damme, B. J. C., Fleuren, G. J., Bakker, W. W., Vernier, R. L. and Hoedemaeker, Ph. J. (1978). Experimental glomerulonephritis in the rat induced by antibodies directed against tubular antigens. V. Fixed glomerular antigens in the pathogenesis of heterologous immune complex nephritis. *Lab. Invest.*, **38**, 502–510

28. Couser, W. G., Steinmuller, D. R., Stilmant, M. M., Salant, D. J. and Lowenstein, L. M. (1978). Experimental glomerulonephritis in the isolated perfused rat kidney. *J. Clin. Invest.*, **62**, 1275–1287

29. Couser, W. G. and Salant, D. (1980). In-situ immune complex formation and glomerular injury. *Kidney Int.*, **17**, 1–13

30. Naruse, T., Fukasawa, T. and Miyakawa, Y. (1975). Laboratory model of membranous glomerulonephritis in rats induced by pronase-digested homologous renal tubular epithelial antigen. *Lab. Invest.*, **33**, 141–152

31. Makker, S. P. and Singh, A. K. (1984). Characterization of the antigen (gp600) of Heymann nephritis. *Lab. Invest.*, **50**, 287–293

32. Ronco, P., Neale, T. J., Wilson, C. B., Galceran, M. and Verroust, P. (1986). An immunopathological study of a 330 kD protein defined by monoclonal antibodies and reactive with anti-RTEa5 antibodies and kidney eluates from active Heymann nephritis. *J. Immunol.*, **136**, 125–130

33. Grupe, W. E. and Kaplan, M. H. (1969). Demonstration of an antibody to proximal tubular antigen in the pathogenesis of experimental autoimmune nephrosis in rats. *J. Lab. Clin. Med.*, **74**, 400–409

34. Miettinen, A., Törnroth, T., Tikkanen, I., Virtanen, I. and Linder, E. (1980). Heymann nephritis induced by kidney brush border glycoproteins. *Lab. Invest.*, **43**, 547–555

35. Kerjaschki, D. and Farquhar, M. G. (1982). The pathogenic antigen of Heymann nephritis is a glycoprotein of the renal proximal tubule brush border. *Proc. Natl Acad. Sci. USA*, **79**, 5557–5561

36. Ronco, P., Melcion, C., Geniteau, E., Ronco, L., Reininger, P., Galceran, P. and Verroust,

P. (1984). Production and characterization of monoclonal antibodies against rat brush border antigens of the proximal convoluted tubule. *Immunology*, **53**, 78–95

37. Ronco, P., Allegri, L., Melcion, C., Pirotsky, E., Appay, M. D., Bariety, J., Pontillon, F. and Verroust, P. (1984). A monoclonal antibody to brush borders and passive Heymann nephritis. *Clin. Exp. Immunol.*, **55**, 319–332

38. Miettinen, A., Törnroth, T. and Vartio, T. (1984). Expression of three brush border membrane polypeptides of high molecular weight in rat kidney and other epithelia. *J. Cell Biol.*, **99**, 106a (Abstract)

39. Bhan, A. K., Schneeberger, E. E., Baird, L. G., Collins, A. B., Kamata, K., Bradford, D., Erikson, M. E. and McCluskey, R. T. (1985). Studies with monoclonal antibodies against brush border antigens in Heymann nephjritis. *Lab. Invest.*, **53**, 421–432

40. Kamata, K., Baird, L. G., Erikson, M. E., Collins, A. B. and McCluskey, R. T. (1986). Characterization of antigen and antibody specificities involved in Heymann nephritis. *J. Immunol.*, **135**, 2400–2412

41. Chatelet, F., Brianti, E., Ronco, P., Roland, J. and Verroust, P. (1986). Ultrastructural localization by monoclonal antibodies of brush border antigens expressed by glomeruli. I. Renal distribution. *Am. J. Pathol.*, **122**, 500–511

42. Behar, M., Katz, A. and Silverman, M. (1986). Biochemical characterization of brush border membrane antigens implicated in the pathogenesis of Heymann nephritis. *Kidney Int.*, **30**, 421–430

43. Goodyear, P. R., Mills, M. and Kaplan, B. S. (1985). Analysis of the Heymann nephritogenic glycoprotein in rat, mouse and human kidney. *Biochem. Cell Biol.*, **64**, 441–449

44. Behar, M., Katz, A. and Silverman, M. (1987). A rat cell hybridoma model for study of autologous immune complex nephritis. *Kidney Int.*, **31**, 165a (Abstract)

45. Neale, T. J. and Wilson, C. B. (1982). Glomerular antigens in Heymann nephritis: Reactivity of eluted and circulating antibody. *J. Immunol.*, **128**, 323-330

46. Kerjaschki, D., Sawada, H. and Farquhar, M. G. (1986). Immunoelectron microscopy in kidney research: Some contributions and limitations. *Kidney Int.*, **30**, 229–245

47. Kerjaschki, D. and Farquhar, M. G. (1983). Immunocytochemical localization of the Heymann nephritis antigen (gp330) in glomerular epithelial cells of normal Lewis rats. *J. Exp. Med.*, **157**, 667–686

48. Goldstein, J. L., Anderson, R. G. W. and Brown, M. S. (1979). Coated pits, coated vesicles, and receptor mediated endocytosis. *Nature*, **279**, 679–683

49. Chatelet, F., Brianti, E., Ronco, P., Roland, J. and Verroust, P. (1986). Ultrastructural localization by monoclonal antibodies of brush border antigens expressed by glomeruli: I. Renal distribution. *Am. J. Pathol.*, **122**, 500–511

50. Doxsey, S. D., Kerjaschki, D. and Farquhar, M. G. (1983). A large membrane glycoprotein (gp330) is a resident of coated pits of several absorptive epithelia. *J. Cell Biol.*, **97**, 178a (Abstract)

51. Chatelet, F., Brianti, E., Ronco, P., Roland, J. and Verroust, P. (1986). Ultrastructural localization by monoclonal antibodies of brush border antigens expressed by glomeruli: II. Extrarenal distribution. *Am. J. Pathol.*, **122**, 512–519

52. Kerjaschki, D., Noronha-Blob, L., Sacktor, B. and Farquhar, M. G. (1984). Microdomains of distinctive glycoprotein composition in the kidney proximal tubule brush borders. *J. Cell Biol.*, **98**, 1505-1513

53. Leung, C. C. K. (1982). Isolation, partial characterization and localization of a rat renal tubular glycoprotein. Antibody-induced birth defects. *J. Exp. Med.*, **156**, 372–384

54. Sahali, D., Mulliez, N., Chatelet, F., Dupuis, R., Ronco, P. and Verroust, P. (1988). Characterization of a 280 kD protein restricted to the coated pits of the renal brush border and the epithelial cells of the yolk sac: Teratogenic effect of the specific monoclonal antibodies. *J. Exp. Med.*, **167**, 213–218

55. Kerjaschki, D. and Farquhar, M. G. (1985). Pathogenic antigen of Heymann nephritis (gp330): Identification, isolation, and localization. In Robinson, R. R. (ed.) *Nephrology*, Vol. 1, pp. 560–574. (Berlin: Springer)

56. Kanalas, J. J. and Makker, S. P. (1988). A possible ligand of serum origin for the kidney autoantigen of Heymann nephritis. *J. Immunol.*, **141**, 4152–4157

57. Schreiner, G. F. and Unanue, E. R. (1976). Membrane and cytoplasmic changes in B lymphocytes induced by ligand–surface immunoglobulin interaction. In Dixon, F. J. and Kunkel, H. G. (eds) *Advances in Immunology*, p. 32. (New York: Academic Press)

58. Camussi, G., Brentjens, J. R., Noble, B., Kerjaschki, D., Malavasi, F., Roholt, O. A., Farquhar, M. G. and Andres, G. A. (1985). Antibody-induced redistribution of Heymann antigen on the surface of cultured glomerular visceral epithelial cells: Possible role in the pathogenesis of Heymann glomerulonephritis. *J. Immunol.*, **135**, 2409–2416

59. Camussi, G., Noble, B., Van Liew, J., Brentjens, J. and Andres, G. A. (1986). Pathogenesis of passive Heymann nephritis: Chlorpromazine inhibits antibody-mediated redistribution of cell surface antigens and prevents development of the disease. *J. Immunol.*, **136**, 2127–2135

60. Agodoa, L. Y. C., Gauthier, V. J. and Mannik, M. (1983). Precipitating antigen-antibody systems are required for the formation of subepithelial electron dense immune deposits in rat glomeruli. *J. Exp. Med.*, **158**, 1259–1272

61. Mannik, M., Agodoa, L. Y. C. and David, K. A. (1983). Rearrangement of immune complexes in glomeruli leads to persistence and development of electron dense deposits. *J. Exp. Med.*, **157**, 1516–1528

62. Vogt, A. (1984). New aspects of the pathogenesis of immune complex glomerulonephritis: Formation of subepithelial deposits. *Clin. Nephrol.*, **21**, 15–20

63. Allegri, L., Brianti, E., Chatelet, F., Manara, G. C., Ronco, P. and Verroust, P. (1986). Polyvalent antigen-antibody interactions are required for the formation of electron dense immune deposits in passive Heymann nephritis. *Am. J. Pathol.*, **126**, 1–6

64. Natori, Y., Hyakawa, I. and Shibata, S. (1986). Passive Heymann nephritis with acute and severe proteinuria induced by heterologous antibody against renal tubular brush border glycoprotein gp108. *Lab. Invest.*, **55**, 63–70

65. Jeraj, K., Vernier, R. L., Sisson, S. P. and Michael, A. F. (1984). A new glomerular antigen in passive Heymann's nephritis. *Br. J. Exp. Pathol.*, **65**, 485–498

66. Bagchus, W. M., Vos, J. T. W. M., Hoedemaeker, Ph. J. and Bakker, W. W. (1986). The specificity of nephritogenic antibodies. III. Binding of anti-Fx1A antibodies in glomeruli is dependent on dual specificity. *Clin. Exp. Immunol.*, **63**, 639–645

67. Assmann, K. J. M., Ronco, P., Tangelder, M. M., Lange, W. P. H., Verroust, P. and Koene, R. A. P. (1985). Comparison of the antigenic targets involved in antibody-mediated glomerulonephritis in the mouse and in the rat. *Am. J. Pathol.*, **121**, 112–119

68. Ronco, P., Van Leer, E. H. G., Chatelet, F., Tauc, M. and Verroust, P. (1987). Brush border hydrolases expressed by glomerular epithelial cells are target antigens for the formation of immune deposits. *Kidney Int.*, **31**, 329a (Abstract)

69. Natori, Y., Hayakawa, I. and Shibata, S. (1987). Identification of gp108, a pathogenic antigen of passive Heymann nephritis, as dipeptidyl peptidase IV.l *Clin. Exp. Immunol.*, **70**, 434–439

70. Natori, Y., Hayakawa, I. and Shibata, S. (1989). Role of dipeptidyl peptidase IV (p108) in passive Heymann nephritis. *Am. J. Pathol.*, **134**, 405–410

71. Abrass, C. K. (1986). Evaluation of sequential glomerular eluates from rats with Heymann nephritis. *J. Immunol.*, **137**, 530–537

72. Hogendoorn, P. C. W., Bruijn, J. A., van der Broek, L. J. C. M., deHeer, E., Foidart, J. M., Goedemaeker, Ph. J. and Fleuren, G. J. (1988). Antibodies to purified renal tubular epithelial antigens contain activity against laminin, fibronectin and type IV collagen. *Lab. Invest.*, **58**, 278–286

73. Naruse, T., Kitamura, D., Miyakawa, Y. and Shibata, S. (1973). Deposition of renal tubular epithelial antigens along the renal glomerular capillary walls of patients with membranous glomerulonephritis. *J. Immunol.*, **110**, 1163–1169

74. Zanetti, M., Mandet, C., Duboust, A., Bedrosiian, J. and Bariety, J. (1981). Demonstration of a passive Heymann-nephritis like mechanism in human kidney transplants. *Clin. Nephrol.*, **15**, 272–288

75. Douglas, M. F. S., Rabideau, D. P., Schwartz, M. M. and Lewis, E. J. (1981). Evidence on autologous immune complex nephritis. *New Engl. J. Med.*, **305**, 1326–1329

76. Whitworth, J., Liebowitz, S., Kennedy, M., Cameron, J., Evans, D., Glassock, R. and Schoenfeld, L. (1976). Absence of glomerular renal epithelial antigen in membranous glomerulonephritis. *Clin. Nephrol.*, **5**, 159–167

77. Zager, R. A., Couser, W. G., Andrews, B. S., Bolton, W. K. and Pohl, M. A. (1979). Radioimmunologic search for anti-tubular epithelial antibodies and circulating immune complexes in patients with membranous nephropathy. *Nephron*, **24**, 10–16

78. Collins, A. D., Andres, G. A. and McCluskey, R. T. (1981). Lack of evidence for a role of renal tubular antigen in human membranous glomerulonephritis. *Nephron*, **27**, 297–301

79. Kerjaschki, D., Horvat, R., Binder, S., Susani, M., Dekan, G., Ojha, P. P., Hillemanns, P., Ulrich, W. and Donini, U. (1987). Identification of a 400-kD protein in the brush borders of human kidney tubules that is similar to gp330, the nephritogenic antigen of rat Heymann nephritis. *Am. J. Pathol.*, **129**, 183–191

80. Natori, Y., Hayakawa, I. and Shibata, S. (1988). Heymann nephritis in rats induced by human renal tubular antigens: Characterization of antigen and antibody specificities. *Clin. Exp. Immunol.*, **69**, 33–40

81. Hoedemaeker, Ph. J. and Weening, J. J. (1989). Relevance of experimental models for human nephropathy. *Kidney Int.*, **33**, 1015–1025

4
Immune Complex Handling in Systemic Lupus Erythematosus

K. A. DAVIES and M. J. WALLPORT

Systemic lupus erythematosus (SLE) has long been regarded as the paradigm for autoimmune disease mediated by immune complexes. The idea that SLE was an 'immune-complex disease' came from a variety of observations. Firstly, antigen–antibody complexes could be found in the serum of patients with active disease[1]. Secondly, active disease was frequently associated with hypocomplementaemia, thought to be due to systemic activation of the classical complement pathway by immune complexes. Thirdly, there was evidence for the deposition of immune complexes (ICs) in a number of organs, including joints, lung, brain and kidney. More specifically, localization of DNA–anti-DNA complexes in kidneys was described in a number of studies[2-4]. Based on the work of Cochrane, Germuth, Dixon and colleagues, in a variety of models of serum-sickness in the late 1950s and 1960s[5], a hypothesis was developed—that the interaction of antigens and antibodies results in the formation of circulating immune complexes, and that deposition of such complexes in the tissues, with local activation of complement and other inflammatory mediators, produces injury. The observation in SLE of both circulating and tissue bound ICs fitted well with this hypotheses. However, recent studies of the immunopathological basis of antibody- and IC-mediated damage have suggested a more complex explanation for the role of immune complexes in SLE[6]. Similarly, in recent years, a g_eater understanding of the role of complement and complement receptors in the processing of immune complexes[7], and the recognition that inherited complement deficiency[8,9] predisposes to SLE, has led to new hypotheses to account for the development of this condition.

THE MEASUREMENT OF CIRCULATING IMMUNE COMPLEXES

The tenet that SLE is an immune complex disease is based on observations of 'immune deposits' (IDs) at sites of tissue injury, and of circulating species containing polymeric immunoglobulin and complement, often with the capacity to bind to Clq[1,10] in many but not all patients with active disease. A variety of different assay systems has been described for the detection of immune complexes[11]. The majority have been based on the binding of complexes to Clq[12-14], though other assays have used different ligands—e.g. conglutinin[15], Raji cells[15,16], neoantigens of C3[17], or precipitation with polyethylene glycol[18]. An increased prevalence of circulating ICs has been documented in patients with SLE by many workers[12,13,15,18-21]. There is also evidence that higher levels of circulating immune complexes are correlated with the severity of disease. Abrass and co-workers[13] studied serial serum samples from 48 patients with SLE, measuring levels of C3, anti-DNA antibody, and circulating ICs. The latter were measured using both fluid-phase and solid-phase Clq binding assays[13]. Elevations of IC levels measured by the solid-phase method were associated with manifestations of active disease, including renal disease and arthritis, as well as an increase in disease activity which prompted a change in therapy. However, a number of patients with neither active renal disease nor arthritis had positive results in the solid-phase assay. There was no correlation with the fluid-phase assay system, and both assays were consistently negative in patients with cutaneous involvement only. Other workers have failed, in similar studies, to correlate the presence or level of circulating IC with disease activity. In the study of Tron and colleagues, who used a polyethylene glycol precipitation assay, only some patients with clinically severe lupus had high levels of circulating IC[18]. Davis and coworkers measured anti-DNA antibodies, C3, and circulating IC (using Clq precipitation in gel, platelet aggregation and anti-complementary activity) in SLE patients. No correlation between any serological parameter and disease activity was demonstrable[22]. Cano and associates[19] also failed to find any correlation between disease activity and IC measurements.

In addition to the variable correlation with disease activity, there is a further problem which complicates the interpretation of Clq-binding assays. A number of investigators have shown that a proportion of the IgG binding to Clq is of monomeric size[23-25]. $F(ab')_2$ fragments of the IgG containing the Clq-binding material were able to bind Clq[24], and this material bound to the collagen-like region of Clq, not to the globular heads of the molecule, which bind to immune complexes[26]. These observations suggest that the Clq-binding IgG, which co-sediments with normal IgG, consists of autoantibodies to Clq, and this has subsequently been confirmed[27]. These findings cast doubt on the interpretation of studies of 'immune complexes' measured by assays using Clq.

Much experimental effort has been directed towards determination of the composition and size of immune complexes in SLE. Although antibodies to many intracellular constituents are readily demonstrable in serum, there is little convincing evidence of their participation in circulating immune complexes. Antibodies to both double-stranded and single-stranded DNA have been detected in sera from patients with SLE[28,29]. However, the presence of circulating IC comprising DNA and anti-DNA antibody is a subject of controversy[30,31] and has recently been critically reviewed by Fournié[32]. C3 has been identified and quantified in circulating IC in a range of autoimmune diseases, including SLE[33], and assay systems for IC have been developed using conglutinin or anti-C3 antibodies as ligands[15,17]. Immune complex size in SLE has been studied by Tung and coworkers[14] using sucrose density gradient centrifugation. Small (just above 7S) complexes were found in patients with cerebral involvement, while in patients with membranous glomerulonephritis (GN) only larger complexes (>19S) were detected. Patients without renal disease, or with a diffuse proliferative GN, had both small and large complexes. In this study, there was an overall correlation between disease activity and circulating complex levels.

IMMUNE COMPLEXES AND TISSUE INJURY IN SLE

Immune complexes and complement proteins have long been regarded as major factors in producing local tissue damage in lupus. Two primary mechanisms have been postulated: (a) the deposition of circulating immune complexes; (b) antibody binding to local antigen at the cell surface, in the tissue matrix, or released from damaged cells.

Localization of immune complexes to kidneys

A diverse range of renal lesions is seen in SLE. Immune deposits may be found in the mesangium, or in subendothelial or subepithelial locations. The first two are associated with proliferative glomerular lesions, while subepithelial deposits are characteristic of membranous glomerulonephritis (see Figure 1). Glomerular pathology in association with SLE is often complex, and mixed lesions are common. Mesangial and subendothelial deposits may be found with the more usual extensive subepithelial deposits[34]. Subepithelial immune deposits are probably the result of *in situ* immune complex formation[35], while the origin of mesangial and subendothelial sites is less certain.

Subepithelial immune complexes

An understanding of the basis of *in situ*, subepithelial, immune deposit formation has arisen primarily from the study of the Heymann nephritis model of membranous nephropathy in the rat. In this model, subepithelial granular IC deposits result from the binding of free antibody to an antigen expressed on the surface of glomerular epithelial cells[36]. Complement-dependent (C5–C9) tissue injury results[37]. This type of glomerular lesion can result from IC formation with either 'fixed' or 'planted' glomerular antigens[6]. The true Heymann nephritis model involves a 'fixed' glomerular antigen—a glycoprotein (gp330) localized along the epithelial cell membrane in endoplasmic reticulum and coated pits[38]. Divalent antibody binding is thought to cause antigenic modulation and redistribution of the IC on the surface of the cell, with resultant capping and shedding of the aggregates into the nearby slit pore areas and lamina rara externa[39,40]. A very similar mechanism is likely to operate in idiopathic membranous nephritis in man[41], and it will be interesting to see whether this will also apply to lupus. In animal models, polyspecific anti-DNA antibodies have been found to bind directly to cell membrane antigens[42] or to localize in glomeruli[43].

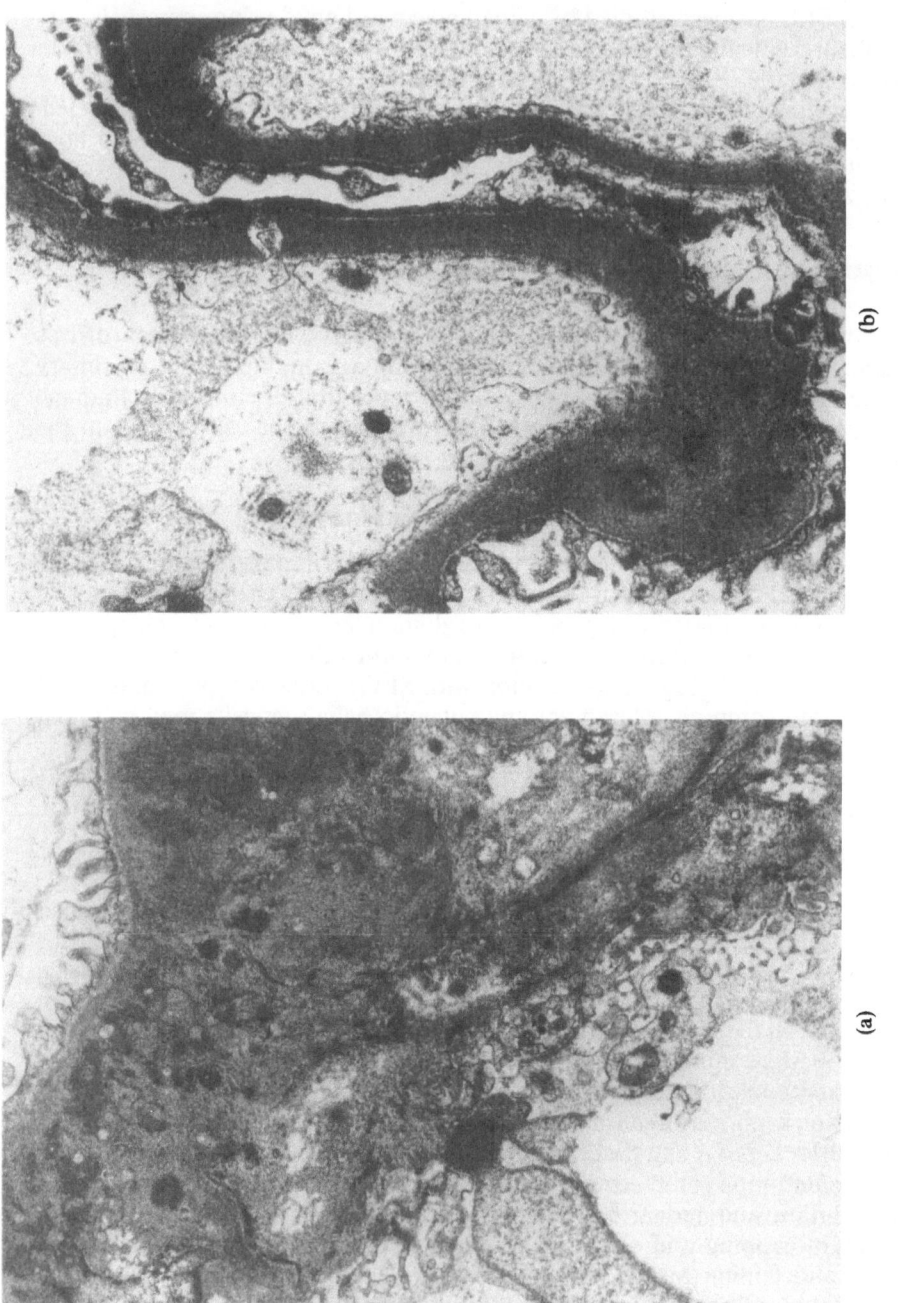

(b)

(a)

Figure 1 Immune complex nephritis: (a) extensive mesangial immune deposits, ×16 000; (b) SLE nephritis with epimembranous and intramembranous immune deposits, ×75 000

It is very difficult to induce the formation of subepithelial deposits containing exogenous antigens by the infusion of immune complexes[44]. Highly cationic, preformed ICs can produce this picture[45], possibly owing to the attraction of cationic antigens or antibodies to anionic glomerular structures. Subepithelial localization of immune deposits may result from filtration forces, while granularity may result from condensation of IC containing polyvalent antigens into larger deposits detectable by electron microscopy[46]. In SLE, one of the primary candidate antigens for involvement in IC formation is dsDNA, an anionic antigen. Izui and colleagues showed localization of injected DNA to glomeruli[47]. The cationic nature of anti-DNA antibodies may also be important. Ebling and Hahn[48] eluted cationic anti-DNA antibodies from mice with lupus nephritis, and similar observations have been made by other workers[49]. However, Gay and coworkers[50] demonstrated the preferential binding of DNA to type V collagen, independently of charge, and this may explain the localization of DNA to glomeruli observed by Izui and colleagues[47].

Subendothelial and mesangial complex formation

These locations are much more readily accessible to macromolecules in the circulation, and trapping of circulating IC may have an important role in immune deposit formation at these sites. Many experiments have demonstrated mesangial and subendothelial deposition after injection of immune complexes. In the traditional animal models of serum sickness, it has always been difficult to distinguish deposition of circulating IC from local immune deposit formation[51]. Injected IC may localize to the mesangium in certain circumstances, but little glomerular damage results[39,52]. However, Mauer and colleagues have shown that if antigen localization to the mesangium is followed by further accretion of antibody, immune deposit formation occurs and a focal proliferative GN may result[53]. Direct antibody-induced mesangial cell damage has also been demonstrated experimentally[54].

Experimental nephritis in association with subendothelial deposits is similarly difficult to induce by the injection of pre-formed IC[44]. It is possible to produce subendothelial deposit formation experimentally by induction of antigen expression on the endothelial cell surface, followed by infusion of an appropriate antibody[55], but such deposits are rapidly shed into the circulation. As postulated above, direct cellular damage by anti-endothelial cell antibodies may play a role. Such antibodies have been described in lupus[56].

Mechanisms of inflammatory damage

A number of mechanisms of glomerular injury in immune complex nephritis have been characterized. Glomerular injury may be induced by complement alone, or by complement and cells. In models of membranous nephropathy, and in lupus nephritis associated with subepithelial immune deposits, the membrane attack complex (MAC)—C5–C9—has been shown to play a pathogenetic role[57]. There is evidence that both complement (C5a) and polymorphonuclear cells are directly involved in the mediation of glomerular damage in many forms of experimental nephritis[58].

Complement activation also has an important role to play in the mediation of cellular injury to blood vessels in SLE[59]. 'Vasculitis' may occur in many different sites in patients with SLE, and direct vascular injury may be important in the mediation of damage in both the kidney and other organs. Both endothelial damage and the deposition of IC appear to be required. Deposition of immune complexes within vessel walls results in complement activation and the release of chemotactic factors, notably C5 fragments. Intravascular aggregation of neutrophils may result, and the resulting inflammatory response may lead to proliferation of endothelial cells, an increase in vascular permeability, and tissue necrosis. Localization of neutrophils to the pulmonary circulation is well described in a variety of situations associated with IC formation and complement activation[60,61], and in certain circumstances may result in leukostatic occlusion of the pulmonary arterioles[59].

Immune complexes and other organs

In the skin, immune deposits in SLE occur typically at the dermo–epidermal junction. A murine experimental model has been described in which mice were immunized with UV-treated DNA, and subsequently exposed to UV light. Specific antibodies to the altered DNA resulted, and immune deposits containing DNA–anti-DNA developed in the skin[62]. As in the kidney, charge may be an important factor in the localization of immune deposits at this site. The dermo–epidermal junction possesses a fixed negative charge. Joselow and coworkers demonstrated that the injection of pre-formed IC, made in antigen excess with cationic antibodies, could induce the formation of immune deposits at this site after 1–4 hours[63]. Similar results could be produced by the chronic immunization of mice with cationized rabbit IgG. In humans, Landry found antibodies to structural components of the dermo–epidermal junction, and also antinuclear antibodies in material eluted from skin[64].

Immune complexes have been implicated in causing inflammation in cardiac disease in SLE. In pericarditis, immune complexes, complement activation by the classical and alternative pathways, anti-nuclear and anti-DNA antibodies have all been detected in pericardial fluid[65–68]. SLE myocarditis may be associated with focal interstitial infiltrates, or areas of necrosis[69]. Immunologically mediated disease of coronary arteries may predispose to immune complex deposition, causing a coronary arteritis[70], and endothelial damage may predispose to the development of atheroma[71], as has been described in experimental animals[72]. Immunoglobulins and complement components have also been demonstrated in cardiac valvular lesions in SLE[73]. In the lung, there is conflicting evidence relating to the importance of immune complexes in the mediation of acute pneumonitis, pulmonary haemorrhage, and chronic interstitial lung disease[74–80].

In the CNS, a variety of disease processes may occur in SLE. Infarction or haemorrhage can result from IC-mediated vasculitis[81]. Hypercoagulability due to the presence of anti-cardiolipin antibodies may have a role in precipitating thrombotic events[82]. Both antibodies and immune complexes (including DNA–anti-DNA complexes) have been demonstrated in the choroid plexus of patients with CNS lupus, but similar observations have been made in asymptomatic patients, suggesting that non-specific IC trapping or formation may occur at this site[83-85]. Depression of C4 levels[86,87] and raised levels of fluid-phase C5b–C9 (MAC) have been described in the CSF of SLE patients with CNS disease[88]. Seibold and coworkers have reported the presence of immune complexes in the CSF of 33 or 34 patients with definite cerebral SLE, compared with one of 12 patients without CNS disease, and 4 of 90 multiple sclerosis patients[89]. Other investigators have described DNA–anti-DNA complexes in the CSF[90]. The relevance of these findings to the immunopathogenesis of cerebral SLE remains unclear at present.

IMMUNE COMPLEX CLEARANCE MECHANISMS IN LUPUS

A failure of the normal physiological clearance mechanisms for immune complexes has been suggested as one hypothesis for the aetiology of SLE in humans. The majority of the evidence suggests that it is the fixed mononuclear phagocytes of the liver and spleen which are normally responsible for IC clearance. Carriage of IC bound to erythrocyte complement receptor type 1 may also be important. Persistence of IC could lead to the stimulation of autoimmunity by autoantigens, either directly, or as a consequence of IC-mediated tissue injury. The idea that abnormal function of the mononuclear phagocytic system might result in failure of IC clearance, and the subsequent deposition of complexes in tissues, results from experimental work demonstrating 'reticulo-endothelial saturation'. Complement has important roles in the processing of immune complexes, and the observation that null genes for certain complement proteins (C1q, C2 and C4) constitute strong disease susceptibility genes for the development of lupus has been interpreted as further evidence for the importance of abnormal IC clearance in the pathogenesis of the disease.

Immune complexes and complement

The complement system affects IC formation and processing in two very important and potentially beneficial ways. Firstly, complement prevents the formation of immune complexes with large lattices. Secondly, the binding of C3 to immune complexes allows their interaction with a range of complement receptors on different cells. In some circumstances these interactions may provoke the uptake and disposal of complexes by cells of the mononuclear phagocytic system. However, in tissues, ligation of immune complexes by specific receptors on leukocytes may have pro-inflammatory consequences.

The ability of complement to inhibit immune precipitation was first described in 1941 by Heidelberger[91]. Miller and Nussenzweig[92], 34 years later, described the ability of complement to solubilize pre-formed immune precipitates, and in 1980 it was demonstrated that complement-mediated inhibition of immune precipitation required classical pathway function[93]. Covalent binding of C3 fragments to IC is essential for keeping IC in solution[94]. C3b may interfere with Ag–Ab bonds by affecting Fc–Fc interactions[95] or by reducing antibody and antigen valency[96]. The capacity of complement to render IC hydrophilic may well be important in influencing solubility[7]. During the early stages of IC formation, C1q can inhibit immune precipitation[97], but it is activation of C3 that is of primary importance[7]. Sera deficient in C2 or C4 cannot inhibit precipitation of IC, as no classical pathway C3 convertase enzyme can be formed[98].

Binding of complement to immune complexes also allows the binding of such ICs to cell surface complement receptors, particularly those for C3b, iC3b and C4b. The process by which opsonized immune complexes bind to CR1 on erythrocytes is commonly described as 'immune adherence'. As long ago as 1915 it was observed that microorganisms would bind to mouse platelets in the presence of normal serum and that the phenomenon was abolished by inactivation of serum by heating[99]. Similar observations were made in 1930[100], and later by Nelson in 1953[101], in experiments in which microorganisms were shown to adhere to human erythrocytes in a complement-dependent manner. More recently, the human erythrocyte C3b receptor (CR1) has been extensively characterized[102]. CR1 is also found on B lymphocytes, subsets of T lymphocytes, neutrophils, monocytes, macrophages, glomerular epithelial cells and follicular dendritic cells[103]. The receptor is a single-chain glycoprotein found in four allotypic forms ranging from 160 to 290 kD[104,105] and binds to C3b, iC3b and C4b.

There is evidence that CR1 on erythrocytes may play a role in the processing of immune complexes, and abnormalities of CR1 expression in patients with SLE have stimulated research into a possible role for deficiency of the receptor in pathogenesis. The size, capacity to activate complement, and structure of immune complexes all influence binding to CR1. Generally, larger complexes bind most efficiently[106-108]. This is illustrated in the case of the binding of tetanus toxoid (TT)–anti-TT complexes to human erythrocytes (Figure 2).

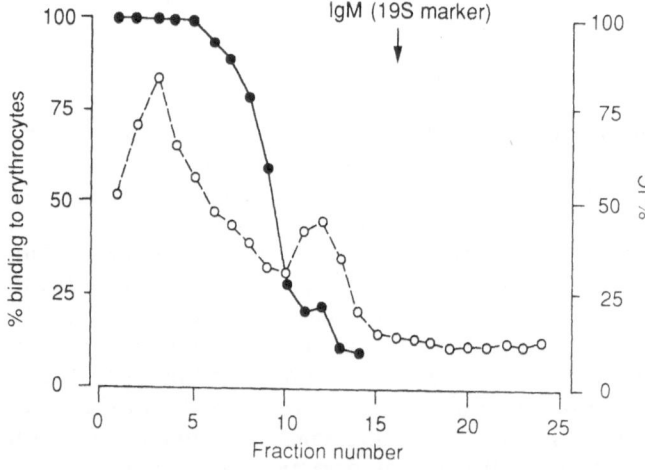

Figure 2 Size and reactivity of tetanus toxoid(TT)–anti-TT immune complexes, centrifuged on a 10–50% sucrose gradient. Radioactivity of fractions is expressed as a percentage of total activity recovered in the gradient (○). The binding of each fraction to erythrocytes was determined (●), larger complexes binding more efficiently than smaller ones. (From Schifferli et al.[108], with permission)

DNA–anti-DNA complex binding to erthrocyte CR1 *in vitro* hs also been studied in detail[106]. Maximum binding was observed with complexes incorporating DNA fragments of 1500 base pairs or more, resulting in a final complex size of about 10 000 kD (equivalent to a sedimentation coefficient of $\geqslant 100$ S). Immune complexes formed *in vitro*, in the presence of complement, bind much less efficiently to erythrocyte CR1[109] than those formed in the absence of complement, and there is evidence to suggest that when ICs are formed *in vivo* only a relatively small proportion bind to CR1[60].

Clearance of immune complexes

Abnormal mononuclear phagocytic function — 'Reticulo-endothelial saturation'

The concept of 'reticulo-endothelial saturation' first developed from the experiments of Biozzi on the fate of different doses of colloidal carbon particles injected into the circulation of rabbits[110]. Haakenstadt and Mannik[111] demonstrated that injection of immune complexes into rabbits resulted in saturable hepatic uptake followed by spillover into other organs. It is a matter of contention whether such saturation of the mononuclear phagocytic system is a factor in human disease.

The function of the mononuclear phagocyte system in both normal volunteers and patients with IC disease has been extensively studied using both erythrocytes coated with anti-rhesus IgG (E-IgG), and more recently aggregated immunoglobulin or soluble immune complexes[112–114]. E-IgG are largely removed from the circulation by the spleen, clearance being mediated by Fc receptors[112,115]. In both human and animal models, opsonized IgM-coated erythrocytes[116] are, on the other hand, largely cleared in the liver[117,118], and evidence suggests that the liver is also the site of soluble IC clearance in man[60] (see below). Many investigators have examined E-IgG clearance specifically in SLE. In the study by Frank and coworkers[119], the clearance half-times ($t_{1/2}$) in patients with SLE correlated with disease activity, and with levels of circulating immune complexes. The same workers subsequently performed a longitudinal study in individual SLE patients, and reported a fall in the clearance half-times of E-IgG *pari passu* with a reduction in disease activity[120]. However, Kimberly and colleagues failed in a similar study[121], to demonstrate any correlation between the $t_{1/2}$ of antibody-coated erythrocytes and circulating immune complex levels. Two other groups have also failed to demonstrate any convincing correlation between circulating IC levels and E-IgG clearance[122,123]. An important factor in the clearance of IgG-coated red cells appears to be splenic blood flow[124], and this factor may be important in the disease-associated handling of coated cells.

Soluble immune complex clearance, complement and erythrocyte CR1

Lobatto and colleagues have recently developed an alternative system for assessing 'mononuclear phagocyte function' in different disease states[125], involving the infusion of radiolabelled soluble aggregates of IgG (AIgG). This model was employed to compare AIgG clearance in 9 normal controls and

15 patients with SLE. Binding of aggregates to red cells was lower in patients (9.3 ± 8.1%) compared with normals (24 ± 20%), and the clearance half-time in the patients was elevated (58 ± 27 min) compared with that in normals (26 ± 8 min). Liver/spleen (L/S) uptake ratios were also significantly higher in SLE patients than in controls, attributable to lower splenic uptake. No correlation was observed in this study between L/S uptake ratios, or clearance half-time, and circulating IC levels or disease activity.

Schifferli and coworkers have recently investigated soluble immune complex clearance, using ^{125}I-labelled tetanus toxoid–anti-TT complexes[108]. Complexes were prepared in 20-fold antibody excess, and were 45 S in size as measured by sucrose density gradient centrifugation. Either native complexes or ICs opsonized with serum in vitro were injected into subjects. Nine normal controls and 15 patients with IC disease/hypocomplementaemia were studied, including four patients with active SLE. Immune complexes were found to bind to red cell CR1 in a complement-dependent manner. CR1 numbers correlated with their degree of uptake. Two phases of complex clearance were observed. A rapid phase of IC clearance was identified, occurring in the first minute, in subjects with low CR1 (including three of the SLE patients), low binding of complexes to erythrocytes, and low complement. This may represent deposition of complexes outside the reticuloendothelial system (see Figure 3). While this work suggests that complement and erythrocyte CR1 may have a role to play in IC clearance in man, this model is still open to the criticism that very large immune complexes, formed in vitro, were used, which may not be representative of those responsible for the causation of IC disease.

There is conflicting evidence regarding the binding of IC formed in the presence of complement to erythrocyte CR1. Varga and colleagues demonstrated that BSA–anti-BSA IC formed in the presence of serum failed to bind to CR1[109]. However, other workers have shown that the successive infusion of human dsDNA antibodies and dsDNA into rabbits and monkeys leads to rapid formation of immune complexes capable of binding to CR1[126]. The formation and fate of immune complexes formed in vivo in patients receiving radioimmunotherapy has been studied[60]. The successive administration of a radiolabelled mouse anti-tumour antibody and a human anti-mouse antibody resulted in the formation of ICs comprising the two antibody species. Rapid complex clearance was observed, with clearance half-time of 11 minutes, and binding of 8–11% of the complexed material to erythrocyte CR1. Both systemic complement activation and a 30% fall in erythrocyte CR1 numbers were observed. External monitoring indicated that clearance took place primarily in the liver.

In the context of these observations, suggesting that erythrocyte CR1 has an important role to play in IC transport and clearance, the demonstration that erythrocytes from SLE patients exhibited defective immune adherence was of great interest. Miyakawa and coworkers found that red cells from most patients with SLE did not exhibit immune adherence to opsonized microtitre plates[127]. This observation has been confirmed in a number of centres, and is due to a reduction in the numerical expression of erythrocyte CR1[128–134]. It has since become clear that there is an inherited numerical

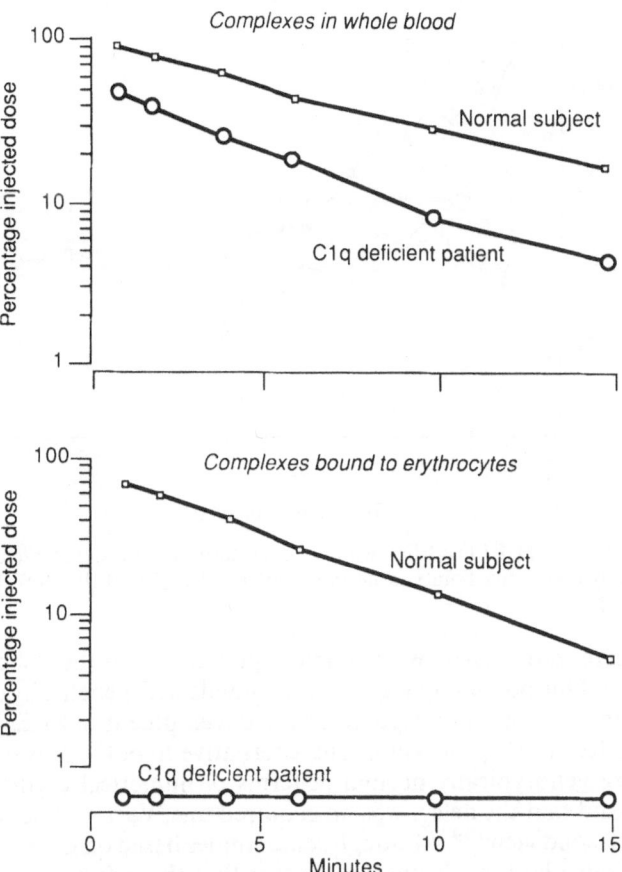

Figure 3 Immune complex elimination rates in a normal individual (□) and an SLE patient with C1q deficiency (○). Percentage of complexes remaining in whole blood is shown in the upper graph, and red cell-bound complexes below. After 1 minute the clearance of IC fitted a monoexponential line. No binding to erythrocyte CR1 was observed in the C1q-deficient lupus patient (see text). (From Schifferli et al.[108], with permission)

polymorphism of CR1 expression on erythrocytes. Early work using immune adherence by Klopstock and coworkers[135], and more recent enumeration of receptors using a radio-ligand binding assay[129], suggest that defective immune adherence is an inherited abnormality encoded by an autosomal recessive gene. Identification of a cDNA clone for CR1 by Wong and colleagues[136,137], has allowed the study of inherited polymorphisms at the genomic level[138]. Using the CR1.1 probe, and HindIII digestion of genomic DNA, two polymorphic bands of 6.9 kb and 7.4 kb were identified. The former correlated with low red cell CR1 expression, and the 7.4 kb band with high CR1 numbers (Figure 4). In family studies, these segregated as alleles at a single locus. Studies using this RFLP showed considerable overlap of numerical expression between 6.9 and 7.4 kb heterozygotes and homozygotes for both the bands, so inference of genotype from phenotype is therefore difficult.

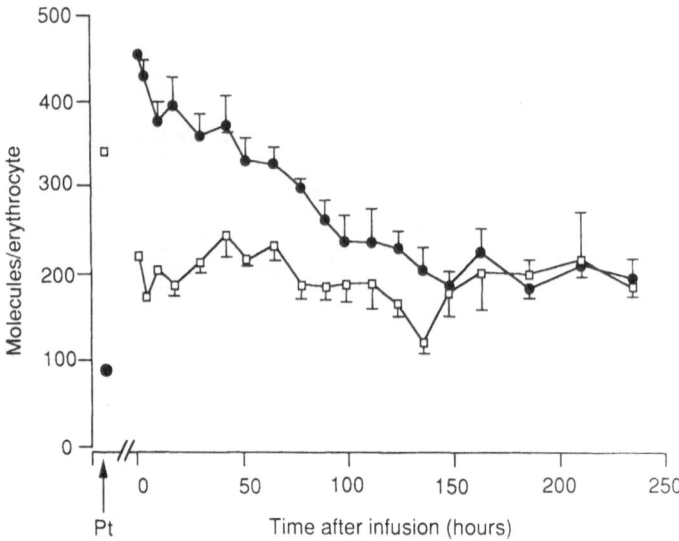

Figure 4 Time course of CR1 loss from two units of erythrocytes transfused into a patient with SLE and haemolytic anaemia. Points are mean ± 1 SE; ● CR1; □ C3d. (From Walport et al.[158], with permission)

In SLE there were clearly two possible explanations for the low erythrocyte CR1 numbers. One possibility was that individuals with genetically determined low CR1 numbers were predisposed to the development of SLE, possibly as a result of defective IC processing. The alternative hypothesis was that lupus patients were genotypically normal in terms of numerical erythrocyte CR1 expression, and that the defect was an acquired one. Various lines of evidence support the second view[139]. Although some studies based on CR1 enumeration in SLE patients and their families suggested that the defect was an inherited one[127,129,140], others have found that the gene frequency of the alleles coding for the 6.9 kb bands (encoding low CR1 expression) and the 7.4 kb bands, was identical in SLE patients and normal controls[141]. Studies of a Boston population, however, showed a slight excess of heterozygotes for the 6.9 and 7.4 kb alleles[40].

Other observations favour the hypothesis that reduced erythrocyte CR1 expression in SLE is mainly acquired. An inverse correlation has been described between the deposition of C3dg molecules on erythrocytes and CR1 numbers[142], and erythrocyte CR1 levels were shown to correlate directly with both elevated ICs and reduced plasma C4[128,130]. Several studies have shown a correlation between CR1 numbers and disease activity in SLE[134,142]. More direct evidence comes from the observation that loss of CR1 from erythrocytes can be demonstrated on cells which are transfused into patients with lupus and/or haemolytic anaemias (Figure 5). A numerical reduction in CR1 has also been described in a variety of other disease states in which ICs are pathogenetically implicated, and/or in which there is abnormal C3 deposition on the cell surface, including paroxysmal nocturnal haemoglobinuria[143], Sjögren's syndrome[144], lepromatous leprosy[145], AIDS[146], autoimmune haemolytic anaemias[142], and juvenile rheumatoid arthritis[147].

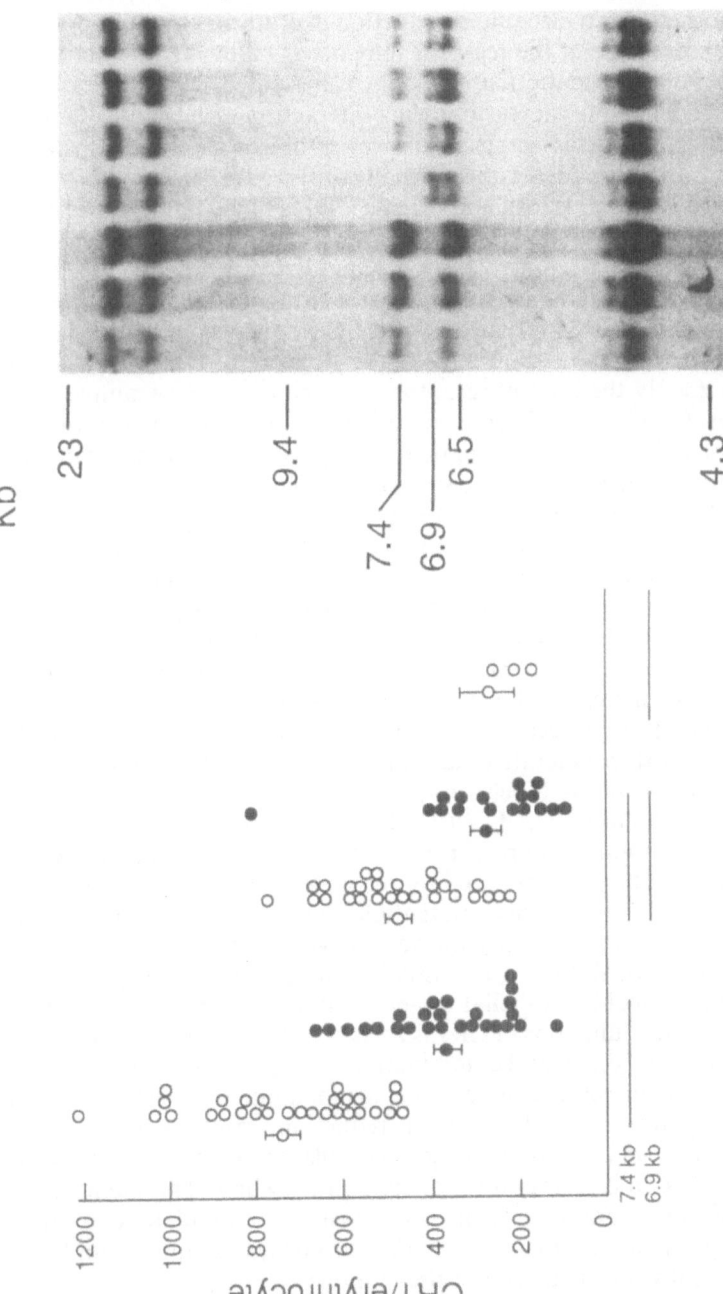

Figure 5 CR1 numbers in normal subjects (open symbols) and SLE patients (solid symbols) according to genotype for 7.4 kb and 6.9 kb alleles defined by a CR1 cDNA probe. The gene frequency of the two alleles does not differ significantly between controls and SLE patients. A Southern blot illustrating the RFLP is shown on the right. (From Moldenhauer et al.[141], with permission)

A transient fall in red cell CR1 numbers was observed in patients with *in vivo* immune complex formation following radioimmunotherapy, *pari passu* with IC clearance and the deposition of C3 and C4 on erythrocytes[60].

A likely hypothesis for the acquired reduction in erythrocyte CR1 numbers in SLE is that proteolysis of the receptor may occur following interaction of red cell-bound IC and hepatic Kupffer cells. C3b-coated erythrocytes have been shown to become spherocytic following interaction with hepatic Kupffer cells *in vivo*[116,148]. In normal subjects, low levels of free CR1 are detectable in plasma[149,150]. In SLE patients, the normally observed relationship between free and red cell CR1 levels is lost, and plasma CR1 is higher in these patients, possibly indicating proteolytic loss from cells[150].

There is evidence for a reduction in CR1 numbers on other cell types in SLE. A number of studies suggest that there is a reduction of CR1 expression on both neutrophils and lymphocytes from SLE patients[151,152]. However, the state of neutrophil activation and the temperature of their preparation may influence greatly the level of receptor expression[153]. For example, Mir and colleagues found no difference in the levels of CR1 expression on neutrophils isolated at 4°C in SLE patients compared with normal controls, but did detect a difference in cells prepared at room temperature, or stimulated with FMLP[154]. In this study, neutrophil CR1 expression was normal in consanguineous relatives of the 22 SLE patients, though abnormalities in the ingestion of EIgGC3b by both monocytes and neutrophils in patients and their relatives were described. These observations remain as yet unexplained, but have been reported in other studies[155]. It would seem likely that the reduction in neutrophil CR1 numbers in SLE is also an acquired defect, and may be related to an increase in receptor turnover, possibly due to IC binding. CR1 numbers are also reduced on the surface of glomerular epithelial cells in lupus patients with proliferative nephritis[156,157], though the significance of this observation as far as IC clearance is concerned is not clear.

The acquired reduction in red cell CR1 in SLE may have a number of consequences for immune complex processing and the potential of IC to cause tissue injury. The carriage of IC on red cells in the jet-stream of small blood vessels may prevent their potentially phlogistic interaction with vascular endothelium. A reduction in the pool of available CR1 on erythrocytes may increase the probability of potentially harmful IC escaping efficient clearance by the reticuloendothelial system, and causing tissue damage at other sites. One of the functions of CR1 is as a co-factor to Factor I-mediated cleavage of iC3b to C3dg. iC3b-coated immune complexes can bind to CR1 and CR3 on phagocytic cells, again resulting in inflammatory effects. A vicious circle may result from IC-induced CR1 reduction, resulting in defective clearance of new, and possibly larger, complexes which may lead to inflammation in blood vessels in the kidneys and elsewhere. This could cause the release of more antigens, which in turn can stimulate continued autoantibody production and the formation of further immune complexes, either systematically, or at the site of tissue injury.

SUMMARY

Our understanding of the role of immune complexes in SLE has increased rapidly in recent years, but the value of their routine measurement in the day-to-day management of the disease is still a matter for debate. Tissue damage may result from the deposition of circulating IC, but it is now clear that local formation of complexes at sites of inflammation may be of equal importance, particularly in the kidney. Defects in Fc-mediated and complement receptor-mediated clearance have been implicated in pathogenesis. Complement has a vital part to play, in the physicochemical modification of IC, in the facilitation of complex binding to erythrocytes to enable their delivery to the reticuloendothelial system, and in the mediation of cellular injury in the disease. There is good evidence for an acquired reduction in the numerical expression of erythrocyte CR1 in SLE, and this may predispose to abnormal biological processing of IC and the perpetuation of IC-mediated tissue damage.

References

1. Agnello, V., Koffler, D., Eisenberg, J. W., Winchester, R. J. and Kunkel, H. G. (1971). C1q precipitins in the sera of patients with systemic lupus erythematosus and other hypocomplementemic states: characterisation of high and low molecular weight types. *J. Exp. Med.*, **134**(3), 228–241
2. Koffler, D., Schur, P. and Kunkel, H. G. (1967). Immunological studies concerning the nephritis of systemic lupus erythematosus. *J. Exp. Med.*, **126**, 607
3. Krishnan, C. and Kaplan, M. H. (1967). Immunopathologic studies of systemic lupus erythematosus. II. Anti-nuclear reaction of gamma-globulin eluted from homogenates and isolated glomeruli of kidneys from patients with lupus nephritis. *J. Clin. Invest.*, **46**, 569
4. Koffler, D., Agnello, V., Thoburn, R. and Kunkel, H. G. (1971). Systemic lupus erythematosus: Prototype of immune complex nephritis in man. *J. Exp. Med.*, **134**, 169–179
5. Cochrane, C. G. (1971). Mechanisms involved in the deposition of immune complexes in tissues. *J. Exp. Med.*, **134**(3), 75–89
6. Couser, W. G. (1986), In situ formation of immune complexes and the role of complement activation in glomerulonephritis. In Carpenter, C. B. (ed.) *Clinics in Immunology and Allergy—Renal Immunology*, pp. 287–306. (London: W. B. Saunders)
7. Schifferli, J. A. and Ng, Y. C. (1988). The role of complement in the processing of immune complexes. In Kazatchkine, M. D. (ed.) *Baillière's Clinical Immunology and Allergy—Complement and Immunological Disease*, pp. 319–334. (London: Baillière Tyndall)
8. Atkinson, J. P., Kaine, J. L., Holers, V. M. and Chan, A. C. (1986). Complement and the rheumatic diseases. In Ross, G. D. (ed.) *Immunobiology of the Complement System*, pp. 197–211. (London: Academic Press)
9. Fielder, A. H., Walport, M. J., Batchelor, J. R., Rynes, R. I., Black, C. M., Dodi, I. A. and Hughes, G. R. V. (1983). Family study of the major histocompatibility complex in patients with systemic lupus erythematosus: importance of null alleles of C4A and C4B in determining disease susceptibility. *Br. Med. J.*, **286**, 423–428
10. Muller-Eberhard, H. J. and Calcott, M. A. (1966). Interaction between C1q and gamma globulin. *Immunochemistry*, **3**, 500.
11. Theofilopoulos, A. N. and Dixon, F. J. (1979). The biology and detection of immune complexes. *Adv. Immunol.*, **28**, 89–220
12. Hay, F. C., Nineham, L. J. and Roitt, I. M. (1976). Routine assay for the detection of immune complexes of known immunoglobulin class using solid phase C1q. *Clin. Exp. Immunol.*, **24**, 396–400
13. Abrass, C. K., Nies, K. M., Louie, J. S., Border, W. A. and Glassock, R. J. (1980). Correlation and predictive accuracy of circulating immune complexes with disease activity in patients with systemic lupus erythematosus. *Arthritis Rheum.*, **23**(3), 273–282

14. Tung, K. S. K., DeHoratius, R. J. and Williams, R. C. (1981). Study of circulating immune complex size in systemic lupus erythematosus. *Clin. Exp. Immunol.*, **43**, 615–625
15. Casali, P., Bossus, A., Carpenter, N. A. and Lambert, P. H. (1977). Solid phase immunoassay or radioimmunoassay for the detection of immune complexes based on their recognition by conglutinin: conglutinin binding test: a comparative study with 125-I labelled C1q binding and Raji cell RIA tests. *Clin. Exp. Immunol.*, **29**, 342–354
16. Muso, E., Sekita, K., Doi, T., Kuwahara, T., Yoshida, H., Tamura, T., Kawai, C. and Hamashima, Y. (1984). Immunopathological correlation between mesangial C3d-deposition and C3d-fixing circulating immune complexes in lupus nephritis. *Clin. Immunol. Immunopathol.*, **32**, 351–358
17. Iida, K., Mitomo, K., Fujita, T. and Tamura, N. (1987). A solid-phase anti-C3 assay for detection of immune complexes in six distinguished forms. *J. Immunol. Meth.*, **98**, 23–28
18. Tron, J. F. and Bach, J. F. (1977). Tests immunologiques pour le diagnostic et le prognostic du lupus erythemateux dissemine avant traitement. *Nouv. Presse Med.*, **6**, 2573–2578
19. Cano, P. O., Jerry, L. M., Sladowski, J. P. and Osterland, C. K. (1977). Circulating immune complexes in systemic lupus erythematosus. *Clin. Exp. Immunol.*, **29**, 187–204
20. Agnello, V., Koffler, D. and Kunkel, H. G. (1973). Immune complex systems in the nephritis of systemic lupus erythematosus. *Kidney Int.*, **3**, 90–99
21. Nydegger, U. E., Lambert, P. H., Gerber, H. and Miescher, P. A. (1974). Circulating immune complexes in the serum in systemic lupus erythematosus and in carriers of hepatitis-B antigen. *J. Clin. Invest.*, **54**, 297–30·9
22. Davis, P., Cumming, R. H. and Verrier-Jones, J. (1977). Relationship between antiDNA antibodies, complement consumption and circulating immune complexes in systemic lupus erythematosus. *Clin. Exp. Immunol.*, **28**, 226–232
23. Robinson, M. F., Roberts, L. J., Jones, J. V. and Lewis, E. J. (1979). Circulating immune complexes in patients with lupus and membranous glomerulonephritis. *Clin. Immunol. Immunopathol.*, **14**, 348–360
24. Uwatoko, S., Aotsuka, S., Okawa, M., Egusa, Y., Yokohari, R. and Aizawa, C. (1984). Characterization of C1q-binding IgG complexes in systemic lupus erythematosus. *Clin. Immunol. Immunopathol.*, **30**, 104–116
25. Uwatoko, S., Aotsuka, S., Okawa, M., Egusa, Y., Yokohari, R. and Aizawa, C. (1984). C1q solid-phase radioimmunoassay: binding properties of solid-phase C1q and evidence that C1q-binding IgG complexes in systemic lupus erythematosus are not bound to endogenous C1q. *J. Immunol. Meth.*, **73**, 67–74
26. Uwatoko, S., Aotsuka, S., Okawa, M., Egusa, Y., Yokohari, R., Aizawa, C. and Suzuki, K. (1987). Ciq solid phase radioimmunoassay: evidence for detection of antibody directed against the collagen-like region of C1q in sera from patients with systemic lupus erythematosus. *Clin. Exp. Immunol.*, **69**, 98–106
27. Uwatoko, S. and Mannik, M. (1988). Low-molecular weight C1q-binding immunoglobulin G in patients with systemic lupus erythematosus consists of autoantibodies to the collagen-like region of C1q. *J. Clin. Invest.*, **82**, 816–824
28. Koffler, D., Agnello, V.l and Winchester, R. (1973). The occurrence of single-stranded DNA in the serum of patients with SLE and other diseases. *J. Clin. Invest.*, **52**, 198–204
29. Tan, E. M., Schur, P. H., Carr, R. I. and Kunkel, H. G. (1966). Deoxyribonucleic acid (DNA) and antibodies to DNA in the serum of patients with systemic lupus erythematosus. *J. Clin. Invest.*, **45**, 1732–1740
30. Harbeck, R. J., Bardana, E. J., Kohler, P. F. and Carr, R. I. (1973). DNA:antiDNA complexes: their detection in systemic lupus erythematosus sera. *J. Clin. Invest.*, **52**, 789–795
31. Izui, S., Lambert, P. H. and Miescher, P. A. (1977). Failure to detect circulating DNA–anti-DNA complexes by four radioimmunological methods in patients with systemic lupus erythematosus. *Clin. Exp. Immunol.*, **30**, 384
32. Fournié, G. J. (1988). Circulating DNA and lupus nephritis. *Kidney Int.*, **33**(2), 487–497
33. Nilsson, B., Bjelle, A., Loof, L. and Nilsson, U. R. (1987). Quantitation and antigenic characterization of bound C3 of circulating immune complexes in systemic lupus erythematosus, rheumatoid arthritis, and primary biliary cirrhosis. *J. Clin. Immunol.*, **7**, 420–426
34. Appel, G. B., Silva, F. G. and Pirani, C. L. (1978). Renal involvement in systemic lupus erythematosus (SLE): a study of 56 patients emphasising histologic classification. *Medicine*, **57**, 371–410

35. Mannik, M. (1987). Mechanisms of tissue deposition of immune complexes. *J. Rheumatol.*, **14**, 35–42
36. Van Damme, B. J. C., Fleuren, G. J., Bakker, W. W., Vernier, R. L.l and Hoedemaeker, P. J. (1978). Experimental glomerulonephritis in the rat induced by antibodies to tubular antigens. IV. Fixed glomerular antigens in the pathogenesis of heterologous immune complex glomerulonephritis. *Lab. Invest.*, **38**, 502–510
37. Salant, D. J., Belok, S., Madaio, M. P. and Couser, W. G. (1980). A new role for complement in experimental membranous nephropathy in rats. *J. Clin. Invest.*, **66**, 1339–1350
38. Kerjaschki, D. and Farquar, M. G. (1983). Immunocytochemical localisation of the Heymann nephritis antigen (GP330) in glomerular epithelial cells of normal Lewis rats. *J. Exp. Med.*, **157**, 667–685
39, Barba, L. M., Caldwell, P. R. B. and Downie, G. H. (1983). Lung injury mediated by antibodies to epithelium. I. In the rabbit repeated interaction of heterologous anti-angiotensin converting enzyme antibodies with alveolar epithelium results in resistance to immune injury through antigenic modulation. *J. Exp. Med.*, **158**, 2141–2158
40. Camussi, G., Brentjens, J. R. and Noble, B. (1985). Antibody-induced redistribution of Heymann's antigen on the surface of cultured glomerular visceral epithelial cells: possible role in the pathogenesis of Heymann glomerular nephritis. *J. Immunol.*, **135**, 2409–2416
41. Wilson, C. B. and Dixon, F. J. (1986). Renal response to immunological injury. In Brenner, B. M. and Rector, F. C. (eds) *The Kidney*, pp. 800-890. (Philadelphia: W. B. Saunders)
42. Shoenfeld, Y., Rauch, J., Massicotte, H., Datta, S. K., André-Schwartz, J., Stollar, B. D. and Schwartz, R. S. (1983). Polyspecificity of monoclonal lupus autoantibodies produced by human-human hybridomas. *N. Engl J. Med.*, **308**, 414–420
43. Madaio, M. P., Carlson, J., Cataldo, J., Ucci, A., Miblorini, P. and Pankewycz, O. (1987). Murine monoclonal anti-DNA antibodies bind directly to glomerular antigens and form immune deposits. *J. Immunol.*, **138**(9), 2883–2889
44. Couser, W. G. and Salant, D. J. (1980). In-situ immune complex formation and glomerular injury. *Kidney Int.*, **17**, 1–13
45. Caulin-Glaser, T., Gallo, G. R. and Lamm, M. E. (1983). Non-dissociating cationic immune complexes can deposit in glomerular basement membrane. *J. Exp. Med.*, **158**, 1561–1572
46. Agodoa, L. Y. C., Gauthier, V. J. and Mannik, M. (1983). Precipitating antigen–antibody systems are required for the formation of sub-epithelial electron dense immune deposits in rat glomeruli. *J. Exp. Med.*, **158**, 1259–1271
47. Izui, S., Lambert, P. H. and Miescher, P. A. (1989). *In vitro* demonstration of a particular affinity of glomerular basement antigen and collagen for DNA: A possible basis for a local formation of DNA–anti-DNA complexes in systemic lupus erythematosus. *J. Exp. Med.*, **144**, 428–443
48. Ebling, F. and Hahn, B. H. (1980). Restricted subpopulations of DNA antibodies in kidneys of mice with sytemic lupus. Comparison of antibodies in serum and renal eluates. *Arthritis Rheum.*, **23**, 392–403
49. Dang, H. and Harbeck, R. J. (1982). Comparison of anti-DNA antibodies from serum and kidney eluates of NZB X NZW F1 mice. *J. Clin. Lab. Immunol.*, **9**, 139–145
50. Gay, S., Losman, M. J., Koopman, W. J. and Miller, E. J. (1985). Interaction of DNA with connective tissue matrix proteins reveals preferential binding to type V collagen. *J. Immunol.*, **135**, 1097–1100
51 Germuth, F. G. and Rodriguez, E. (1973). *Immunopathology of the Renal Glomerulus: Immune Complex Deposit and Anti-basement Membrane Disease*, 1st Edn. (Boston: Little, Brown)
52. Couser, W. G. and Salant, D. J. (1982). Immunopathogenesis of glomerular capillary wall injury in nephrotic states. *Contemp. Issues Nephrol.*, **9**, 47–83
53. Mauer, S. M., Sutherland, D. E. R. and Howard, R. J. (1973). The glomerular mesangium. III. Acute immune mesangial injury: a new model of glomerulonephritis. *J. Exp. Med.*, **137**, 553–570
54. Yamamoto, T. and Wilson, C. B. (1986). Antibody-induced mesangial damage: the model, functional alterations and effects of complement. *Kidney Int.*, **29**, 296
55. Matsuo, S., Caldwell, P., Brentjens, J. and Andres, G. (1985). Nephrotoxic serum glomerulonephritis induced in the rabbit by anti-endothelial cell antibodies. *Kidney Int.*, **27**, 217
56. Cines, D. B., Lyss, A. P., Reeber, M. B. and DeHoratius, R. J. (1984). Presence of complement-fixing anti-endothelial cell antibodies in systemic lupus erythematosus. *J. Clin.*

Invest., **73**, 611–625

57. Biesecker, G., Katz, S. and Koffler, D. (1981). Renal localisation of the membrane attack complex in systemic lupus erythematosus. *J. Exp. Med.*, **154**, 1779–1794

58. Henson, P. M. and Cochrane, C. G. (1975). The effects of complement depletion on experimental tissue injury. *Ann. N.Y. Acad. Sci.*, **256**, 426–440

59. Abramson, S., Belmont, H. M., Hopkins, P., Buyon, J., Winchester, R. and Weissmann, G. (1987). Complement activation and vascular injury in systemic lupus erythematosus. *J. Rheumatol.*, **14**(suppl. 3), 43–46

60. Davies, K. A., Stewart, S., Hird, V. and Walport, M. J. (1988). In vivo formation and clearance of immune complexes in humans. *J. Immunol.*, **144**, 4613–4620

61. Lewis, S. L., Van Epps, D. E. and Chenoweth, D. E. (1986). C5a receptor modulation on neutrophils and monocytes from chronic hemodialysis and peritoneal dialysis patients. *Clin. Nephrol.*, **26**, 37–44

62. Natali, P. G. and Tan, E. M. (1973). Experimental skin lesions in mice resembling systemic lupus erythematosus. *Arthritis Rheum.*, **16**, 579–589

63. Joselow, S. A., Gown, A. and Mannik, M. (1985). Cutaneous deposition of immune complexes in chronic serum sickness of mice induced with cationised or unaltered antigen. *J. Invest. Dermatol.*, **85**, 559–563

64. Landry, M. and Sams, W. M. (1973). Systemic lupus eryuthematosus: studies of the antibodies bound to skin. *J. Clin. Invest.*, **52**, 1871–1880

65. Hunder, C. G., Mullen, B. J. and McDuffie, F. C. (1974). Complement in pericardial fluid of lupus erythematosus: studies of two patients. *Ann. Intern. Med.*, **80**, 453–458

66. Dubois, E. L. (1974). *Lupus Erythematosus: A Review of the Current Status of Discoid and Systemic Lupus Erythematosus and their Variants*, 2nd Edn. (Los Angeles: University of Southern California Press)

67. Goldenberg, D. L., Leff, G. and Grayzel, A. I. (1975). Pericardial tamponade in systemic lupus erythematosus: with absent hemolytic complement activity in pericardial fluid. *N.Y. State J. Med.*, **75**, 910–912

68. Michet, C. J. and Hunder, C. G. (1984). Pericarditis. In Ansell, B. M. and Simkin, P. A. (eds.) *The Heart and Rheumatic Disease*, pp. 1–26. (London: Butterworths International Medical Reviews—Rheumatology)

69. Bulkley, B. H. and Roberts, W. C. (1975). The heart in systemic lupus erythematosus and the changes induced in it by corticosteroid therapy. *Am. J. Med.*, **58**, 243–264

70. Korbet, S. M., Schwartz, M. M. and Lewis, E. J. (1984). Immune complex deposition and coronary vasculitis in systemic lupus erythematosus. Report of two cases. *Am. J. Med.*, **77**, 141–146

71. Bennet, R. M. (1984). Myocardial involvement. In Ansell, B. M. and Simkin, P. A. (eds.) *The Heart and Rheumatic Diseases*, pp. 27–64. (London: Butterworths International Medical Reviews—Rheumatology)

72. Hardin, N. H., Minnick, C. R. and Murphy, G. E. (1973). Experimental induction of atheroarteriosclerosis by the synergy of allergic injury to arteries and lipid-rich diet. *Am. J. Pathol.*, **73**, 301–326

73. Shapiro, R. F., Gamble, C. N. and Wisner, K. B. (1977). Immunopathogenesis of Libman Sacks endocarditis. Assessment by light and immunofluorescent microscopy in two patients. *Ann. Rheum. Dis.*, **36**, 508–515

74. Inoue, T., Kanayana, Y. and Ohe, A. (1979). Immunopathologic studies of pneumonitis in systemic lupus erythematosus. *Ann. Intern. Med.*, **91**, 30–34

75. Pertschuk, L. P., Moccia, L. F. and Rosen, Y. (1977). Acute pulmonary complications in systemic lupus erythematosus—immunofluorescence and light microscopic study. *Am. J. Clin. Pathol.*, **68**, 553–557

76. Churg, A., Franklin, W. and Chan, K. L. (1980). Pulmonary haemorrhage and immune-complex deposition in the lung: Complications in a patient with systemic lupus erythematosus. *Arch. Pathol. Lab. Med.*, **104**, 388–391

77. Castadena, S., Herrero-Beaumont, G. and Abuad, J. M. (1985). Pulmonary hemorrhage in lupus erythematosus without evidence of an immunologic cause. *Arch. Intern. Med.*, **145**, 2128–2129

78. Desnoyers, M. R., Bernstein, S. and Cooper, A. G. (1984). Pulmonary hemorrhage in lupus erythematosus without evidence of an immunologic cause. *Arch. Intern. Med.*, **144**, 1398–1400

79. Marino, C. T. and Pertschuk, L. P. (1981). Pulmonary hemorrhage in systemic lupus erythematosus. *Arch. Intern. Med.*, **141**, 201–203

80. Eisenberg, H., Dubois, E. L. and Sherwin, R. P. (1973). Diffuse interstitial lung disease in systemic lupus erythematosus. *Ann. Intern. Med.*, **79**, 37–45

81. McCune, W. J. and Golbus, J. (1988). Neuropsychiatric lupus. *Rheum. Dis. Clin. North. Am.*, **14**(1), 149–167

82. Harris, E. N., Gharavi, A. E., Boey, M. L., Patel, B. M., Mackworth-Young, C. G., Loizou, S. and Hughes, G. R. V. (1983). Anticardiolipin antibodies: Detection by radioimmunoassay and association with thrombosis in systemic lupus erythematosus. *Lancet*, **2**, 1211–1214

83. Boyer, R. S., Sun, N. C. J. and Verity, A. (1980). Immunoperoxidase staining of the choroid plexus in systemic lupus erythematosus. *J. Rheumatol.*, **7**, 645–650

84. Lambert, P., Garret, R. and Lampert, A. (1977). Ferritin immune complexes in the choroid plexus. *Acta Neuropathol.*, **38**, 83

85. Lampert, P. W. and Oldstone, M. B. A. (1973). Host immunoglobulin G and complement deposits in the choroid plexus during spontaneous immune complex disease. *Science*, **180**, 408

86. Hadler, N. M., Gerwin, R. D., Frank, M. M., Whitaker, J. N., Baker, M. and Decker, J. L. (1973). The fourth component of complement in the cerebrospinal fluid in systemic lupus erythematosus. *Arthritis Rheum.*, **16**, 507–521

87. Petz, L. D., Sharp, G. C. and Cooper, N. R. (1971). Serum and cerbrospinal fluid complement and serum autoantibodies in systemic lupus erythematosus. *Medicine*, **50**, 259

88. Sanders, M. E., Alexander, E. L. and Koski, C. L. (1987). Detection of activated terminal complement (C5b-9) in cerebrospinal fluid from patients with central nervous system involvement of primary Sjögren's syndrome or systemic lupus erythematosus. *J. Immunol.*, **138**, 2095–2099

89. Seibold, J. R., Buckingham, R. B. and Medsger, T. A. (1982). Cerebrospinal fluid immune complexes in systemic lupus erythematosus involving the central nervous system. *Semin. Arthritis Rheum.*, **12**, 68–76

90. Keefe, E. B., Bardana, E. J. and Harbeck, R. J. (1974). Lupus meningitis: Antibody to deoxyribonucleic acid (DNA) and DNA–anti-DNA complexes in cerebrospinal fluid. *Ann. Intern. Med.*, **80**, 58–60

91. Heidelberger, M. (1941). Quantitative chemical studies on complement or alexin. I. A method. *J. Exp. Med.*, **73**, 691–694

92. Miller, G. W. and Nussenzweig, V. (1975). A new complement function: solubilization of antigen-antibody aggregates. *Proc. Natl Acad. Sci. USA*, **72**, 418–423

93. Schifferli, J. A., Bartolotti, S. R. and Peters, D. K. (1980). Inhibition of immune precipitation by complement. *Clin. Exp. Immunol.*, **42**, 387–392

94. Hong, K., Takata, Y., Sayama, K., Konozo, H., Takeda, J., Nakata, Y., Kinoshita, T. and Inoue, K. (1984). Inhibition of immune precipitation by complement. *J. Immunol.*, **133**, 1464–1469

95. Moller, N. P. and Steengaard, J. (1983). Fc mediated immune precipitation. I. A new role of the Fc portion of IgG. *Immunology*, **38**, 631–640

96. Miller, L. J., Bainton, D. F., Borregaard, N. and Springer, T. A. (1987). Stimulated mobilization of monocyte Mac-1 and p150,95 adhesion proteins from an intracellular vesicular compartment to the cell surface. *J. Clin. Invest.*, **80**, 535–544

97. Schifferli, J. A., Steiger, G. and Schapira, M. (1985). The role of C1, C1 inhibitor and C4 in modulating immune precipitation. *Clin. Exp. Immunol.*, **60**, 605–612

98. Schifferli, J. A., Woo, P. and Peters, D. K. (1982). Complement-mediated inhibition of immune precipitation. Role of the classical and alternative pathways. *Clin. Exp. Immunol.*, **47**, 555–562

99. Bull, C. G. (1915). The agglutination of bacteria *in vivo*. *J. Exp. Med.*, **22**, 484–491

100. Duke, L. H. and Wallace, J. M. (1930). 'Red cell adhesion' in trypanosomiasis in man and animals. *Parasitology* **22**, 414–456

101. Nelson, R. A. Jr. (1953). The immune adherence phenomenon: an immunologically specific reaction between micro-organisms and erythrocytes leading to enhanced phagocytosis. *Science*, **118**, 733–737

102. Fearon, D. T. (1980). Identification of the membrane glycoprotein that is the C3b receptor of the human erythrocyte, polymorphonuclear leukocyte, B lymphocyte, and monocyte. *J. Exp. Med.*, **152**, 20–30

103. Cooper, N. R. (1988). Laboratory investigation of complement proteins and complement receptors. In Kazatchkine, M. D. (ed.) *Baillière's Clinical Immunology and Allergy—Complement and Immunological Disease*, pp. 263–293. (London: Baillière Tyndall)

104. Dykman, T. R., Hatch, J. A. and Atkinson, J. P. (1984). Polymorphism of the human C3b/C4b receptor. Identification of a third allele and analysis of receptor phenotypes in families and patients with systemic lupus erythematosus. *J. Exp. Med.*, **159**, 691–703

105. Wong, W. W., Jack, R. M., Smith, J. A., Kennedy, C. A. and Fearon, D. T. (1985). Rapid purification of the human C3b/C4b receptor (CR1) by monoclonal antibody affinity chromatography. *J. Immunol. Methods*, **82**, 303–313

106. Lennek, R., Baldwin, A. S. Jr., Waller, S. J., Morley, K. W. and Taylor, R. P. (1981). Studies of the physical biochemistry and complement-fixing properties of DNA/anti-DNA immune complexes. *J. Immunol.*, **127**, 602–608

107. Horgan, C. and Taylor, R. P. (1984). Quantitative analyses of complement fixation in three immune complex systems. *Immunology*, **52**, 753–759

108. Schifferli, J. A., Ng, Y. C., Estreicher, J. and Walport, M. J. (1988). The clearance of tetanus toxoid/anti-tetanus toxoid immune complexes from the circulation of humans. *J. Immunol.*, **140**, 899–908

109. Varga, L., Thiry, E. and Fust, G. (1988). BSA-anti-BSA immune complexes formed in the presence of human complement do not bind to autologous red blood cells. *Immunology*, **64**, 381–386

110. Biozzi, G., Benacerraf, B.l and Halpern, B. N. (1953). Quantitative study of the granulopectic activity of the reticuloendothelial system II: a study of the granulopectic activity of the RES in relation to the dose of carbon injected. Relationship between the weight of the organs and their activity. *Br. J. Exp. Pathol.*, **34**, 441–457

111. Haakenstad, A. O. and Mannik, M. (1974). Saturation of the reticuloendothelial system with soluble immune complexes. *J. Immunol.*, **112**, 1939–1947

112. Frank, M. M., Lawley, T. J., Hamburger, M. I. and Brown, E. J. (1983). NIH Conference: Immunoglobulin G Fc receptor-mediated clearance in autoimmune diseases. *Ann. Intern. Med.*, **98**, 206–218

113. Lobatto, S., Daha, M. R., Breedveld, F. C., Pauwels, E. K., Evers Schouten, J. H., Voetman, A. A., Cats, A. and van Es, L. A. (1988). Abnormal clearance of soluble aggregates of human immunoglobulin G in patients with systemic lupus erythematosus. *Clin. Exp. Immunol.*, **72**, 55–59

114. Schifferli, J. A., Ng, Y. C., Paccaud, J. P. and Walport, M. J. (1989). The role of hypocomplementemia and low erythrocyte complement receptor type I numbers in determining abnormal immune complex clearance in humans. *Clin. Exp. Immunol.*, **75**, 329–335

115. Kimberly, R. P. and Ralph, P. (1983). Endocytosis by the mononuclear phagocyte system and autoimmune disease. *Am. J. Med.*, **74**, 481–493

116. Atkinson, J. P. and Frank, M. M. (1974). Studies on the in vivo effects of antibody. Interaction of IgM antibody and complement in the immune clearance and destruction of erythrocytes in man. *J. Clin. Invest.*, **54**, 339–348

117. Mannik, M. and Arend, W. P. (1971). Fate of preformed immune complexes in rabbits and rhesus monkeys. *J. Exp. Med.*, **134**, 19–31

118. Veerhuis, R., Krol, M. C., van Es, L. A. and Daha, M. R. (1986). Differences in clearance kinetics of particulate immune complexes and soluble aggregates of IgG in vivo. *Clin. Immunol. Immunopathol.*, **41**, 379

119. Frank, M. M., Hamburger, M. I., Lawley, T. J., Kimberly, R. P. and Plotz, P. H. (1979). Defective reticuloendothelial system Fc-receptor function in systemic lupus erythematosus. *N. Engl J. Med.*, **300**, 518–523

120. Hamburger, M. I., Lawley, T. J., Kimberly, R. P., Plotz, P. H. and Frank, M. M. (1982). A serial study of splenic reticuloendothelial systems Fc-receptor function in systemic lupus erythematosus. *Arthritis Rheum.*, **25**, 48

121. Kimberly, R. P., Parris, T. M., Inman, R. D. and McDougal, J. S. (1983). Dynamics of mononuclear phagocyte system Fc receptor function in systemic lupus erythematosus. Relation to disease activity and circulating immune complexes. *Clin. Exp. Immunol.*, **51**, 261–268

122. Parris, T. M., Kimberly, R. P., Inman, R. D., McDougal, S., Gibofsky, A. and Christian, C. (1982). Defective Fc-receptor mediated function of the mononuclear phagocyte system in lupus nephritis. *Ann. Intern. Med.*, **97**, 526

123. Valentijn, R. M., van Es, L. A. and Daha, M. R. (1984). The specific detection of IgG, IgA and the complement components C3 and C4 in circulating immune complexes. *J. Clin. Lab. Immunol.*, **14**, 81–86

124. Walport, M. J., Peters, A. M., Elkon, K. B., Pusey, C., Lavender, J. P. and Hughes, G. R. V. (1985). The splenic extraction ratio of antibody-coated erythrocytes and its response to plasma exchange and pulse methylprednisolone. *Clin. Exp. Immunol.*, **60**, 465–473

125. Lobatto, S., Daha, M. R., Voetman, A. A., Evers-Schouten, J. H., Van Es, A. A., Pauwels, E. K. J. and van Es, L. A. (1987). Clearance of soluble aggregates of immunoglobulin G in healthy volunteers and chimpanzees. *Clin. Exp. Immunol.*, **68**, 133

126. Edberg, J. C., Kujala, G. A. and Taylor, R. P. (1987). Rapid immune adherence reactivity of nascent, soluble antibody/DNA immune complexes in the circulation. *J. Immunol.*, **139**, 1240

127. Miyakawa, Y., Yamada, A., Kosaka, K., Tsuda, F., Kosugi, E. and Mayumi, M. (1981). Defective immune-adherence (C3b) receptor on erythrocytes from patients with systemic lupus erythematosus. *Lancet*, **2**, 493–497

128. Iida, K., Mornaghi, R. and Nussenzweig, V. (1982). Complement receptor (CR1) deficiency in erythocytes from patients with systemic lupus erythematosus. *J. Exp. Med.*, **155**, 1427–1438

129. Wilson, J. G., Wong, W. W., Schur, P. H. and Fearon, D. T. (1982). Mode of inheritance of decreased C3b receptors on erythrocytes of patients with systemic lupus erythematosus. *N. Engl J. Med.*, **307**, 981–986

130. Inada, Y., Kamiyama, M., Kanemitsu, T., Hyman, C. L. and Clark, W. S. (1982). Studies on immune adherence (C3b) receptor activity of human erythrocytes: relationship between receptor activity and presence of immune complexes in serum. *Clin. Exp. Immunol.*, **50**, 189–197

131. Walport, M. J., Ross, G. D., Mackworth Young, C., Watson, J. V., Hogg, N. and Lachmann, P. J. (1985). Family studies of erythrocyte complement receptor type 1 levels: reduced levels in patients with SLE are acquired, not inherited. *Clin. Exp. Immunol.*, **59**, 547–554

132. Uko, G., Dawkins, R. L., Kay, P., Christiansen, F. T. and Hollingsworth, P. N. (1985). CR1 deficiency in SLE: acquired or genetic? *Clin. Exp. Immunol.*, **62**, 329–336

133. Minota, S., Terai, C.l, Nojima, Y., Takano, K., Takai, E., Miyakawa, Y. and Takaku, F. (1984). Low C3b receptor reactivity on erythrocytes from patients with systemic lupus erythematosus detected by immune adherence hemagglutination and radioimmunoassays with monoclonal antibody. *Arthritis Rheum.*, **27**, 1329–1335

134. Holme, E., Fyfe, A., Zoma, A., Veitch, J., Hunter, J. and Whaley, K. (1986). Decreased C3b receptors (CR1) on erythrocytes from patients with systemic lupus erythematosus. *Clin. Exp. Immunol.*, **63**, 41–48

135. Klopstock, A., Schwartz, J., Bleiberg, Y., Adam, A., Szeinberg, A. and Schlomo, J. (1965). Hereditary nature of the behaviour of erythrocytes in immune adherence—haemagglutination phenomenon. *Vox. Sang.*, **10**, 177–187

136. Wong, W. W., Klickstein, L. B., Smith, J. A., Weis, J. H. and Fearon, D. T. (1985). Identification of a partial cDNA clone for the human receptor for complement fragments C3b/C4b. *Proc. Natl Acad. Sci. USA*, **82**, 7711–7715

137. Wong, W. W., Kennedy, C. A., Bonnacio, E. T., Wilson, J. G., Klickstein, L. B., Weis, J. H. and Fearon, D. T. (1986). Analysis of multiple restriction fragment length polymorphisms of the gene for the human complement receptor type 1. *J. Exp. Med.*, **164**, 1531–1546

138. Wilson, J. G., Murphy, E. E., Wong, W. W., Klickstein, L. B., Weis, J. H. and Fearon, D. T. (1986). Identification of a restriction fragment length polymorphism by a CR1 cDNA that correlates with the number of CR1 on erythrocytes. *J. Exp. Med.*, **164**, 50–59

139. Walport, M. J. and Lachmann, P. J. (1988). Erythrocyte complement receptor type 1, immune complexes, and the rheumatic diseases. *Arthritis Rheum.*, **31**, 153–158

140. Wilson, J. G., Wong, W. W., Murphy, E. E., Schur, P. H. and Fearon, D. T. (1987). Deficiency of the C3b/C4b receptor (CR1) of erythrocytes in systemic lupus erythematosus: analysis of the stability of the defect and of a restriction fragment length polymorphism of the CR1 gene. *J. Immunol.*, **138**, 2708–2710

141. Moldenhauer, F., David, J., Fielder, A. H., Lachmann, P. J. and Walport, M. J. (1987). Inherited deficiency of erythrocyte complement receptor type 1 does not cause susceptibility to systemic lupus erythematosus. *Arthritis Rheum.*, **30**, 961–966

142. Ross, G. D., Yount, W. J., Walport, M. J., Winfield, J. B., Parker, C. J., Taylor, R. P., Myones, B. L. and Lachmann, P. J. (1985). Disease-associated loss of erythrocyte complement receptors (CR1, C3b receptors) in patients with systemic lupus erythematosus

and other diseases involving autoantibodies and/or complement activation. *J. Immunol.*, **135**, 2005–2014

143. Pangburn, M,. K., Schreiber, R. D., Trombold, J. S. and Müller-Eberhard, H. J. (1983). Paroxysmal nocturnal hemoglobinuria: deficiency in factor H-like functions of the abnormal erythrocytes. *J. Exp. Med.*, **157**, 1971–1980

144. Thomsen, B. S., Oxholm, P., Manthorpe, R. and Nielsen, H. (1986). Complement C3b receptors on erythrocytes, circulating immune complexes, and complement C3 split products in patients with primary Sjögren's syndrome. *Arthritis Rheum.*, **29**, 857–862

145. Tausk, F. A., Schreiber, R. D. and Gigli, I. (1984). CR1 deficiency in patients with Hansen's disease. *Trans. Assoc. Am. Physicians*, **97**, 346–352

146. Tausk, F. A., McCutchan, J. A., Spechko, P., Schreiber, R. D. and Gigli, I. (1986). Altered erythrocyte C3b receptor expression, immune complexes, and complement activation in homosexual men in varying risk groups for acquired immune deficiency syndrome. *J. Clin. Invest.*, **78**, 977–982

147. Thomsen, B. S., Heilmann, C., Jacobsen, S. E. H., Pedersen, F. K., Morling, N., Jakobsen, B. K., Svejgaard, A. and Nielsen, H. (1987). Complement C3b receptors on erythrocytes in patients with juvenile rheumatoid arthritis. *Arthritis Rheum.*, **30**, 967–971

148. Brown, D. L., Lachmann, P. J. and Dacie, J. V. (1970). The in vivo behavior of complement-coated red cells: studies in C6-deficient, C3-depleted, and normal rabbits. *Clin. Exp. Immunol.*, **7**, 401–402

149. Ripoche, J. and Sim, R. B. (1986). Loss of complement receptor type 1 (CR1) on ageing of erythrocytes. Studies of proteolytic release of the receptor. *Biochem. J.*, **235**, 815–821

150. Yoon, S. H. and Fearon, D. T. (1985). Characterization of a soluble form of the C3b/C4b receptor (CR1) in human plasma. *J. Immunol.*, **134**, 3332–3338

151. Wilson, J. G., Ratnoff, W. D., Schur, P. H. and Fearon, D. T. (1986). Decreased expression of the C3b/C4b receptor (CR1) and the C3d receptor (CR2) on B lymphocytes and of CR1 on neutrophils of patients with systemic lupus erythematosus. *Arthritis Rheum.*, **29**, 739–747

152. Fyfe, A., Holme, E. R., Zoma, A. and Whaley, K. (1987). C3b receptor (CR1) expression on the polymorphonuclear leukocytes from patients with systemic lupus erythematosus. *Clin. Exp. Immunol.*, **67**, 300–308

153. Fearon, D. T. and Collins, L. A. (1983). Increased expression of C3b receptors on polymorphonuclear leukocytes by chemotactic factors and purification procedures. *J. Immunol.*, **130**, 370–375

154. Mir, A., Porteu, F., Levy, M., Lesavre, P. and Halbwachs Mecarelli, L. (1988). C3b receptor (CR1) on phagocytic cells from SLE patients: analysis of the defect and familial study. *Clin. Exp. Immunol.*, **73**, 461–466

155. Hurst, N. P., Nuki, G. and Wallington, T. (1984). Evidence for intrinsic cellular defects of 'complement' receptor-mediated phagocytosis in patients with systemic lupus erythematosus (SLE). *Clin. Exp. Immunol.*, **55**, 303–312

156. Kazatchkine, M. D., Fearon, D. T., Appay, M. D., Mandet, C. and Bariety, J. (1982). Immunohistochemical study of the human glomerular C3b receptor in normal kidney and in seventy-five cases of renal diseases: loss of C3b receptor antigen in focal hyalinosis and in proliferative nephritis of systemic lupus erythematosus. *J. Clin. Invest.*, **69**, 900–912

157. Emancipator, S. N., Iida, K., Nussenzweig, V. and Gallo, G. R. (1983). Monoclonal antibodies to human complement receptor (CR1) detect defects in glomerular diseases. *Clin. Immunol. Immunopathol.*, **27**, 170–175

158. Walport, M. J., Ng, Y. C. and Lachmann, P. J. (1987). Erythrocytes transfused into patients with SLE and haemolytic anaemia lose complement receptor type 1 from their cell surface. *Clin. Exp. Immunol.*, **69**, 501–507

5
The Membrane Attack Complex of Complement in Renal Injury

G. M. HÄNSCH

The complement system, originally described as the bactericidal entity of serum, is now well accepted as an inflammatory mediator system. When complement is activated, e.g. by antigen–antibody complexes (classical pathway) or bacterial or cell surfaces (alternative pathway), mediators with pro-inflammatory activities are generated (Figure 1, Table 1). The most important mediator appears to be C5a, known for its chemotactic activity and its ability to trigger the release of secondary mediators from neutrophils and monocytes. Furthermore, C3b is generated, which for a short time has the capacity to bind covalently to cell surfaces. There, it triggers C3b receptor-carrying cells such as neutrophils or monocytes to release mediators and proteolytic enzymes. In the Arthus reaction (a classical model of inflammation), complement deposits indicating complement activation are seen at the site of antigen–antibody reaction, together with neutrophil infiltration (for review see refs. 1, 2).

In glomerulonephritis, similar mechanisms have been proposed, and in affected glomeruli, complement deposits are seen as well as accumulation of neutrophils[3,4]. Information on the causative role of complement and neutrophils

Table 1 Biologically active split products of the complement system

C4a, C3a, C5a	'Anaphylatoxins'
C5a	Chemotactic for leukocytes
C5a	Activation of leukocytes – release of oxygen radicals – release of granular enzymes – stimulation of eicosanoid metabolism (?)
C3b	'Opsonin' (enhancement of phagocytosis and frustrated phagocytosis) Activation of the alternative pathway of complement activation

81

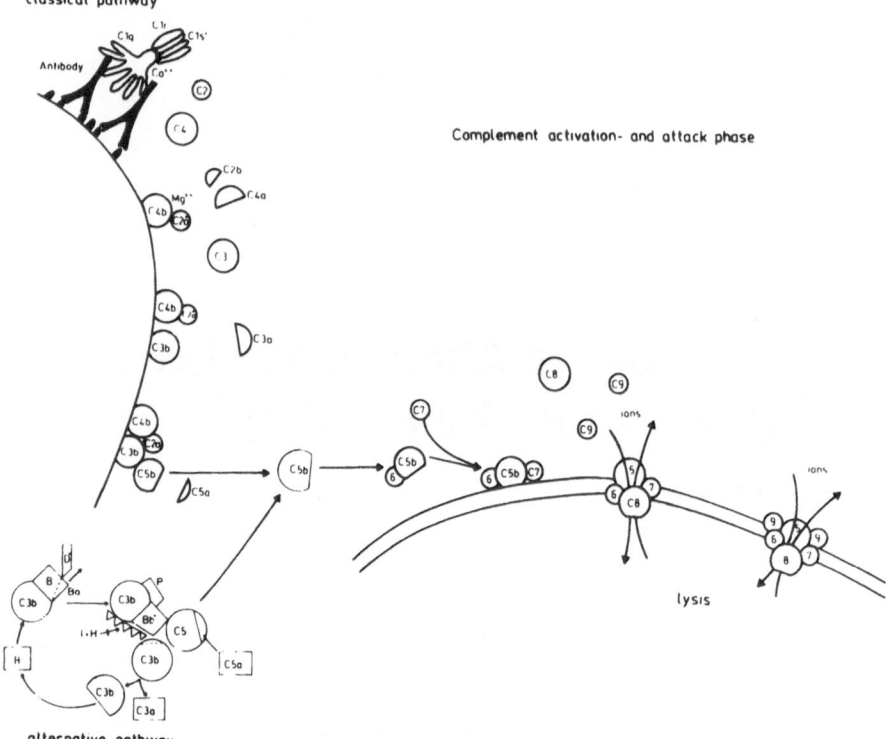

Figure 1 *Complement activation and attack phase.* The first component C1q is bound to two adjacent antibodies. Activation of C1s ensues ('C1 esterase'), which in turn cleaves the complement proteins C2 and C4. The resulting membrane-bound C42 enzyme ('classical C3-convertase') cleaves C3 and C5, the latter only when a C3b-molecule serves as a binding site. The letters a and b refer to the complement split products generated by enzymatic cleavage. The smaller C4, C3 and C5 cleavage products C4a, C3a and C5a, known as anaphylatoxins, are released and C4b and C3b bind covalently to the membrane. As an opsonin, C3b earmarks particles for phagocytosis by C3b receptor-carrying cells. Cleaved C5, i.e. C5b, subsequently binds the components C6-9. These components arrange to form a transmembrane pore. At the C5b-8 stage ion flux through the pore is seen. In the absence of antibodies, complement is also activated on 'permissive' surfaces ('alternative pathway'). Pre-formed C3b binds factor B, resulting in cleavage and activation by a serum enzyme, factor D. If the C3bBb complex stabilized by properdin (P) is bound to the 'permissive' surface, more C3 is cleaved. 'Permissive' surfaces are defined by their ability to prevent the immediate cleavage of bound C3b by the factors H and I. On other surfaces, further activation of the alternative pathway will not ensue. C3b provides a binding site for C5, which in turn is cleaved by the C3bBb enzyme. After C5 is cleaved the assembly of C5-9 will follow in the same way as in classical pathway activation. Upon complex formation, C5b-9 inserts into the membrane. There, these components form a transmembrane pore, allowing ions and water to enter the cells

derived first from experimentally induced anti-glomerular basement membrane (anti-GBM) nephritis. The development of proteinuria, the first indicator of kidney disease, did not occur when the animals were depleted of neutrophils or complement; moreover, when the animals were depleted of complement, no neutrophil infiltration was seen[3-6]. Thus, the attraction of leukocytes and their release of proteolytic enzymes appeared to be the main role of complement in the development of some forms of glomerulonephritis (GN)[7,8].

It was subsequently recognized that complement split products, especially C5a and C3b, also stimulated release of oxygen radicals or eicosanoids from neutrophils and monocytes respectively (Table 1) (for review see refs. 9, 10). These mediators may also activate further effector cells and mediator systems, leading to a potentiation of the initial reaction.

After elimination of the initial provoking agent, e.g. the immune complexes, the inflammatory reaction usually ceases and the tissue is repaired. For unknown reasons, in some instances, the acute inflammation develops into a chronic form, leading to extensive tissue damage and to scar formation from repair processes.

Even though the function of complement-derived mediators could account for many of the phenomena seen in glumerulonephritis, it might not be the only way in which complement is involved. In some forms of glomerulonephritis, e.g. IgA-GN or membranous GN, leukocyte infiltrates are not regularly seen. Moreover, in experimentally induced glomerular injury, e.g. experimental membranous nephropathy in the rat, damage occurs in the absence of neutrophil infiltrates. Since complement is required, other complement-derived activities might be involved[11-15]. For several reasons, the terminal complement components, C5b-9, attracted more interest: (1) deposits of C5b-9 were found in many forms of glomerulonephritis[16-18]; (2) in some forms of experimentally induced glomerulonephritis a dependency of proteinuria on C5b-9 was found[19,20]. The role of C5b-9, however, was not understood, since the only known function of C5b-9 at that time was its ability to kill cells. Complement-mediated killing, however, was not observed in glomerulonephritis.

ACTIVATION OF COMPLEMENT AND FORMATION OF THE C5b-9 COMPLEX

In recent years, the activation and mode of action of the terminal complement components have been studied extensively (for review see refs. 21, 22). Activation of complement, either by the classical pathway or by the alternative pathway, results in the production of enzymes, the C3/C5-convertases, which cleave the complement component C5. Cleavage of C5 results in release of C5a, the chemotactic peptide, and C5b, which for a rather short time has the capacity to bind the following component C6. There is also evidence for a C5-convertase-independent C56-complex formation, e.g. by other proteolytic enzymes[23], by oxygen radicals[24], and also by physicochemical alterations, such as pH-shift[25] or freezing and thawing[26]. The generation of the activated C5b6 (or of C56) is the crucial event in the activation of the terminal complement components. Once C5b6 is formed, it can bind to virtually all membranes in the vicinity of the complement activation site. This binding is reversible, but by uptake of C7 a C5b67 complex is formed that irreversibly binds to lipid membranes or lipoproteins. The stable C5b67 complex binds the component C8 and the resulting C5-8 complex in turn binds C9. One C5b-8 complex can bind multiple C9 molecules. Upon complex formation, the complement proteins exert hydrophobic domains and insert into the lipid bilayer. They form a transmembrane pore with a hydrophilic interior, thus allowing the passage of ions and water. Even in the C5b-8 state, a transmembrane pore is formed and lysis occurs in erythrocytes (Figure 1). Binding of C9 increases the efficiency of lysis by enlarging or stabilizing the pore. In erythrocytes, one functional channel is sufficient to cause lysis. After C5b-9 pore formation, swelling of the erythrocytes is seen, in line with the concept of colloid osmotic lysis. An important aspect of the action of C5b-9 is that once C5b6 is formed it does not necessarily bind directly to the activation site, e.g. to the activating immune complex, but attaches to membranes in the vicinity ('deviated lysis'[27]; 'innocent bystander lysis'[28]) independently of a receptor or an acceptor structure. The action of C5b-9 is limited by the short half-life of its membrane binding site[28]. By binding to fluid phase C5b-9, several serum proteins, especially S-protein (vitronectin)[29,30], prevent its attachment to the membrane. In consequence, fluid-formed C5b-9 complexes are usually associated with S-protein, and are therefore also termed S-C5b-9. Furthermore, intrinsic membrane proteins species specifically inhibit the complement attack by homologous complement[31,32]. Thus, due to the inhibitory proteins and the short half-life of the C3/C5 convertases, the formation of a functional C5b-9 is rather inefficient[33]. However, under pathological conditions large amounts of complement are activated, and C5b-9 or S-C5b-9 complexes are found, even in the peripheral blood[34,35].

THE INTERACTION OF COMPLEMENT WITH NUCLEATED CELLS

The interaction of complement with nucleated cells is a very complex reaction. More complement is needed to cause cell death and, in contrast to erythrocyte lysis, one single channel is not sufficient for killing[36]. Furthermore, it is questionable whether the killing of nucleated cells is due to the loss of osmotic control, or whether metabolic reactions are involved[37]. As reason for the large amounts of complement required for cell killing, membrane repair mechanisms, dependent on an intact lipid metabolism, have been proposed[38,39]. Elimination of complement complexes from nucleated cells was studied as a possible repair mechanism[40]. Nucleated cells internalize membrane-bound C5b-7, C5b-8, or even sublethal amounts of C5b-9, thus enabling them to survive a limited number of complement channels. A further repair mechanism, in granulocytes and platelets, was shown to be shedding of C5b-9[41,42]. The transmembrane signals triggering the repair are not yet understood. In response to C5b-9, however, several membrane-associated events are observed, e.g. Ca^{2+} flux[43,44], membrane depolarization[45], and degradation and synthesis of membrane lipids[46-48]. The correlation of these membrane events to the killing of nucleated cells, and to repair mechanisms, is still under investigation.

THE C5b-9 COMPLEX AS A MEDIATOR

Alteration of membrane lipids in response to complement has long been observed[39,46-48]. Of special interest was the C5b-9-dependent cleavage of phosphatidyl choline with release of free fatty acids, e.g. arachidonic acid[49,50].

Table 2 Biological activity of the terminal complement proteins C5b-8 or C5b-9

Function elicited	Target cells
Eicosanoid synthesis	Macrophages[49,51], monocytes[58], platelets[54], Kupffer cells[52], granulocytes[53], mesangial cells[57], oligodendrocytes[55]
Oxygen radicals	Granulocytes[56,58], mesangial cells[59]
Interleukin-1 synthesis	Monocytes[58], mesangial cells[57]
Collagen synthesis	Podocytes[60]

Since free arachidonic acid is the precursor molecule of the eicosanoids, the question was raised whether C5b-9 would, in addition to killing, also modulate cell functions.

To study the effect of non-lytic amounts of complement, the terminal complement proteins were purified from human plasma. Isolated C5 and C6 were mixed and activated by an immobilized C3/C5 convertase, yielding a rather stable fluid phase C5b6 complex. Together with isolated C7, C8 and C9, it caused lysis of erythrocytes with the amount of C5b6 determining the number of C5b-9 complexes formed on the target cell. When C5b6 in various amounts was added to monocytes together with an excess of purified C7, C8 and C9, release of arachidonic acid was observed, followed by the release of prostaglandin E. Several other cell types have also been studied, including macrophages[49,51], Kupffer cells[52], neutrophils[53], platelets[44,54], and oligodentrocytes[55]. In all cases, release of eicosanoids was seen in response to sublethal doses of C5b-9 (Table 2). In addition to eicosanoid synthesis, C5b-9 also stimulated other metabolic pathways, including generation of oxygen radicals[56-58] and synthesis of interleukin-1[57,58].

C5b-9 AS A STIMULATOR OF GLOMERULAR CELLS

There is now good evidence for the stimulation of neutrophils and cells of the monocyte/macrophage lineage by C5b-9. More recent data show interaction of C5b-9 with tissue cells. Of interest is the interaction of sublytic doses of C5b-9 with cultured glomerular cells. Mesangial cells respond to C5b-9 with the release of arachidonic acid derivatives and interleukin-1[57]. The early data derived from studies with rat mesangial cells, but more recent data show that cultured human mesangial cells are equally responsive. In all experiments, stimulation was seen with complement doses that did not cause cell death. Assembly of C5b-9 on the membrane was required; when one component was missing, or when pre-formed C5b-9 complexes or S-C5b-9 complexes were used (which do not have a membrane binding site), no stimulation occurred (Figure 2). In the absence of C9, C5b-8 was almost equally efficient as C5b-9, suggesting that stimulation occurs irrespectively of pore size, which, at least in erythrocytes and lipid membranes, is determined by the number of C9 molecules. In addition to interleukin-1, human mesangial cells also released tumour necrosis factor (unpublished observations), prostaglandin E[57] and oxygen radicals[59].

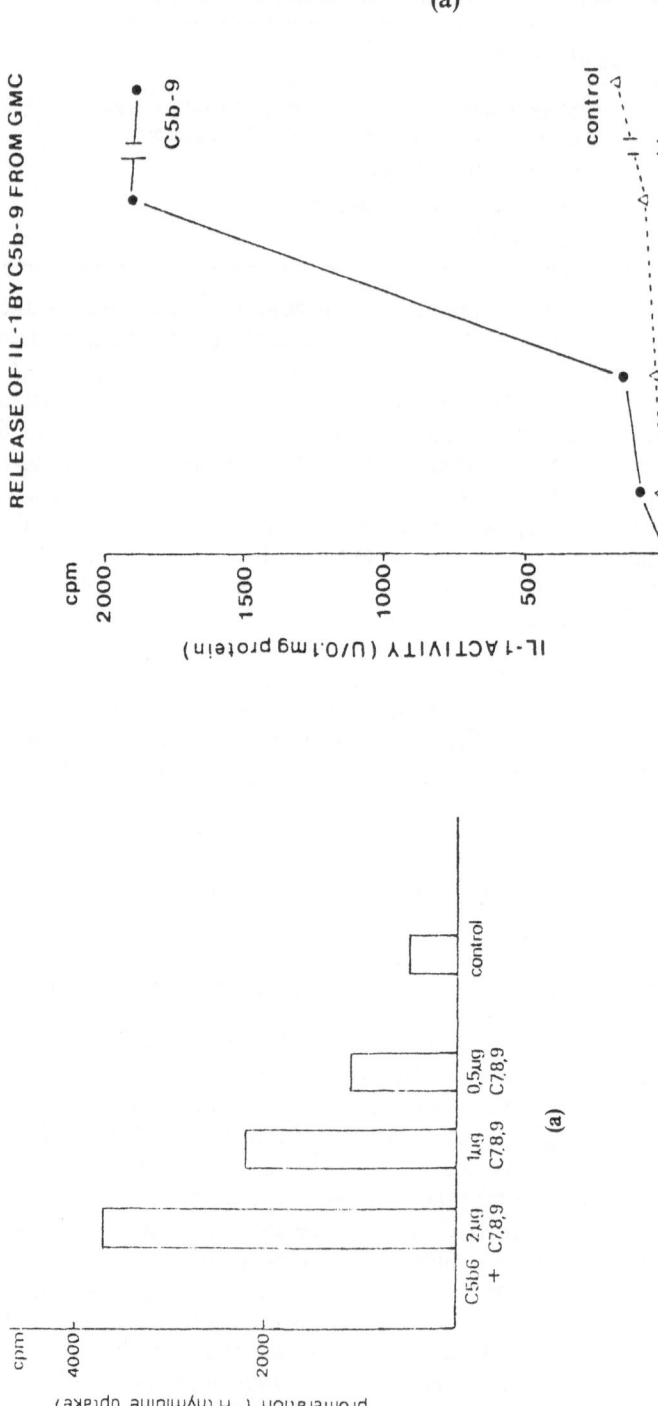

Figure 2 *Stimulation of interleukin-1 (IL-1) synthesis in human glomerular mesangial cells by C5b-9.* **(a)** Cultivated glomerular cells were incubated with highly purified pre-activated C5b6 in various concentrations for 5 min at room temperature. Isolated C7 (1 μg), C8 (2 μg) and C9 (1 μg) were subsequently added. After 20 min the supernatants were removed and the cells were further incubated for 24 h. In the supernatants, IL-1 activity was quantitated using a thymocyte proliferation assay. As a control, C5b-9 incubated for 30 min at 37°C prior to addition to the cells was used. **(b)** In a similar system, IL-1 synthesis was followed kinetically. As a control, inactivated C5b-9 was again used

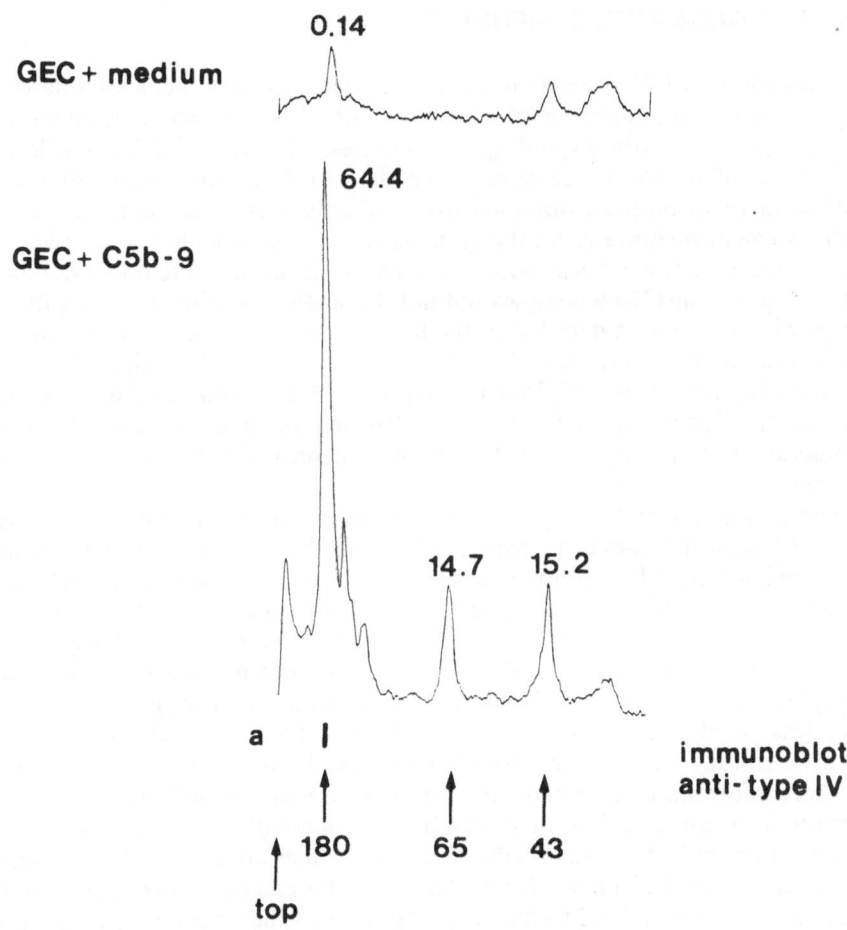

Figure 3 *Induction of collagen synthesis in human podocytes by C5b-9.* Podocytes (GEC) were cultivated in the presence of β-aminoisoproprionitrile and vitamin C to prevent cross-linking of the collagen. As a collagen precursor, [³H]proline was added to culture. The cells were incubated with C5b-9 for 24 h. Supernatants were separated by SDS–polyacrylamide gel electrophoresis under reducing conditions and autoradiographed. A scan of the autoradiograph shows radioactivity in two major bands with apparent molecular weights of 180 and 170 kD. In addition, minor bands appeared at 65 and 43 kD. With a specific antibody to collagen type IV, the 180–170 kD bands could be identified by immunoblotting. Without stimulation (i.e. in medium), GEC produced only a small amount of collagen under our culture conditions

C5b-9 also altered the collagen synthesis of cultured visceral epithelial cells (podocytes)[60] (Figure 3). Enhanced collagen synthesis by podocytes might cause the thickening and spike formation of the basement membrane, as seen in some forms of chronic nephritis[61]. Enhanced collagen synthesis by other glomerular cells might lead to sclerosis, as seen in association with chronic glomerular diseases. Association of C5b-9 deposits with sclerotic areas supports the concept of a complement-dependent increase in matrix production[62].

C5b-9 IN GLOMERULONEPHRITIS

The finding that C5b-9, aside from its lytic function, also has a stimulatory capacity raises the question of whether or not C5b-9 might participate in physiological or pathophysiological processes. The first hint for a role of C5b-9 in inflammatory reactions was derived from immunohistological studies of renal biopsies obtained from patients with epimembranous and anti-basement-membrane antibody nephritis[16]. When C5b-9 assembles, a neoantigen is expressed. Antibodies against the neoantigen are now available and recognize the C5b-9 complex but not the single components. Using these antibodies, C5b-9 was detected in the biopsies with a similar distribution to the immunoglobulins (Figure 4). In subsequent studies, C5b-9 deposits were described in many forms of glomerulonephritis (data summarized in Table 3). Moreover, C5b-9 deposits were also detected in experimentally-induced glomerulonephritis, e.g. passive Heymann nephritis[63] or chronic serum sickness[64].

Deposition of C5b-9, however, does not necessarily mean that it is actively involved in the inflammatory process. Moreover, by histological examination, it is difficult to differentiate between the association of C5b-9 with cell membranes, which is a prerequisite for cell stimulation, and S-C5b-9 deposits in the immediate vicinity of the cells, probably as the result of a trapping of the large complex[65]. On the other hand, free (i.e. not membrane-associated) complexes might have been shed from the membrane after triggering the cells to release mediators. Shedding of C5b-9 might be dependent on the same transmembrane signal as the stimulation of mediator release.

More information on the involvement of C5b-9 in inflammatory processes derives from another line of research, experimentally induced glomerular injury in animals. Use was made of rabbits, which are genetically deficient in C6. Owing to the lack of C6, no C5b-9 complex can be formed, but normal amounts of C3b and C5a can be generated[66]. When serum sickness was induced in these animals by repeatedly injecting cationic BSA, proteinuria did not occur in the C6-deficient animals, even though immune complexes of cationic BSA and anti-BSA were found as deposits in the kidney[19]. Comparable data were obtained in rats with reduced C6 plasma levels in passive Heymann nephritis (PHN)[67]. After partial removal of C6 by an anti-C6 antibody, proteinuria did not occur, in spite of fixation of the antigen[67]. Experiments with isolated perfused kidneys showed essentially similar data; proteinuria was only seen with normal serum, but not with serum lacking C8[68]. In these experiments, as in the PHN-model, proteinuria occurred independently of infiltrating cells[68], but was dependent on the terminal complement components. The conclusion from these and similar experiments was that, at least under the experimental conditions used, C5b-9 can cause proteinuria[67-70]. So far, the underlying mechanism is still unclear. Direct interaction of C5b-9 with the basement membrane appears to be possible, e.g. change of surface charges, but also interaction of C5b-9 with glomerular cells, leading to the release of mediators that in turn could attack the basement membrane. In PHN, a direct interaction of C5b-9 with podocytes has been shown; C5b-9 is internalized by podocytes, transported

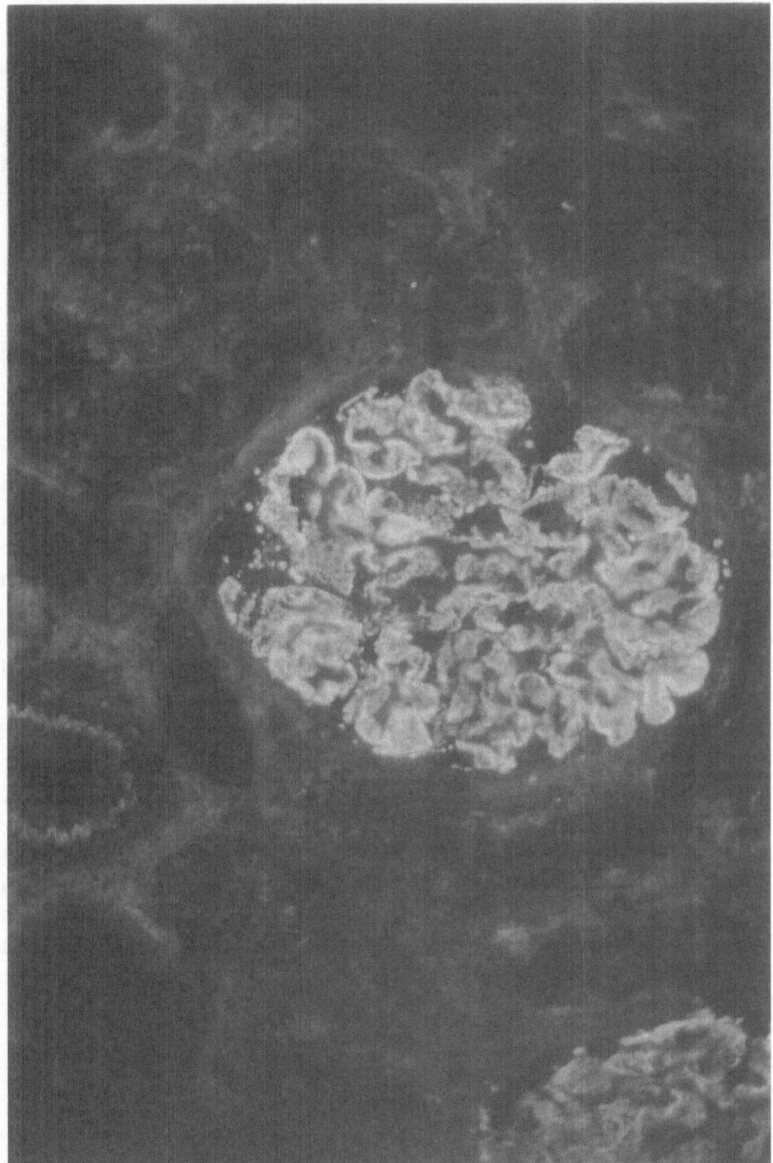

Figure 4 *Deposits of terminal complement components in the glomeruli of a patient suffering from membranous nephropathy.* With an antibody to the C5b-9 neoantigen, deposits of C5b-9 could be demonstrated. (Photograph courtesy of Dr E. W. Rauterberg, Institut für Immunologie der Universität Heidelberg)

through the cells, and appears in the urine[71]. C5b-9 complexes were also detected in the urine of patients suffering from various forms of glomerulo-nephritis, pointing to a possible involvement of C5b-9 in human disease[72,73].

Table 3 Deposits of the terminal complement proteins in various forms of glomerulonephritis

Form of GN	Location of deposits
Lupus nephritis	Glomerular basement membrane, peritubular basement membrane
Membranous glomerulonephritis	Subepithelial in glomerular capillary wall
Goodpasture syndrome	Linear deposits in glomerular basement membrane (GBM)
IgA nephritis	Mesangial and peripheral
Henoch–Schönlein purpura nephritis	Mesangial and peripheral
Post-streptococcal GN	Subendothelial and mesangial
Membranoproliferative glomerulonephritis types I and II	Predominantly in peripheral glomerular capillary wall

Data taken in part from ref. 82

Aside from this observation, study of the role of complement in glomerulonephritis is mostly restricted to the involvement of early complement components. In patients suffering from C3-nephritic factor-positive mesangioproliferative nephritis, complement consumption is seen due to uncontrolled complement activation by the C3-nephritic factor-stabilized C3/C5 convertase (for review see ref. 74 and Chapter 10). Furthermore, studies with patients genetically deficient in one of the early complement components revealed a high coincidence with glomerulonephritis of systemic lupus erythematosus[75,76]. As a possible mechanism, reduced immune complex clearance has been discussed (see Chapter 4). With regard to the terminal complement proteins, there are a few case reports of C7-[77] or C8-[78] deficient patients suffering from glomerulonephritis, indicating that glomerular damage can occur in the absence of C5b-9. These reports, however, are not representative, since deficiencies in the terminal complement components are either rare or are rarely detected. Defects in the terminal sequence do not necessarily lead to clinical manifestations. In some patients with C7 or C8 deficiency, recurrent bacterial infections, especially with *Neisseria*, have been observed (for review see ref. 76).

SUMMARY

The analysis of renal biopsies, the data derived from experimentally induced glomerulonephritis, and the studies of the interaction of C5b-9 with cultivated glomerular cells suggest the participation of C5b-9 in glomerulonephritis. Complement components C5b-9 could contribute to the inflammatory response by stimulating eicosanoid and interleukin-1 production, inducing mesangial cell proliferation, causing tissue damage due to oxygen radical and TNF production, and triggering the synthesis of matrix material (Figure 5).

Compared to other mediators, C5b-9 has an important property: once activated, it can bind independently of a receptor to virtually all types of

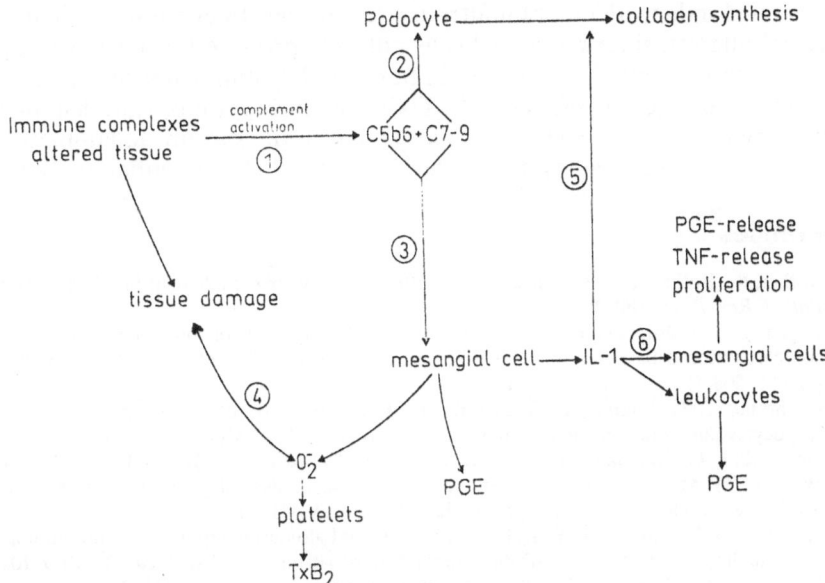

Figure 5 *C5b-9-mediated reactions in the glomerulus.* (**1**) When complement is activated, e.g. by immune complexes, C5b6 is generated. Depending on the site of generation and on the concentration, it may bind together with C7, C8 and C9 to podocytes (**2**), where it triggers collagen synthesis. Alternatively, when C5b-9 bind to mesangial cells (**3**), they respond by release of oxygen radicals, PGE or interleukin-1 (IL-1). Oxygen radicals have multiple biological functions, e.g. stimulation of platelets or tissue damage (**4**). On damaged tissue, complement is activated, thereby probably potentiating the initial reaction. Mesangial cell-derived IL-1 can stimulate podocytes to synthesize collagen (**5**), or trigger leukocytes or other mesangial cells (**6**). Mesangial cells proliferate and release PGE and tumour necrosis factor in response to IL-1.

cells in the vicinity of the activation site. In all cells tested so far, C5b-9 can elicit a response. Its activity is limited to sites of C-activation by the short half-life of its membrane-binding site, by serum proteins, such as LDL or S-protein[29,30], and by membrane proteins which protect cells against attack by homologous complement (for review see ref. 32). However, when large amounts of complement are activated, e.g. when a large number of immune complexes are present, these regulatory mechanisms might be insufficient and cell activation could occur.

In inflamed or destroyed tissue, complement is readily activated. Damaged cells activate complement[81]; and enzymes released from damaged or infiltrating cells are potential activators of the terminal complement components, as are oxygen radicals. Thus, in areas of tissue injury, complement activity can be generated continuously, and this, in turn, by affecting local cells and leukocytes, modulates inflammatory processes.

From studies with cultivated cells it was also learnt that glomerular cells are not mere by-standers in inflammatory reactions. Podocytes, and to an even greater degree mesangial cells, respond to inflammatory mediators by changing their metabolism. Furthermore, mesangial cells also secrete inflammatory mediators, e.g. in response to C5b-9 or interleukin-1 (for review see refs. 79, 80). Thus, within the glomerulus, inflammatory mediators can be generated independently of infiltrating leukocytes. Interleukin-1 might be of special interest, since mesangial cells not only produce this mediator, e.g. after stimulation with LPS or C5b-9, but are also stimulated by it, e.g. to proliferate and to release eicosanoids, TNF, and probably more interleukin-1. Locally synthesized mediators could enhance or sustain inflammatory reactions, eventually leading to the development of chronic inflammation.

References

1. Rother, K., Rother, U. and Hänsch, G. M. (1985). The role of complement in inflammation. *Pathol. Res. Prac.*, **180**, 117–124
2. Fligiel, S. E. G., Johnson, K. J. and Ward, P. A. (1988). The role of complement in immune complex induced tissue injury. In Rother, K. and Till, G. (eds.) *The Complement System*, pp. 487–504. (New York: Springer)
3. Cochrane, C. J., Unanue, E. R. and Dixon, F. J. (1965). A role of polymorphonuclear leukocytes and complement in nephrotoxic nephritis. *J. Exp. Med.*, **122**, 99–116
4. Germuth, F. G., Rodriguez, E., Shah, H. J., Lorelle, K., McGee, S., Milano, L. and O'Lester Wise (1978). Antibasement membrane disease. II. Mechanism of glomerular injury in an accelerated model of Masugi nephritis. *Lab. Invest.*, **39**, 421–427
5. Hammer, D. K. and Dixon, F. J. (1963). Experimental glomerulonephritis. II. Immunologic events in the pathogenesis of nephrotoxic serum nephritis in the rat. *J. Exp. Med.*, **117**, 1019–1043
6. Unanue, E. and Dixon, F. J. (1964). Experimental glomerulonephritis. IV. Participation of complement in nephrotoxic nephritis. *J. Exp. Med.*, **119**, 965–982
7. Cochrane, C. G. (1969). Mediation of immunologic glomerular injury. *Transplant. Proc.*, **1**, 949–958
8. Goldstein, J. M. (1976). Polymorphonuclear leukocyte lysosomes and immune tissue injury. *Progress in Allergy*, **20**, 301
9. Hartung, H. P. and Hadding, U. (1983). Synthesis of complement by macrophages and modulation of their function through complement activation. *Springer Semin. Immunopathol.*, **6**, 283–326
10. Bitter-Suermann, D. (1988). The anaphylatoxins. In Rother, K. and Till, G. (eds.) *The Complement System*, pp. 359–367. (New York: Springer)
11. Naish, P. F., Thompson, N. M., Simpson, I. J. and Peters, D. K. (1975). The role of polymorphonuclear leukocytes in the autologous phase of nephrotoxic nephritis. *Clin. Exp. Immunol.*, **22**, 102–109
12. Hunsicker, L. G. (1975). The role of complement in glomerulonephritis. *Milit. Med.*, **140**, 614–618
13. Salant, D. J., Darby, C. and Couser, W. G. (1980). Experimental membranous glomerulonephritis in rats. Quantitative studies of glomerular deposit formation in isolated glomeruli and whole animals. *J. Clin. Invest.*, **66**, 71–81
14. Salant, D. J., Belok, S., Madaio, M. P. and Couser, W. G. (1980). A new role for complement in experimental membranous nephropathy in rats. *J. Clin. Invest.*, **66**, 1339–1350
15. Couser, W. G., Baker, P. J. and Adler, S. (1985). Complement and the direct mediation of glomerular injury: a new perspective. *Kidney Int.*, **2**, 79–890
16. Rauterberg, E. W., Gehrig, T. and Kohl, P. (1981). The attack complex of complement in epimembranous and anti-basement membrane antibody glomerulonephritis. (Abstract) *Kidney Int.*, **20**, 160
17. Biesecker, G., Katz, S. and Koffler, D. (1981). Renal localization of the membrane attack complex in systemic lupus erythematosus nephritis. *J. Exp. Med.*, **154**, 1779–1794
18. Rauterberg, E. W., Liebknecht, H.-M., Wingen, A.-M. and Ritz, E. (1987). Complement membrane attack (MAC) in idiopathic IgA-glomerulonephritis. *Kidney Int.*, **31**, 820–829
19. Groggel, G. C., Adler, S., Rennke, H. G., Couser, W. G. and Salant, D. J. (1983). Role of the terminal complement pathway in experimental nephropathy in the rabbit. *J. Clin. Invest.*, **71**, 1948–1957
20. Groggel, G. C., Salant, D. J., Darby, C., Rennke, H. and Couser, W. G. (1985). Role of terminal complement pathway in the heterologous phase of antiglomerular basement membrane nephritis. *Kidney Int.*, **27**, 643–651
21. Hänsch, G. M. (1988). The complement attack phase. In Rother, K. and Till, G. (eds.) *The*

Complement System, pp. 202–230. (New York: Springer)

22. Shin, M. L. and Carney, D. F. (1988). Cytotoxic action and other metabolic consequences of the terminal complement proteins. In Shin, M. L. (ed.) *Cytotoxic Mediators of Inflammation and Host Defense*. Progress in Allergy, No. **40**, pp. 44–81

23. Wetsel, R. A. and Kolb, W. P. (1982). Complement-independent activation of the fifth component (C5) of human complement: limited trypsin digestion resulting in the expression of biologic activity. *J. Immunol.*, **128**, 2209–2216

24. Vogt, W., von Zabern, I., Hesse, D., Nolte, R. and Haller, Y. (1986/87). Generation of an activated form of human C5 (C5b like C5) by oxygen radicals. *Immunology Letters*, **14**, 209–215

25. Rother, U., Hänsch, G. M., Rauterberg, E. W., Jungfer, H. and Rother, K. (1978). Deviated lysis. Lysis of unsensitized cells by complement. V. Generation of the activity by low pH and low ionic strength. *Z. Immun. Forsch.*, **155**, 118–129

26. Dessauer, A., Rother, U. and Rother, K. (1984). Freeze thaw activation of the complement attack phase. I. Separation of two steps in the formation of the active C56 complex. *Acta Pathol. Microbiol. Scand., Supplement 284*, 75–81

27. Rother, U., Hänsch, G. M., Menzel, J. and Rother, K. (1974). Deviated lysis: transfer of complement lytic activity to unsensitized cells. I. Generation of the transferable activity on the surface of complement resistant bacteria. *Z. Immun. Forsch.*, **148**, 172–186

28. Götze, O. and Müller-Eberhard, H. J. (1970). Lysis of erythrocytes by complement in the absence of antibody. *J. Exp. Med.*, **132**, 898–915

29. Lint, T. F., Behrends, C. L. and Gewurz, H. (1977). Serum lipoproteins and C567-INH-activity. *J. Immunol.*, **119**, 883–888

30. Podack, E. R. and Müller-Eberhard, H. J. (1978). Binding of deoxycholate phosphatidyl cholin vesicles, lipoprotein or S-protein to complexes of terminal complement components. *J. Immunol.*, **121**, 1025–1030

31. Shin, M. L., Hänsch, G. M., Hu, V. and Nicholson-Weller, A. (1986). Membrane factors responsible for the homologous species restriction of complement-mediated lysis: evidence for a factor other than DAF operating at the stage of C8 and C9. *J. Immunol.*, **136**, 1777–1782

32. Hänsch G. M. (1989). The homologous species restriction of the complement attack. In Podack, E. (ed.) *Cytotoxic Effector Mechanisms. Current Topics in Microbiology and Immunology*, pp. 109–118. (New York: Springer)

33. Bhakdi, S., Fassbender, W., Hugo, F., Careno, M.-P., Berstecher, C., Malasit, P. and Kazatchkine, M. D. (1988). Relative inefficiency of terminal complement activation. *J. Immunol.*, **141**, 3117–3122

34. Mollness, T. E., Lea, T., Froland, S. S. and Harboe, M. (1985). Quantitization of the terminal complement complex by an enzyme-linked immunosorbent assay based on monoclonal antibodies against a neoantigen of the complex. *Scand. J. Immunol.*, **22**, 197–202

35. Koski, C. L., Sanders, M. E., Swoveland, P. T., Lawley, T. J., Shin, M. L., Frank, M. M. and Joiner, K. A. (1987). Activation of the terminal components of complement in patients with Guillain-Barré syndrome and other demyelinating neuropathies. *J. Clin. Invest.*, **80**, 1492–1497

36. Koski, C. L., Ramm, L. E., Hammer, C. H., Mayer, M. M. and Shin, M. L. (1983). Cytolysis of nucleated cells by complement: cell death displays multi-hit characteristics. *Proc. Natl Acad. Sci.*, **80**, 3816–3820

37. Kim, S. H., Carney, D. F., Hammer, C. H. and Shin, M. L. (1987). Nucleated cell killing by complement: effects of C5b-9 channel size and extracellular Ca^{++} and the lytic process. *J. Immunol.*, **138**, 1530–1536

38. Burakoff, S. J., Martz, E. and Benacerraf, B. (1978). Is the primary complement lesion insufficient for lysis? Failure of cells damaged under osmotic protection to lyse in EDTA or at low temperature after removal of osmotic protection. *Clin. Immunol. Immunopathol.*, **4**, 108–126

39. Ohanian, S. H. and Schlager, S. I. (1981). Humoral immune killing of nucleated cells: mechanism of complement-mediated attack and target cell defense. *CRC Crit. Rev. Immunol.*, **1**, 165–209

40. Carney, D., Hammer, C. and Shin, M. L. (1986). Elimination of the terminal complement intermediates from the plasma membrane of nucleated cells: the rate of disappearance differs for cells carrying C5b-7 or C5b-8 or a mixture of C5b-8 and a limited number of C5b-9. *J. Immunol.*, **134**, 1804–1809

41. Morgan, P. B., Dankert, J. R. and Esser, A. F. (1986). Recovery of human neutrophils from complement attack: removal of the membrane attack complex by endocytosis and exocytosis. *J. Immunol.*, **138**, 246–253

42. Sims, P. J. and Wiedmer, T. (1986). Repolarization of the membrane potential of blood platelets after complement damage: evidence for a Ca^{++} dependent exocytotic elimination of C5b-9 pores. *Blood*, **68**, 556–561

43. Campbell, A. K., Daw, R. A. and Luzio, J. P. (1979). Rapid increase in intracellular free Ca^{++} induced by antibody and complement. *FEBS Lett.*, **107**, 55–60

44. Betz, M., Seitz, M. and Hänsch, G. M. (1987). Thromboxane synthesis in human platelets induced by the late complement components C5b-9. *Int. Arch. Allergy Appl. Immunol.*, **82**, 313–316

45. Wiedmer, T. and Sims, P. J. (1985). Effect of complement proteins C5b-9 on blood platelets. Evidence for reversible depolarisation of membrane potential. *J. Biol. Chem.*, **260**, 8014–8019

46. Güttler, F. and Clausen, J. (1969). Changes in lipid pattern of Hela cells exposed to immunoglobulin G and complement. *Biochem. J.*, **115**, 959–968

47. Schlager, S., Ohanian, S. H. and Borsos, T. (1979). Identification of lipid synthesized and released by tumor cells under attack by antibody and complement. *J. Immunol.*, **120**, 1644–1650

48. Hänsch, G. M., Betz, M. and Shin, M. L. (1984). Cytolysis of nucleated cells by complement: inhibition of transmethylation enhances killing by C5b-9. *J. Immunol.*, **132**, 1440–1444

49. Imagawa, D., Osifchin, N. E., Paznekas, W. A., Shin, M. L. and Mayer, M. M. (1983). Consequence of cell membrane attack by complement: release of arachidonate and formation of inflammatory derivates. *Proc. Natl Acad. Sci. USA*, **80**, 6647–6651

50. Betz, M. and Hänsch, G. M. (1984). Release of arachidonic acid: a new function of the late complement components. *Immunobiology*, **166**, 473–479

51. Hänsch, G. M., Seitz, M., Martinotti, G., Betz, M., Rauterberg, E. W. and Gemsa, D. (1984). Macrophages release arachidonic acid, prostaglandin E2 and thromboxane in response to the late complement components. *J. Immunol.*, **133**, 2145–2150

52. Zachariou, Z., Reichel, M., Seitz, M., Hänsch, G. M. and Rauterberg, E. W. (1986). Spontaneous and complement membrane attack (MAC) induced release of prostanoids from Kupffer and liver endothelial cells. In Knook, D. I. and Wisse, E. (eds.) *Proceedings of the 3rd International Kupffer Cell Symposium*, pp. 335–336. (Amsterdam: Elsevier)

53. Seeger, W., Suttorp, N., Hellwig, A. and Bhakdi, S. (1986). Noncytolytic terminal complement complexes might serve as calcium gates to elicit leukotriene B4 generation in human polymorphonuclear leukocytes. *J. Immunol.*, **137**, 1286–1293

54. Hänsch, G. M., Gemsa, D. and Resch, K. (1985). Induction of prostanoid synthesis in human platelets by the late complement components C5b-9 and channel-forming antibiotic nystatin: inhibition of reacylation of liberated arachidonic acid. *J. Immunol.*, **135**, 1320–1324

55. Shirazi, Y., Imagawa, D. K. and Shin, M. L. (1987). Release of arachidonic-acid derived inflammatory mediators from sublethally injured oligodentrocytes by terminal complement proteins C5b-9. *J. Neurochem.*, **48**, 271–278

56. Hallett, M. B., Luzio, P. and Campbell, A. K. (1981). Stimulation of Ca^{++} dependent chemiluminescence in rat polymorphonuclear leukocytes by polysterene beads and the nonm-lytic action of complement. *Immunology*, **44**, 569–576

57. Lovett, D., Hänsch, G. M., Goppelt, M. and Resch, K. (1987). Activation of glomerular mesangial cells by the terminal membrane attack complex of complement. *J. Immunol.*, **138**, 2473–2480

58. Hänsch, G. M., Seitz, M. and Betz, M. (1987). Effect of the late complement components C5b-9 on human monocytes: release of prostanoids, oxygen radicals and of a factor inducing cell proliferation. *Int. Arch. Appl. Immunol.*, **82**, 317–320

59. Adler, S., Baker, P. J., Johnson, R. J., Ochi, R. F., Pritzl, P. and Couser, W. G. (1986). Complement membrane attack complex stimulates production of reactive oxygen metabolites by cultured rat mesangial cells. *J. Clin. Invest.*, **77**, 762–767

60. Torbohm, I., Wingen, A.-M., Berger, B., Rother, K. and Hänsch, G. M. (1990). The terminal complement component C5b-9 modulate the type IV collagen production of human glomerular epithelial cells in culture. *Kidney Int.*, 1098–1104

61. Striker, L. M., Killen, P. D., Chi, E. and Striker, G. E. (1984). The composition of glomerulosclerosis and membranoproliferative glomerulonephritis. *Lab. Invest.*, **51**, 181–196

62. Adler, S., Striker, L. J., Striker, G. E., Perkinson, T. E., Hibbert, B. A. and Couser, W. G.

(1986). Studies on the glomerular sclerosis in the rat. *Am. J. Pathol.*, **123**, 553–562

63. Adler, S., Baker, P. J., Pritzl, P. and Couser, W. G. (1984). Detection of the terminal complement components in experimental glomerular injury. *Kidney Int.*, **26**, 830–837

64. Koffler, D., Biesecker, G., Noble, B., Andres, G. A. and Martinez-Hernandez, A. (1983). Localization of the membrane attack complex (MAC) in experimental immune complex glomerulonephritis. *J. Exp. Med.*, **157**, 1885–1905

65. Bariety, J., Hinglais, N., Bhakdi, S., Mandet C., Rouchon, M. and Kazatchkine, M. (1989). Immunohistochemical study of complement S protein (Vitronectin) in normal and diseased human kidneys: relationship to neoantigens of the C5b-9 terminal complex. *Clin. Exp. Immunol.*, **75**, 76–81

66. Rother, U. and Rother, K. (1961). Über einen angeborenen Komplementdefekt bei Kaninchen. *Z. Immun. Forsch. Exp. Ther.*, **121**, 224–232

67. Baker, P. J., Ochi, R., Adler, S., Johnson, R. and Couser, W. G. (1985). C6 depletion abolishes proteinuria in experimental membranous nephropathy. *Clin. Res.*, **33**, 474A

68. Cybulski, A. V., Rennke, H. G., Feintzeig, I. D. and Salant, D. (1986). Complement-induced glomerular epithelial cell injury. Role of the membrane attack complex in rat membranous nephropathy. *J. Clin. Invest.*, **77**, 1096–1107

69. Quigg, R. J., Cybulsky, A. V., Jacobs, J. B. and Salant, D. J. (1988). Anti-Fx1A produces complement-dependent cytotoxicity of glomerular epithelial cells. *Kidney Int.*, **34**, 43–52

70. Camussi, G., Salvidio, G., Biesecker, G., Brentjens, J. and Andres, G. (1987). Heymann antibodies induce complement-dependent injury of rat glomerular visceral epithelial cells. *J. Immunol.*, **139**, 2906–2914

71. Kerjashki, D., Schulze, M., Binder, S. and Couser, W. G. (1989). Transcellular transport and membrane insertion of the C5b-9 membrane attack complex of complement by glomerular epithelial cells in experimental membraneous nephropathy, *J. Immunol.*, **143**, 546–552

72. Schulze, M., Baker, P. J., Johnson, R. J., Pruchno, C. J., Donadio, J. V. and Couser, W. G. (1989). Increased urinary excretion of C5b-9 distinguishes passive Heymann nephritis in the rat. *Kidney Int.*, **35**, 60–68

73. Schulze, M., Baker, P. J., Johnson, R. J., Pruchno, C. J., Donadio, J. V., Götze, O. and Couser, W. G. (1988). Erhöhte Urin-Ausscheidung von Complement-C5b-9-Komplexen bei Patienten mit membranöser Nephropathie. *Nieren- und Hochdruckkrankheiten*, Heft **9**, 353

74. Daha, M. R. (1988). C3 nephritis factor. In Rother, K. and Till, G. O. (eds.) *The Complement System*, pp. 463–469. (New York: Springer)

75. Schifferli, J. A. and Peters, D. K. (1983). Complement, the immune-complex lattice, and the pathophysiology of complement-deficiency syndromes. *Lancet*, **2**, 957

76. Rother, K. and Rother, U. (1986). Hereditary and acquired complement deficiencies in animal and man. *Progress in Allergy*, No. 39.

77. Nemerow, G. R., Gewurz, H., Osofsky, S. G. and Lint, T. F. (1978). Inherited deficiency of the seventh components of complement associated with nephritis. *J. Clin. Invest.*, **61**, 1602–1610

78. Jasin, H. E. (1977). Absence of the eighth component of complement in association with systemic lupus erythematosus-like disease. *J. Clin. Invest.*, **60**, 709–715

79. Ardaillou, R., Baud, L. and Sraer, J. (1987). Role of arachidonic acid metabolites and reactive oxygen species in glomerular immune-inflammatory process. *Springer Semin. Immunopathol.*, **9**, 371–385

80. Lovett, D. H. and Sterzel, R. B. (1986). Cell culture approaches to the analysis of glomerular inflammation. *Kidney Int.*, **30**, 246–254

81. Baker, P. J., Osofsky, S. G. (1980). Activation of human complement by heat-killed human kidney cells grown in culture. *J. Immunol.*, **124**, 81–86

82. Rauterberg, E. W. (1987). Demonstration of complement deposits in tissue. In Rother, K. and Till, G. (eds.) *The Complement System*, pp. 287–326. (New York: Springer)

6
Cell-mediated Immunity in Glomerulonephritis

S. R. HOLDSWORTH and P. G. TIPPING

Human glomerulonephritis is generally regarded as being initiated by immunological stimuli within glomeruli. This view of the initiation of glomerulonephritis has grown largely from immunohistological studies of human renal biopsies in the 1960s. These studies revealed humoral immune reactants, principally antibody and complement, deposited in the majority of diseased glomeruli. Developments in cellular immunology also allowed *in vitro* assessment of T lymphocyte sensitization to glomerular antigens. Studies using a variety of glomerular antigenic preparations demonstrated that specifically sensitized circulating T lymphocytes were present in patients with glomerulonephritis. These findings raised the possibility that cell-mediated immunity may also be involved in the initiation or the perpetuation of immune glomerular injury.

In the late 1960s, however, the involvement of cell-mediated immunity in glomerulonephritis was generally discounted. A major reason for this was that effector elements of cell-mediated immunity (lymphocytes and monocytes) could not be demonstrated in glomeruli of affected patients. In addition, the functional importance of humoral effector mechanisms—anti-glomerular basement membrane (anti-GBM) antibody, immune complexes and complement—was established in experimental models of glomerulonephritis. These observations, together with the prominence of humoral immune reactants in human renal biopsies, emphasized the potential for humoral immunity alone to account for the mediation of injury in glomerulonephritis. Recent human and experimental evidence has led to a re-examination of the role of cell-mediated immunity in glomerulonephritis. In this chapter, this evidence will be reviewed.

DEFINITION AND CLASSIFICATION OF CELL-MEDIATED IMMUNITY

The essential element of cell-mediated immunity following antigen recognition in sensitized hosts is that the effector response involves the local actions of

Table 1 Patterns of cell-mediated immunity

---

1 Delayed type hypersensitivity
    MHC restricted
    Effector cells are T cells and monocytes

2 Cell-mediated cytotoxicity
    MHC restricted, cytotoxic T lymphocytes
    Natural killer cytotoxicity (not MHC restricted)

3 Antibody-dependent cell-mediated cytotoxicity
    Not MHC restricted
    Effector cells are monocytes and T lymphocytes

---

mononuclear inflammatory cells. Antibody and other humoral mediators play only a minor role in these responses. The separation of immune responses into cell-mediated and humorally mediated is somewhat artificial in that antigen-presenting cells and T helper cells are an integral part of antibody production, and cell-mediated responses are unlikely to occur in the total absence of antibodies. However, there are several different immunological responses which are considered to be predominantly cell-mediated immune reactions[1,2] (Table 1).

Delayed type hypersensitivity

The delayed type hypersensitivity reaction which occurs after intradermal injection of antigen in presensitized recipients is perhaps the classical example of cell-mediated immunity[3]. This response is characterized by local lymphocyte and macrophage accumulation and fibrin deposition causing induration. Persistent antigenic stimulation may lead to granuloma formation. Local release of cytokines by specifically sensitized lymphocytes and activated macrophages contributes to injury in this type of response. Recent evidence suggests that this form of cell-mediated immunity may be involved in those types of glomerulonephritis with prominent fibrin deposition.

Antibody dependent cell-mediated cytotoxicity

Antibody-dependent cell-mediated cytotoxicity (ADCC) involves Fc receptor binding of effector cells to antibody-coated targets[4]. Effector cells include monocytes/macrophages, lymphocytes and neutrophils. Binding is not MHC restricted and is mediated by IgG (usually IgG1 and IgG3) specifically bound to the target. This mechanism has been described most extensively for lysis of red blood cells, but lysis of tumour cells and virally infected cell lines by this mechanism has also been described.

Direct cellular cytotoxicity

This form of injury may be mediated by cytotoxic T lymphocytes or cells exhibiting 'natural killer' activity. Cytotoxic T cells bind to target cells in an MHC restricted manner, and directly induce cytolysis by a number of mechanisms which may involve lymphotoxins and pore-forming proteins[5,6].

Natural killer activity may also be considered as a form of direct cellular cytotoxicity, although this is not MHC restricted[7].

The potential for these three effector mechanisms of cell-mediated immunity to play a role in the mediation of injury in glomerulonephritis will be considered further.

REQUIREMENTS FOR DEMONSTRATION OF CELL-MEDIATED IMMUNITY IN GLOMERULONEPHRITIS

Historically, a role for humoral immunity in glomerulonephritis was established because of the recognition that glomerular injury could be induced experimentally by immune complex deposition[8], and by injection of heterologous antibody to glomerular basement membrane antigens[9,10]. The demonstration using immunofluorescence techniques that immunoglobulin and complement were deposited in glomeruli further reinforced this view[11,12]. Recognition of the presence of elements of cellular immunity in glomerulonephritis has occurred more recently, and has generated renewed interest in the possible effector role of cell-mediated immunity in glomerulonephritis.

To establish a functional role for cell-mediated immunity in glomerulonephritis, several criteria must be met (Table 2). First, the essential cellular elements of cell-mediated immunity should be demonstrated at the site of injury; that is, T helper and/or cytoxic T lymphocytes and macrophages should be present within glomeruli. Second, the timing of the influx of the effectors of cell-mediated immunity should be such that they are present at the initiation of injury (e.g. proteinuria), or at a time that would allow them to contribute to the perpetuation or evolution of inflammatory reactions in the glomerulus — e.g. intrinsic cell proliferation, glomerular fibrin deposition, crescent formation or glomerulosclerosis. Third, there should be evidence that the potential effector cells are activated at the site of injury, and that they express functional activities relevant to the development of glomerular injury—e.g. cytokines with mitogenic actions on intrinsic cells and fibroblasts, mediators capable of causing structural or functional glomerular injury, or factors stimulating local fibrin deposition. Fourth, T lymphocytes initiating and directing the immune response should be specifically sensitized to antigens, either endogenous or planted, that are present within the glomerulus, and the transfer of specifically sensitized T lymphocytes to naive recipients in relevant experimental models of glomerulonephritis should be able (at least partly) to initiate injury.

Table 2 Requirements for demonstration of cell-mediated immunity in glomerulonephritis

1 Cellular elements of cell-mediated immunity present in diseased glomeruli

2 Influx of effector cells temporally correlated with glomerular injury

3 Evidence of functional activation of effector cells within glomeruli

4 Evidence of specific sensitization of glomerular T cells to relevant antigens and the ability to reproduce injury in naive recipients by transfer of sensitized cells (for delayed type hypersensitivity)

5 Depletion of relevant effector cells should ameliorate injury

Fifth, depletion of relevant effector cells should ameliorate injury. Recent studies in both human and experimental glomerulonephritis have addressed many of these requirements.

DEMONSTRATION OF EFFECTOR CELLS OF CELL-MEDIATED IMMUNITY IN NEPHRITIC GLOMERULI

Monocytes/macrophages

Characteristic of cell-mediated immune inflammation is the recruitment of cells of the monocyte/macrophage lineage. In the late 1970s, the appreciation of glomerular monocyte accumulation in patients with glomerulonephritis was a major stimulus for the reassessment of the role of cell-mediated immunity in glomerulonephritis. Occasional reports as early as 1951[13] recognized the involvement of monocytes in glomerulonephritis, but their general lack of distinguishing features by light-microscopy meant that little attention was paid to their accumulation in human renal biopsies. In the 1970s, rigorous electron-microscopic analysis of crescentic and proliferative experimental glomerulonephritis suggested that cells with ultrastructural features of monocytes/macrophages were present in glomerular lesions[14-16].

At the same time, a number of specialized histological techniques were used to assess the presence of monocytes in glomeruli. These techniques included histochemistry[17-19], chromosomal analysis[20], tissue culture appearances[21,22], and monoclonal antibodies[23-25]. Several studies assessing macrophage accumulation in human glomerulonephritis have now been performed[20,21,24-31]. Monocytes are present in many different types of glomerulonephritis, but they are most numerous in the proliferative forms, in particular in crescentic glomerulonephritis (Table 3). They are observed in diseases thought to be initiated by immune complex deposition, e.g. systemic lupus erythematosus[25], cryoglobulinaemia[29] and endocarditis, and are also present in large numbers in anti-GBM antibody-associated glomerulonephritis[21]. Monocytes are also prominent in glomerulonephritis where immunoglobulin deposition is not apparent, so-called 'idiopathic' or 'immune negative' glomerulonephritis[32,33].

At the same time as macrophage involvement in human glomerulonephritis was appreciated, examintion of animal models using similar techniques revealed that macrophages were also prominent in proliferative and crescentic

Table 3 Types of human glomerulonephritis with prominent macrophage involvement

Post-infectious
Cryoglobulinaemia
Proliferative lupus nephritis
Mesangiocapillary
Crescentic
Type I—anti-GBM antibody-associated
Type II—immune complex-associated
Type III—immune-negative

experimental glomerulonephritis. These observations were confirmed in a variety of species, including mouse[34], rat[19,23,25], rabbit[22,36], sheep[22] and avian glomerulonephritis[37,38]. Monocyte accumulation occurs in anti-GBM antibody-initiated glomerulonephritis[19,22,23], as well as immune complex[16,36] and spontaneously occurring models[34]. There appears to be a relationship between the intensity of monocyte influx and the degree of proliferation observed histologically.

T lymphocytes

T lymphocytes, like macrophages, are difficult to identify by light-microscopy. Recognition of glomerular T lymphocytes has relied on electron-microscopic ultrastructural evaluation and on the use of immunohistochemical techniques. Several studies have commented on the presence of cells with the ultrastructural appearances of lymphocytes in experimental models of glomerulonephritis, including acute serum sickness[16] and anti-GBM antibody-induced glomerulonephritis[19,35,39].

More comprehensive studies of the participation of T lymphocytes in glomerulonephritis have been performed using specific monoclonal antibodies reacting with cell surface antigenic markers found on T lymphocytes and their subsets. These studies have focused mainly on human glomerulonephritis, because of its clinical importance and the availability of well-characterized reagents. A number of such studies have now been published[32,33,40-43] and the results are summarized in Table 4.

There have been fewer immunohistochemical studies of the presence of T lymphocytes in experimental glomerulonephritis. In the rat, well-characterized reagents have allowed the identification of T lymphocytes and their subsets in anti-GBM antibody-initiated glomerulonephritis[44]. In the rabbit, there are preliminary reports of T lymphocytes in acute serum sickness[45] and crescentic anti-GBM antibody-initiated glomerulonephritis[46]; however, the

Table 4 Studies of T lymphocytes in human glomerulonephritis

Authors	Ref.	Crescentic glomerulonephritis AntiGBM CIC IN			Proliferative glomerulonephritis	Non-proliferative glomerulonephritis
Bolton et al.	[33]	+ +	+ +	+ +	ND	ND
Nolasco et al.	[40]	+ +	+ +	+ +	+/−*	−
Hooke et al.	[43]	−	−	−	−	−
Neale et al.	[42]	+ +	+ +	+ +	+/−*	−
Stachura et al.	[32, 41]	+ +	+ +	+ +	+/−*	Membranous + +

Anti-GBM—anti-glomerular basement membrane antibody associated
CIC—circulating immune complex
IN—'immune negative'
ND—not done

* Mesangiocapillary, SLE and post-infectious glomerulonephritis are associated with increased T lymphocytes, while IgA, Henoch–Schonlein purpura, minimal-change disease and membranous glomerulonephritis (except for Stachura et al.) are not associated with T lymphocyte influx

lack of availability of suitable reagents has prevented T lymphocyte subset analysis in these models. Experimental studies have allowed assessment of the timing of the T lymphocyte influx in relation to the development of injury, which is not feasible in human glomerulonephritis. These studies have helped to elucidate the functional role of T lymphocytes in glomerulonephritis and are discussed in detail later.

In human glomerulonephritis, T lymphocytes are most prominent in crescentic disease. This is true for all causes of crescentic glomerulonephritis, including anti-GBM antibody-induced, immune complex-associated, and those with no evidence of humoral immune reactant deposition. Only in a single study has T lymphocyte accumulation not been confirmed in crescentic glomerulonephritis[43]. Analysis of T lymphocyte subsets confirms a predominance of CD4 positive helper cells in most studies, although Neale et al.[42] found a predominance of CD8 (cytotoxic/suppressor) positive cells. Lymphocytes are observed in both crescents and glomerular tufts. All authors comment on the dense periglomerular infiltration of T lymphocytes surrounding crescentic glomeruli, although the pathogenic significance of this infiltrate is unknown.

The presence of glomerular T lymphocytes is correlated closely with the degree of proliferation and presence of crescents. Only in one study has T lymphocyte influx been reported in non-proliferative glomerulonephritis[41]. In non-crescentic proliferative glomerulonephritis, T lymphocyte influx varies. Most reports indicate the presence of T lymphocytes in mesangiocapillary glomerulonephritis and proliferative lupus nephritis. Although only a few cases of post-infectious glomerulonephritis have been reported, a small T lymphocyte influx has been observed in most. It is of interest that in studies of a large number of biopsies demonstrating IgA nephritis, T lymphocytes have not been observed and monocytes are uncommon. T lymphocytes are also absent in minimal-change disease and most reported cases of membranous glomerulonephritis.

Glomerular B lymphocyte presence has also been assessed, but significant accumulation has not been observed in human or experimental glomerulonephritis. A number of studies have correlated T lymphocyte presence with monocyte influx[33,40,41,43]. The presence of T lymphocytes generally appears to parallel the presence of monocytes. In one study, a correlation was sought between T lymphocytes and monocyte accumulation and fibrin deposition[42]. A close association was observed between the presence of these immune effector components, as is also seen in delayed type hypersensitivity responses.

Cytotoxic T lymphocytes and natural killer activity

Phenotypic analysis of T cell surface markers allows identification of helper and suppressor/cytotoxic subsets in humans, rats and mice. Natural killer cells are identified by their functional capacity to directly lyse tumour cells rather than by any unique morphological criteria; there are no simple markers to identify them in tissues.

Using monoclonal antibodies, cells bearing phenotypic markers of cytotoxic/suppressor T lymphocytes have been identified in human and experimental glomerulonephritis, but these generally constitute a minority of the glomerular T lymphocytes. The participation of cells with natural killer activity has not been studied.

Intrinsic glomerular cells

Accumulated data indicate that intrinsic glomerular cells have the potential to act as effector cells of injury in glomerulonephritis.

Mesangial cells

Recently, the development and exploitation of mesangial cell culture has allowed the demonstration of the potential for mesangial cells to act as inflammatory mediators (see Chapter 7). Mesangial cells can produce interleukin-1[47–49], platelet-derived growth factor[50], proteolytic enzymes[51–53], reactive oxygen species[54], eicosanoids[55], leukotrienes[55,56], and prostaglandins[57–59]. Platelet-activating factor has been shown to be produced by isolated rat kidney cells[60]. Macrophage products, principally interleukin-1[51,61,62], have been shown to be capable of stimulating mesangial cell inflammatory effector functions. There is little evidence of T lymphocyte-directed mesangial activation. Similarly, there is as yet little *in vivo* evidence for a role for mesangial cells as inflammatory effector cells in immune glomerular injury.

Recent data suggest that within the mesangium are a population of bone marrow-derived mononuclear cells with features of monocytes. These cells have been most convincingly shown in rat glomeruli[63]. They express Ia antigens and are capable of antigen presentation to T lymphocytes in a genetically restricted manner, and thus can potentially initiate or participate in cell-mediated immune responses within glomeruli. The lack of features which allow them to be distinguished from other macrophage populations makes it difficult to dissect their role in inducing glomerular injury in models of proliferative glomerulonephritis in which rapid glomerular localization of circulating mononuclear leukocytes occurs. Studies suggesting a pathogenetic role for these resident glomerular macrophages in non-proliferative models of glomerulonephritis are not yet available.

Epithelial cells

Glomerular epithelial cells can also potentially respond to pro-inflammatory cytokines. Proliferation of these cells has been observed in response to leukotriene C4[64]. These cells also express receptors for C3b[65]. Epithelial cell proliferation can contribute to glomerular crescent formation[18,66,67]; however, their other contributions to injury in glomerulonephritis have not been assessed.

Endothelial cells

In vitro studies of endothelial cells suggest that they have the potential to participate in cell-mediated immunity. Endothelial cells express MHC Class I antigens under standard culture conditions[68], and can be stimulated to express MHC Class II antigens by γ-interferon released from lymphocytes[69,70].

Expression of MHC Class II antigens may allow endothelial cells to act as antigen-presenting cells

Endothelial cells also respond to cytokines such as interleukin-1 and tumour necrosis factor released from mononuclear cells. These cytokines enhance the expression of procoagulant molecules[71-73], inhibit tissue plasminogen activator expression[74,75], and increase the synthesis of prostaglandin I_2, which inhibits platelet aggregation[76]. The net effect of these alterations in endothelial cell activation is to promote local coagulation and fibrin deposition. Further, cytokines promote expression of endothelial leukocyte adhesion molecules and intercellular adhesion molecules. These molecules promote leukocyte localization on endothelium within inflammatory foci[77]. These *in vitro* observations demonstrate the potential for endothelial cells to participate in cell-mediated immunity; however, the relative contribution of these mechanisms to injury in glomerulonephritis is unknown.

MACROPHAGES AS MEDIATORS OF GLOMERULAR INJURY

Once the presence of the major cellular participants of cell-mediated immunity—T lymphocytes and macrophages—had been demonstrated in both human and experimental glomerulonephritis, studies of the timing of their appearance, their functional capacities, and the effects of depletion and repletion were needed to define their functional role in the induction of glomerular injury.

Timing of glomerular macrophage accumulation

Indirect evidence for the functional contribution of macrophages to glomerular injury has been provided by studies demonstrating the temporal relationship of their appearance to the development of injury in experimental models of glomerulonephritis. Studies in anti-GBM antibody-induced glomerulonephritis in rats[19-23] and rabbits[22,78,79], and in acute[16,36,79] and chronic serum sickness[79], have demonstrated macrophage ingress coincident with the initiation of proteinuria and glomerular hypercellularity. Similar studies have demonstrated a close relationship between glomerular macrophage accumulation and the onset of proteinuria in autoimmune Steblay nephritis[22] in sheep.

Macrophage infiltration has also been shown to precede fibrin deposition and crescent formation in anti-GBM glomerulonephritis, and to coincide with increased expression of procoagulant activity by glomeruli[80]. Macrophage ingress is also correlated temporally with the *in vitro* release of cytokines by glomeruli from nephritic animals[81,82].

In human glomerulonephritis, the temporal relationship between macrophage ingress and injury is more difficult to establish. Macrophages are plentiful in glomeruli from patients with rapidly progressive crescentic glomerulonephritis biopsied in the acute phase of their disease[21,31]. There is a relationship between the presence of macrophages and indices of disease activity such as the extent of cellular proliferation, the presence of neutrophils, and cellular crescents. Macrophages are less numerous in glomeruli with evidence of chronic damage such as segmental or global sclerosis[31].

Granulomata are recognized as a manifestation of a cell-mediated immune response to persistent antigen. Formation of granulomata involves transformation of monocytes to histiocytes and giant cells, and may be mediated via cytokines such as interleukin-4[83]. The development of crescents within glomeruli shows many features similar to those of granuloma formation[84,85]. Studies assessing the timing of macrophage accumulation and the development of cellular crescents suggest that macrophage transformation to epitheloid and giant cells may be involved in crescent formation[20,18,66,85,86].

Macrophage depletion and transfer studies

Macrophage depletion and repletion studies provide evidence for the functional role of macrophages in the mediation of glomerular injury in experimental glomerulonephritis. Depletion experiments have been performed with alkylating agents[87] and irradiation[19]. In these studies, depletion of circulating monocytes and abrogation of glomerular macrophage accumulation was associated with significant reduction of glomerular injury. These agents, however, deplete other bone marrow-derived leukocytes in addition to monocytes. This is relevant because neutrophils are also potential mediators of glomerular injury[88,89] and are commonly observed infiltrating diseased glomeruli at the same time as macrophages[36]. The conclusions drawn from these non-specific depletion experiments have been strengthened in some studies by observing that injury can partially be restored by passive transfer of monocytes to leukocyte-depleted animals[87].

Studies using anti-macrophage sera have allowed the specific induction of macrophage depletion without affecting neutrophil numbers or their potential to induce glomerular injury. These experiments have shown that abrogation of macrophage accumulation in experimental anti-GBM antibody-induced glomerulonephritis[79], and immune complex-induced glomerulonephritis[79,90], is associated with significantly reduced proteinuria and histological amelioration of injury, despite deposition of disease-initiating antibody or immune complexes.

An alternative approach has been the development of a 'passive autologous' model of anti-GBM antibody-induced glomerulonephritis[79]. This model can be induced by the passive administration of low doses of homologous antibody directed at a planted glomerular antigen, and it has two significant advantages. First, by using subnephritogenic doses of heterologous anti-GBM antibody as the planted antigen, glomerular neutrophil accumulation does not occur. Second, when the disease-inducing antibodies are administered passively, the potential of depleting agents to affect the development of disease by reducing the host antibody response can be eliminated. Specific monocyte depletion with anti-macrophage serum demonstrates that glomerular hypercellularity and proteinuria in this model are dependent on monocyte accumulation[79].

This model has allowed assessment of the role of monocytes/macrophages on other aspects of glomerular injury as well as the development of proteinuria. Recent studies have demonstrated that the onset of glomeruloneph-

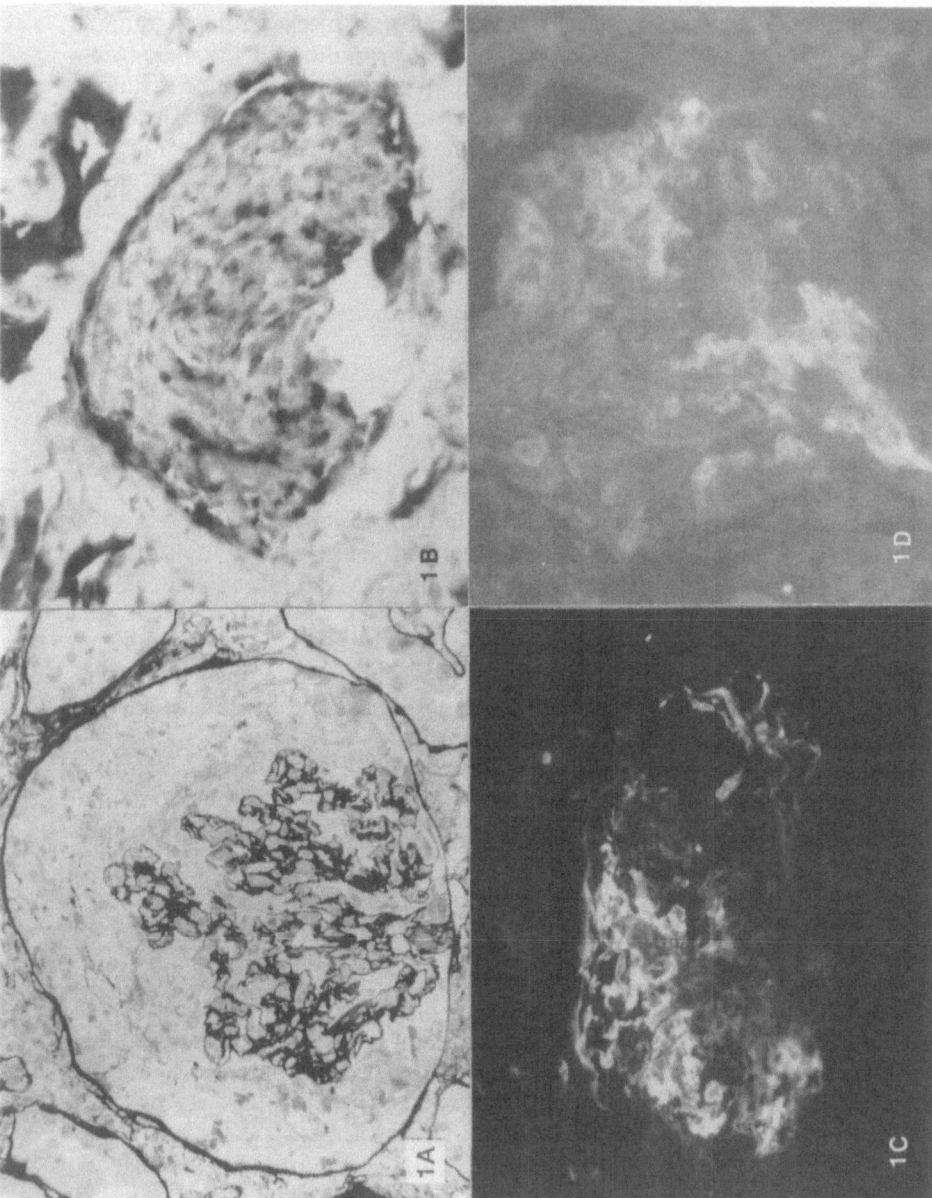

Figure 1 Photomicrographs of glomeruli from a patient with crescentic glomerulonephritis demonstrating a cellular crescent (**A**), esterase-positive macrophages in the glomerular tuft and crescent (**B**), and fibrin (**C**) and tissue factor (**D**) within the glomerulus demonstrated by immunofluorescence

ritis is associated with a marked enhancement of glomerular procoagulant activity and glomerular fibrin deposition, which is macrophage dependent[87]. Cultured nephritic glomeruli release pro-inflammatory macrophage cytokines, interleukin-1 and tumour necrosis factor *in vitro*[81,82,91,92]. Macrophage depletion demonstrates that interleukin-1 production is dependent on monocyte accumulation within glomeruli[92]. *In vitro* studies suggest that monocyte products may stimulate mesangial cell proliferation[48,61,93,94], and such proliferation has been observed in association with monocyte accumulation *in vivo*[62]. The lack of glomerular proliferation after monocyte depletion in experimental glomerulonephritis would support the potential role of monocytes in the induction of mesangial cell proliferation.

Glomerular fibrin deposition is a prominent feature of the most severe forms of human and experimental crescentic glomerulonephritis. The importance of fibrin as a mediator of injury has been demonstrated by studies of the protective effects of defibrination and fibrinolytic agents in experimental[94-98] and human[99] glomerulonephritis. Defibrination preserves glomerular filtration and prevents crescent formation. Macrophage depletion studies in experimental anti-GBM antibody-induced glomerulonephritis have demonstrated that glomerular macrophages, by their expression of procoagulant molecules, can initiate glomerular fibrin deposition[87]. The potential of macrophage-derived cytokines to increase procoagulant molecules on endothelial cells[71-73] may also contribute to the initiation of fibrin deposition by macrophages in glomerulonephritis.

Effector functions and activation status of glomerular macrophages

Although depletion studies have confirmed the importance of macrophages in the mediation of glomerular injury, these studies do not allow insight into the cellular mechanisms by which macrophages induce injury. Macrophages have a vast array of pro-inflammatory effector functions[100], and have the potential to interact with intrinsic glomerular cells, to release cytokines and other mediators of injury, and to express cell surface molecules which may also modulate glomerular injury (Table 5). Studies of these aspects of macrophage function in glomerulonephritis are limited.

The potential of macrophage cytokines such as interluekin-1 to influence the proliferation of mesangial cells has been demonstrated *in vitro*[48,63,93,94]; however, the contribution of this effect to intrinsic cell proliferation *in vivo* has not been assessed. Macrophages isolated from glomeruli of mice developing spontaneous 'lupus' nephritis have been shown to have enhanced expression of mRNA for interleukin-1 and tumour necrosis factor[82]. The expression of mRNA for these cytokines was significantly greater in glomerular monocytes than in cultured mesangial cells from the same nephritic mice. Macrophage cytokines also influence endothelial cell function *in vitro*[76], but no studies have addressed these potential interactions in glomerulonephritis.

A recent approach to determination of the effector functions and activation status of glomerular macrophages is the isolation of pure populations of these cells from diseased glomeruli. Techniques have now been described for isolating glomerular macrophages by exploiting their adherence properties[101],

107

Table 5 Potential effector functions of macrophage products relevant to injury in glomerulonephritis

---

A *Alterations in glomerular permselectivity*
    Reactive oxygen species
    Cyclo-oxygenase products
    Lipo-oxygenase products
    Proteolytic enzymes
    Lysosomal acid hydrolases
    Platelet-activating factor
    Tumour necrosis factor

B *Recruitment of inflammatory cells and intrinsic cell proliferation*
    Interleukin-1
    Tumour necrosis factor
    Colony-stimulating factors
    Platelet-derived growth factor
    Transforming growth factor β

C *Fibrin deposition*
    Tissue factor
    Prothrombinase
    Clotting factors
    Plasminogen activator
    Plasminogen activator inhibitors
    Interleukin-1
    Tumour necrosis factor

D *Crescent formation and glomerulosclerosis*
    Fibroblast growth factor
    Fibroblast activating factor
    Interleukin-4
    Fibronectin
    Collagenase inhibitor

---

and by fluorescence-activated cell sorting of cells released after enzymatic digestion of glomeruli[102].

Isolated glomerular macrophages have been demonstrated to release reactive oxygen species[103,104]. Glomerular macrophages also express enhanced procoagulant activity[105]. It has been demonstrated that the release of reactive oxygen species and expression of procoagulant activity by glomerular macrophages is significantly augmented as compared with circulating monocytes from the same animals. These data indicate that glomerular macrophages are activated and that this activation occurs within diseased glomeruli[103,105].

Studies of the expression of cell surface molecules in tissue sections of nephritic glomeruli, using semiquantitative staining techniques, have demonstrated increased MHC Class II antigen expression on macrophages[104,106]. This observation also suggests that glomerular macrophages are activated.

Regulation of glomerular macrophage activation

Macrophage activation can occur through a variety of mechanisms. These include interaction with antibody and complement, non-immunological stimuli such as endotoxin, and interaction with specifically sensitized T lymphocytes. The participation of macrophages in glomerulonephritis, together with T lymphocytes, deposited immunoglobulin and activated complement, provide ample potential for local macrophage activation. The relative contributions of each of these potential stimuli have not yet been assessed. In 'immune negative' glomerulonephritis, T lymphocytes and macrophages are observed in the absence of humoral immune reactants[32,33]. In this setting, the potential for activation of macrophages by sensitized T cells alone may represent the clearest demonstration of cell-mediated immunity in human glomerulonephritis.

Exacerbations of severe crescentic glomerulonephritis have been reported in association with bacterial sepsis[107]. As endotoxin may activate macrophages, and as these forms of glomerulonephritis are characterized by a significant glomerular macrophage presence, it is possible that endotoxin-induced macrophage activation may account for this association.

T LYMPHOCYTES AS INITIATORS AND MEDIATORS OF INJURY

The functional role of T lymphocytes in the initiation and perpetuation of injury in glomerulonephritis has not received the same attention as that of macrophages. Initial studies relied on ultrastructural appearances to identify T lymphocytes; however, more recently monoclonal antibody technology has greatly facilitated identification of T lymphocytes in glomeruli.

Using electron microscopy, Kreisburg et al.[35] observed a transient glomerular influx of cells with the ultrastructural appearances of lymphocytes, preceding localization of monocytes, in the heterologous phase of anti-GBM antibody-induced glomerulonephritis in rats. This influx is unlikely to represent cell-mediated immunity, as these animals had not previously been sensitized to the disease-initiating heterologous anti-GBM antibody. Hunsicker et al.[16] noted the glomerular co-localization of monocytes and lymphocytes in serum sickness nephritis by electron microscopy, but did not further delineate the timing of the T lymphocyte appearance.

The application of monoclonal antibody technology has facilitated studies of the timing of T lymphocyte infiltration in glomerulonephritis. Using this technique, T lymphocyte presence has been established in experimental anti-GBM antibody-induced glomerulonephritis[44,46], and preliminary studies suggest that they may be present in acute serum sickness[45]. T lymphocytes appear to arrive prior to macrophage ingress and the development of proteinuria in augmented anti-GBM antibody-induced glomerulonephritis in rats[44], suggesting that they may have a role in directing macrophage recruitment into glomeruli. This view is supported by demonstration of the release of macrophage migration-inhibition factor from T lymphocyte-infiltrated glomeruli[108]. Both T cell accumulation and macrophage migration-inhibition factor production were blocked by the use of the anti-T-lymphocyte agent cyclosporin A[108]. Amelioration of injury by cyclosporin A in acute serum sickness[109] also suggests the possibility that T lymphocytes may modulate macrophage accumulation or activation in this disease.

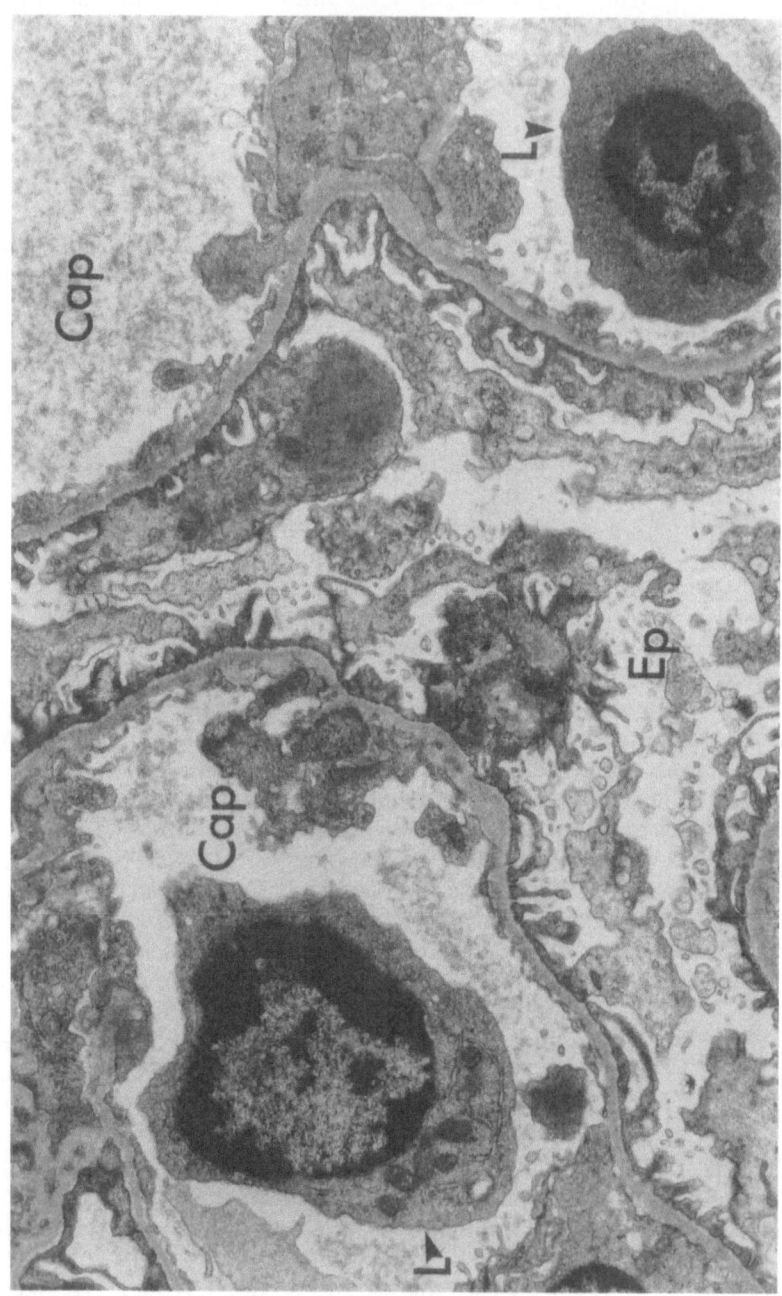

Figure 2 A photoelectronmicrograph of a glomerulus from a rat with anti-GBM antibody-induced glomerulonephritis demonstrating cells with the ultrastructural features of lymphocytes (L) within glomerular capillary loops (Cap) (Reprinted from Kidney International with permission)

Experiments in nude (T lymphocyte-deficient) mice also provide evidence for the importance of an intact immune system in the induction of active anti-GBM antibody and immune complex-initiated glomerulonephritis[110,111]. The resistance of these animals to the development of glomerulonephritis confirms the requirement for competent T lymphocytes in the initiation of immune glomerular injury. Unfortunately, in these studies, humoral immunity to disease-initiating antibodies was also deficient and no firm conclusion as to the direct role of cell-mediated immunity could be drawn.

Adoptive transfer studies have demonstrated the ability of specifically sensitized T lymphocytes to direct mononuclear cell accumulation in the glomerulus. Bhan *et al.* transferred lymph node cells from animals sensitized to heterologous globulin[39] and bovine serum albumin[112] to recipients previously injected with subnephritogenic doses of heterologous anti-GBM globulin- and bovine serum albumin-containing immune complexes respectively. Although the severe injury observed in animals with unmanipulated disease did not occur in animals receiving transferred cells, glomerular mononuclear cells were observed together with some histological appearances of injury. These studies demonstrate the ability of lymphocytes to direct the glomerular localization of the effector cells of cell-mediated immunity.

The ability of cyclophosphamide to induce bursal atrophy in chickens has allowed Bolton *et al.* to study the effects of cell-mediated immunity in the absence of a humoral immune response. These investigators induced 'autoimmune' anti-GBM glomerulonephritis by the injection of heterologous glomerular basement membrane[37,38]. Despite the inability of cyclophosphamide-treated chickens to develop any detectable antibody response to this antigen, a crescentic glomerulonephritis with mononuclear cell proliferation was observed[37]. This study strongly supports the potential for cell-mediated immunity to induce glomerulonephritis. The model can also be induced in naive birds by transfer of avian lymphocytes from birds sensitized to GBM antigens, confirming and extending the evidence that cell-mediated immunity can induce glomerulonephritis[113].

PATTERNS OF CELL-MEDIATED IMMUNITY IN GLOMERULONEPHRITIS

Delayed type hypersensitivity

Proliferative forms of glomerulonephritis, particularly those with prominent glomerular fibrin deposition and crescent formation, show features similar to those seen in delayed type hypersensitivity reactions which occur following intradermal injection of certain antigens. The essential features of these lesions include the infiltration of T lymphocytes and macrophages, and the local deposition of fibrin[114]. Persistent antigen may stimulate granuloma formation. Transfer studies have demonstrated that specifically sensitized T lymphocytes are responsible for the initiation of delayed type hypersensitivity. Release of lymphokines from T lymphocytes at the site of injury promotes macrophage accumulation[115] and activation[115,116], including expression of procoagulant activity[119], a cell-bound lipoprotein which triggers local tissue fibrin deposition. The stimulation of macrophage procoagulant activity in response to antigen *in vitro* has been used as a sensitive index of T lymphocyte sensitization to these antigens[118,119].

Fibrin is an important mediator of injury in delayed type hypersensitivity reactions. The role of fibrin has been highlighted by studies which demonstrate that afibrinogenaemic patients[120] and patients on anticoagulants do not develop skin induration after intradermal testing with antigens for delayed type hypersensitivity[121]. Recent evidence suggests close parallels between this process and glomerulonephritis. Depletion and repletion studies have shown that macrophages are pivotal for the initiation of fibrin deposition in anti-GBM antibody-induced glomerulonephritis[87]. Glomerular injury in crescentic forms of experimental glomerulonephritis is substantially reduced by anticoagulation and defibrination[95-99].

In proliferative glomerulonephritis in humans[122] and animals[87,105,123], the procoagulant activity of isolated glomeruli is greatly augmented. This procoagulant activity has the functional characteristics of tissue factor[123]—a cell surface lipoprotein which binds Factor VII and activates the extrinsic coagulation pathway. Other procoagulants, including a prothrombinase (in splenic macrophages), have been reported in murine lupus nephritis[124]. Glomerular macrophages express augmented procoagulant activity compared with alveolar macrophages and blood monocytes from the same animals[105], indicating that they are locally activated and may significantly contribute to the augmented glomerular procoagulant activity.

Sensitized T lymphocytes have the potential to induce monocyte activation and augment their expression of procoagulant activity[125-127]. The lymphokine responsible for induction of procoagulant activity (macrophage procoagulant inducing factor) has recently been partially purified and characterized[128]. As T lymphocytes have the potential to induce macrophage procoagulant activity and are present in nephritic glomeruli, augmented glomerular macrophage procoagulant activity may be a manifestation of cell-mediated immunity in glomerulonephritis.

The presence of a mononuclear cell infiltrate of T lymphocytes and macrophages expressing tissue factor, together with fibrin deposition, indicates that these proliferative and crescentic forms of glomerulonephritis share many features in common with delayed type hypersensitivity reactions in the skin.

A recent prospective study of renal biopsies from patients with glomerulonephritis showed the presence of the essential elements of cell-mediate immunity—T lymphocytes, macrophages and tissue factor in association with fibrin-positive glomerulonephritis[41]. In contrast, these mediators were not present in fibrin-negative biopsies. This study suggests that cell-mediated immunity may be an important mechanism in the initiation of fibrin deposition in human glomerulonephritis. Further, as fibrin deposition plays an important role in crescent formation[95-98], cell-mediated immunity is also likely to be involved in genesis of glomerular crescents.

Antibody-dependent cell-mediated cytotoxicity

This form of cell-mediated immunity is traditionally regarded as being initiated by specific antibody localization, directing cytotoxic T lymphocyte- or monocyte-mediated cell killing by direct cell contact. The traditional model of antibody-initiated, cell-mediated glomerular injury is that of heterologous phase anti-GBM antibody-induced injury, in which neutrophils are the predominant cellular mediators[88,129]. This is not a classical example of ADCC, because neutrophil accumulation is induced by activated complement components rather than Fc receptor–antibody binding[88,130].

More relevant to human disease is glomerulonephritis induced by homologous antibody, for example acute serum sickness and autologous phase anti-GBM antibody-induced glomerulonephritis, in which the development of proteinuria is independent of complement activation but dependent on monocyte ingress. Monocyte localization appears to be directed by Fc receptor–antibody binding, as Fc-cleaved antibody is incapable of initiating monocyte localization or proteinuria[131]. Therefore, these models demonstrate antibody-dependent cell-mediated glomerular injury. Cell cytotoxicity is not a prominent feature of these models of glomerulonephritis, but the monocyte-dependent induction of proteinuria may involve effector mechanisms of injury similar to those involved in cytotoxicity.

The differences in mediator systems induced by heterologous antibody as opposed to homologous antibody appear to be due to differences in the antibody Fc–inflammatory cell Fc receptor affinity[132]. Complement-activating capacities of homologous and heterologous antibodies are similar. Neutrophils have very low affinity for both heterologous and homologous antibody and require complement for chemoattraction. Monocytes have significantly higher affinity for homologous than heterologous antibody, and are attracted in numbers sufficient to cause injury at antibody doses below that required to cause complement activation and neutrophil chemoattraction. Thus, models initiated by heterologous antibody rely mainly on complement/neutrophil-mediated injury, while homologous antibody preferentially initiates monocyte-induced injury thus representing a form of antibody-dependent cell-mediated cytotoxicity. These observations are directly relevant to human glomerulonephritis where autologous antibody initiates disease.

The mechanisms of monocyte-induced proteinuria remain uncertain. Relevant effector systems may include production of proteases, cytokines and reactive oxygen species. As discussed previously, glomerular monocytes in experimental glomerulonephritis show greatly enhanced capacity for production of reactive oxygen species and tumour necrosis factor. How these monocyte products interfere with the complex cell biology that maintains the integrity of glomerular permselectivity, thereby inducing proteinuria, remains to be elucidated.

Direct cytotoxicity by T lymphocytes and natural killer activity

Cytotoxic T lymphocytes bear CD8 surface markers, and cells with this phenotype have been demonstrated in proliferative glomerulonephritis in humans[32,33,40-42]. Numerically these are not the predominant cell type observed in most studies, and no evidence of direct cytotoxic function in glomeruli is available. In rats, cytotoxic/suppressor cells have also been demonstrated to be present during the initiation of anti-GBM antibody-induced glomerulonephritis[44]. This model exhibits marked cellular proliferation within the glomerulus, and there is as yet no evidence for direct cellular cytotoxicity via T lymphocytes or natural killer activity.

CELL-MEDIATED IMMUNITY IN HUMAN GLOMERULONEPHRITIS

Recent studies have provided data pertinent to the role of cell-mediated immunity in human glomerulonephritis (Table 2). By necessity, these studies are indirect and the evidence is circumstantial. Most evidence involves observation of the presence of immune reactants in diseased glomeruli, and correlation of the timing of their appearance with disease activity. Specific depletion and transfer studies of potential effector cells have not been performed.

A number of studies have now demonstrated that the effector cells of cell-mediated immunity—T lymphocytes and macrophages—participate in glomerulonephritis (see earlier). They also show that these cells are generally present together, and only in association with severe, often acute, glomerular injury. If the presence of T lymphocytes is used as the criterion for the participation of cell-mediated immunity in glomerulonephritis, then this form of immune injury would appear to be limited to the minority of patients who have severe proliferative and crescentic disease.

Determining the time course of cellular events in human glomerulonephritis has obvious limitations, but when T lymphocyte and macrophage presence was correlated with the duration of disease by Nolasco et al.[133], these cells were observed maximally in the initiation phase of glomerulonephritis, with T lymphocyte influx preceding macrophage accumulation. These findings are similar to observations of T lymphocyte/macrophage accumulation in experimental glomerulonephritis, and are consistent with a role for T lymphocytes in initiating monocyte-induced injury. The transient appearance of lymphocytes also means that unless biopsies are examined early in disease participants of cell-mediated immunity will be underestimated.

Evidence has been presented earlier for the participation of delayed hypersensitivity mechanisms in human glomerulonephritis. The demonstration of T lymphocytes, macrophages and augmented glomerular procoagulant activity in fibrin-related glomerulonephritis confirms that the factors involved in delayed type hypersensitivity participate concurrently in active glomerular injury. The association of T lymphocytes and macrophages with crescent formation is also consistent with the participation of cell-mediated immunity in this complex chronic inflammatory response. Crescent formation has histological features, including the presence of epithelioid macrophages and giant cells, consistent with delayed type hypersensitivity.

The association of macrophage accumulation with antibody deposition also potentially allows for the participation of antibody-dependent cell-mediated cytotoxicity mechanisms in human glomerulonephritis. However, it is in those forms of glomerulonephritis without immunoglobulin deposition that the strongest case for cell-mediated immunity is suggested. Several studies have now confirmed the glomerular presence of T lymphocytes and macrophages in so called 'immune negative' glomerulonephritis[32,33]. These forms of glomerulonephritis would perhaps be better termed 'antibody-negative' glomerulonephritis. The presence of effector cells of cell-mediated immunity in the absence of antibody provides a strong basis for suggesting a role for cell-mediated immunity in human glomerulonephritis.

While specific depletion of immune cells has not been performed in human glomerulonephritis, it is relevant to note that those forms of therapy that appear efficacious in severe proliferative human glomerulonephritis have a major effect on reducing cell-mediated immune function. These agents include steroids[134] and alkylating drugs[135,136]. In many types of glomerulonephritis, they may affect both antibody production and effector cells. However, in antibody-negative glomerulonephritis, steroid and alkylating drug responsiveness would support a role for cell-mediated immunity as the effector of injury.

Confirmation of the role of cell-mediated immunity in glomerulonephritis would include evidence for antigen sensitization of glomerular T lymphocytes. These studies are limited by our ignorance of the nature of the initiating antigen in most forms of glomerulonephritis. Although glomerular T lymphocyte sensitization has not yet been assessed, circulating T lymphocyte sensitization to innate glomerular antigens has been demonstrated. This was reported first by Bendixon et al. in 1968[137]. These investigators demonstrated migration-inhibition factor release by lymphocytes in response to fetal kidney homogenate in patients with glomerulonephritis but not in patients with other forms of renal disease.

A number of subsequent studies have confirmed the sensitization of circulating lymphocytes from patients with glomerulonephritis to a variety of glomerular antigens, ranging from crude extracts to purified fractions of glomerular basement membrane[138-141]. Sensitization to glomerular basement membrane was not correlated with the presence of anti-GBM antibodies in one study[139]. These observations are consistent with the involvement of cell-mediated immunity; however, it must be acknowledged that this sensitization may be a secondary response to glomerular injury brought about by other mechanisms. Even so, cell-mediated immunity could potentially be involved in perpetuating such injury.

A variety of perturbations of the immune system have been observed in minimal-lesion glomerulonephritis[142,143]. Lymphocyte production of vascular permeability factors has been described in vitro[144], suggesting a possible mechanism for T lymphocyte-directed changes in glomerular permeability. While this suggests the potential for direct T lymphocyte-induced injury, it is difficult to invoke this as evidence for local cell-mediated glomerular injury, as several studies have demonstrated that T lymphocytes are not present in glomeruli in minimal-change glomerulonephritis[40-43].

A number of recent technical advances offer hope for new developments in the assessment of cell-mediated immunity in human glomerulonephritis. Tissue hybridization with cDNA probes may allow evaluation of gene expression of relevant effector products by glomerular mononuclear inflammatory cells. The recent cloning of T lymphocytes from kidney tissue[145], coupled with polymerase chain reaction expansion of T lymphocyte DNA, will allow further assessment of T lymphocyte sensitization and activation. Ignorance of the initiating antigenic stimuli in most cases of glomerulonephritis limits our capacity to fully evaluate cell-mediated immunity in glomerulonephritis. A number of known antigenic stimuli are currently available for assessment. Examples of these are glomerular basement membrane in anti-GBM antibody-induced glomerulonephritis, DNA in systemic lupus erythematosus, and a variety of microbial antigens in infection-related glomerulonephritis.

SUMMARY

Initial advances in the understanding of the immunopathogenesis of glomerulonephritis demonstrated the potential of humoral immunity to initiate and mediate glomerular injury. This was largely due to the availability of techniques that allowed assessment of antibody and complement. In the last decade, techniques allowing evaluation of cell-mediated immunity have been applied to studies of human and experimental glomerulonephritis. These studies provide evidence that cell-mediated immunity contributes to the initiation and mediation of glomerulonephritis. Cell-mediated immunity may act in association with humoral immunity, or in some situations (e.g. 'immune-negative' glomerulonephritis) may be the only immune effector system present.

The requirements for proof of the role of cell-mediated immunity in glomerulonephritis have been presented (Table 2). Many of these requirements have been fulfilled. The cellular effector elements of cell-mediated immunity have now been shown to be present in the glomerular lesions of experimental models of proliferative and crescentic glomerulonephritis. The time course of their involvement is consistent with a role for these cells in the induction of injury. These cells have also been demonstrated in glomeruli from a subgroup of patients with severe proliferative and crescentic glomerulonephritis. Evidence is emerging that these cells are activated within affected glomeruli and that they express many effector functions relevant to the associated injury. Observation of the effects of specific monocyte and lymphocyte depletion, and induction of glomerular injury by transfer of lymphocytes sensitized to glomerular antigens, strongly supports the potential for cell-mediated immunity in glomerulonephritis.

References

1. Roitt, I., Brostoff, J. and Male, D. (1985). Cell mediated immunity. In *Immunology*, pp. 11.1–11.8 (London: Gower Medical)
2. Pierce, C. W. and Benacerraf, B. (1976). Cellular basis of the immune response. In Miescher, P. A. and Muller-Eberhard, H. J. (eds.) *Textbook of Immunopathology*, Vol. 1, pp. 1–14. (New York: Grune and Stratton)
3. Remold, H. and Davis, J. R. (1976). Cellular or delayed hypersensitivity. In Miescher, P. A. and Muller-Eberhard, H. J. (eds.) *Textbook of Immunopathology*, Vol. 1, pp. 157–172. (New York: Grune and Stratton)

4. Poplack, D. G., Cole, D. E. and Srinivasan, U. (1984). Monocyte mediated antibody-dependent cellular cytotoxicity. In Bellanti, J. A. and Herscowitz, H. B. (eds.) *The Reticuloendothelial System, A Comprehensive Treatise*, Vol. 6, *Immunology*, pp. 303–318. (New York: Plenum Press)
5. Young, J. D. and Lui, C. C. (1988). Multiple mechanisms of lymphocyte mediated killing. *Immunol. Today*, **9**, 140–144
6. Clark, W. R. (1988). Perforin—a primary or auxiliary lytic mechanism? *Immunol. Today*, **9**, 101–104
7. Goldfarb, R. H. (1986). Cell mediated cytotoxic reactions. *Hum. Pathol.*, **17**, 138–145
8. Von Pirquet, C. E. (1911). Allergy. *Arch. Intern. Med.*, **7**, 383–436
9. Lindemann, W. (1900). Sur le mode d'action de certains poisons renaux. *Ann. Inst. Pasteur*, **14**, 49–60
10. Kay, C. F. (1942). The mechanism of a form of glomerulonephritis: Nephrotoxic serum nephritis in rabbits. *Am. J. Med. Sci.*, **204**, 483–490
11. Scheer, R. L. and Grossman, M. A. (1962). Immune aspects of the glomerulonephritis associated with pulmonary haemorrhage. *Ann. Intern. Med.*, **60**, 1009
12. Lachmann, P. J., Müller-Eberhard, H. J., Kunkel, H. G. and Paronetto, F. (1962). The localization of 'in vivo' bound complement in tissue sections. *J. Exp. Med.*, **115**, 63–82
13. Jones, D. B. (1951). Inflammation and repair in the glomerulus. *Am. J. Pathol.*, **27**, 991–1009
14. Kondo, Y. and Shigematsu, H. (1972). Cellular aspects of rabbit Masugi nephritis. I Cell Kinetics in recoverable glomerulonephritis. *Virchows Arch. (Zellpathol.)*, **10**, 40–50
15. Kondo, Y., Shigematsu, H. and Kobayashi, Y. (1972). Cellular aspects of rabbit Masugi nephritis II. Progressive glomerular injuries with crescent formation. *Lab. Invest.*, **27**, 620–631
16. Hunsicker, L. G., Shearer, T. P., Plattner, S. B. and Weisenburger, P. (1979). The role of monocytes in serum sickness nephritis. *J. Exp. Med.*, **150**, 413–425
17. Holdsworth, S. R., Allen, D. E., Thomson, N. M., Glasgow, E. F. and Atkins, R. C. (1980). Histochemistry of glomerular cells in animal models of crescentic glomerulonephritis. *Pathology*, **12**, 339–346
18. Magil, A. B. and Wadsworth, L. D. (1982). Monocyte involvement in glomerular crescents. A histochemical and ultrastructural study. *Lab. Invest.*, **47**, 160–166
19. Schreiner, G. F., Cotran, R. S., Pardo, V. and Unanue, E. R. (1978). A mononuclear cell component in experimental immunological glomerulonephritis. *J. Exp. Med.*, **147**, 369–384
20. Schiffer, M. S. and Michael, A. F. (1978). Renal cell turnover studied by Y chromosome (Y body) staining of the transplanted human kidney. *J. Lab. Clin. Med.*, **92**, 841–848
21. Atkins, R. C., Holdsworth, S. R., Glasgow, E. F. and Matthews, F. E. (1976). The macrophage in human rapidly progressive glomerulonephritis. *Lancet*, **1**, 830–832
22. Holdsworth, S. R., Thomson, N. M., Glasgow, E. F., Dowling, J. P. and Atkins, R. C. (1978). Tissue culture of isolated glomeruli in experimental glomerulonephritis. *J. Exp. Med.*, **147**, 98–109
23. Boyce, N. W., Holdsworth, S. R. and Atkins, R. C. (1987). Quantitation of intraglomerular mononuclear phagocytes in experimental glomerulonephritis in the rat using specific monoclonal antibodies. *Pathology*, **19**, 290–293
24. Hooke, D. H., Hancock, W. W., Gee, D. C., Kraft, N. and Atkins, R. C. (1984). Monoclonal antibody analyis of glomerular hypercellularity in human glomerulonephritis. *Clin. Nephrol.*, **22**, 163–168
25. Atkins, R. C., Holdsworth, S. R., Hancock, W. W., Thomson, N. M. and Glasgow, E. F. (1982). Cellular mechanisms in human glomerulonephritis. The role of mononuclear leukocytes. *Springer Semin. Immunopathol.*, **5**, 269–296
26. Shigematsu, H., Shishido, H., Kuhara, K., Tsushida, H., Suzuki, H., Hirose, K. and Tojo, S. (1978). Participation of monocytes in transient glomerular hypercellularity in post streptococcal glomerulonephritis. *Virchows Arch. (Zellpathol.)*, **12**, 367–370
27. Magil, A. B. and Wadsworth, L. D. (1981). Monocytes in human glomerulonephritis. An electronmicroscopic study. *Lab. Invest.*, **45**, 77–81
28. Monga, G., Mazzucco, G., di Belgiojoso, G. B. and Busnach, G. (1979). The presence and possible role of monocyte infiltration in human chronic glomerulonephritis. Light microscopic, immunofluorescence and histochemical correlations. *Am. J. Pathol.*, **94**, 271–284
29. Monga, G., Mazzucco, G., Coppo, R., Piccoli, G. and Coda, R. (1976). Glomerular findings in mixed IgG-IgM cryoglobulinemia. Light and electronmicroscopic, immunofluorescence and histochemical correlations. *Virchows Arch. (Zellpathol.)*, **20**, 185–196
30. Ferrario, F., Castiglioni, A., Colasanti, G., di Belgiojosa, G. B., Bertoli, S., D'Amico, G.

and Nava, S. (1985). The detection of monocytes in human glomerulonephritis. *Kidney Int.*, **28**, 513–519

31. Atkins, R. C., Glasgow, E. F., Holdsworth, S. R., Thomson, N. M. and Hancock, W. W. (1980). Tissue culture of isolated glomeruli from patients with glomerulonephritis. *Kidney Int.*, **17**, 515–527

32. Stachura, I., Si, L. and Whiteside, T. L. (1984). Mononuclear subsets in human idiopathic crescentic glomerulonephritis. Analysis in tissue sections with monoclonal antibodies. *J. Clin. Immunol.*, **4**, 202–208

33. Bolton, W. K., Innes, D., Sturgill, B. C. and Kaiser, D. L. (1987). T cells and macrophages in rapidly progressive glomerulonephritis. Clinicopathologic correlations. *Kidney Int.*, **32**, 869–876

34. McGiven, A. R., Hunt, J. S., Day, W. A. and Jackson, A. E. (1981). Phagocytic cells in glomerular cultures from NZB/W mice. *Br. J. Exp. Pathol.*, **62**, 59–64

35. Kreisberg, J. I., Wayne, D. B. and Karnovsky, M. J. (1979). Rapid and focal loss of negative charge associated with mononuclear cell infiltration early in nephrotoxic serum nephritis. *Kidney Int.*, **16**, 290–300

36. Holdsworth, S. R., Neale, T. J. and Wilson, C. B. (1980). The participation of macrophages and monocytes in experimental immune complex glomerulonephritis. *Clin. Immunol. Immunopathol.*, **15**, 510–524

37. Bolton, W. K., Tucker, F. L. and Sturgill, B. C. (1984). New avian model of experimental glomerulonephritis consistent with mediation by cellular immunity. Non humorally mediated glomerulonephritis in chickens. *J. Clin. Invest.*, **73**, 1263–1276

38. Bolton, W. K., Tucker, F. L. and Sturgill, B. C. (1984). Experimental autoimmune glomerulonephritis in chickens. *J. Clin. Lab. Immunol.*, **3**, 179–184

39. Bhan, A. K., Schneeberger, E. E., Collins, A. B. and McCluskey, R. T. (1978). Evidence for a pathogenic role of a cell-mediated immune mechanism in experimental glomerulonephritis. *J. Exp. Med.*, **148**, 246–260

40. Nolasco, F. E., Cameron, J. S., Hartley, B., Coelho, A., Hildreth, G. and Reuben, R. (1987). Intraglomerular T cells and monocytes in nephritis. Study with monoclonal antibodies. *Kidney Int.*, **31**, 1160–1166

41. Stachura, I., Si, L., Madan, E. and Whiteside, T. (1984). Mononuclear cell subsets in human renal disease. Enumeration in tissue sections with monoclonal antibodies. *Clin. Immunol. Immunopathol.*, **30**, 362–373

42. Neale, T. J., Tipping, P. G., Carson, S. D. and Holdsworth, S. R. (1988). Participation of cell mediated immunity in deposition of fibrin in glomerulonephritis. *Lancet*, **2**, 421–424

43. Hooke, D. H., Gee, D. C. and Atkins, R. L. (1987). Leukocyte analysis using monoclonal antibodies in human glomerulonephritis. *Kidney Int.*, **31**, 964–972

44. Tipping, P. G., Neale, T. J. and Holdsworth, S. R. (1985). T lymphocyte participation in antibody induced experimental glomerulonephritis. *Kidney Int.*, **27**, 530–537

45. Foster, S. R., Brelje, T. E., Vreede, P. J. and Hunsicker, L. G. (1988). T-lymphocytes in rabbit serum sickness nephritis. *Kidney Int.*, **33**, 314 (Abstract)

46. Eldredge, C. M. and Wiggins, R. C. (1987). T cells in the glomerulus, periglomerular region and around venules early in crescentic nephritis in the rabbit. Evidence for glomerulo-interstitial signals. *Kidney Int.*, **31**, 318 (Abstract)

47. Lovett, D. H., Ryan, J. L. and Sterzel, R. B. (1983). A T lymphocyte activating factor derived from glomerular mesangial cells. *J. Immunol.*, **130**, 1796–1801

48. Lovett, D. H. and Larsen, A. (1988). Cell cycle dependent interleukin 1 gene expression by cultured glomerular mesangial cells. *J. Clin. Invest.*, **82**, 115–122

49. Werber, H. I., Emancipator, S. N., Tykocinski, M. L. and Sedor, J. R. (1987). The interleukin gene is expressed by rat mesangial cells and is augmented in immune complex glomerulonephritis. *Immunology*, **138**, 3207–3212

50. Abboud, H. E., Poptic, E. and DiCorleto, P. (1987). Production of platelet derived growth factor-like protein by rat mesangial cells in culture. *J. Clin. Invest.*, **80**, 675–683

51. Martin, J., Lovett, D. H., Gemsa, D., Sterzel, R. B. and Davies, M. (1986). Enhancement of glomerular mesangial cell neutral proteinase secretion by macrophages. Role of interluekin 1. *J. Immunol.*, **137**, 525–529

52. Lovett, D. H., Ryan, J. L., Kashgarian, M. and Sterzel, R. B. (1982). Lysosomal enzymes in glomerular cells of the rat. *Am. J. Pathol.*, **107**, 161–166

53. Lovett, D. H., Sterzel, R. B., Ryan, J. L. and Kashgarian, M. (1983). Neutral protease

activity produced in vitro by cells of the glomerular mesangium. *Kidney Int.*, **23**, 342–349

54. Baud, L., Hagege, J., Sraer, J., Rondeau, E., Perez, J. and Ardaillou, R. (1983). Reactive oxygen production by cultured rat glomerular mesangial cells during phagocytosis is associated with stimulation of lipooxygenase activity. *J. Exp. Med.*, **158**, 1836–1852

55. Lianos, E. A. (1988). Synthesis of hydroxyeicostetraenoic acids and leukotrienes in rat nephrotoxic serum glomerulonephritis. Role of anti-glomerular basement membrane antibody dose, complement, and neutrophils. *J. Clin. Invest.*, **82**, 427–435

56. Cattell, V., Cook, H. T., Smith, J., Salmon, J. A. and Moncada, S. (1987). Leukotriene B4 production in normal rat glomeruli. *Nephrol. Dial. Transplant.*, **2**, 154–157

57. Scharschmidt, L. A. and Dunn, M. J. (1983). Prostaglandin synthesis by rat glomerular mesangial cells in culture. Effects of angiotensin II and anginine vasopressin. *J. Clin. Invest.*, **71**, 1756–1764

58. Hassis, A., Konieczkowski, M. and Dunn, M. J. (1979). Prostaglandin synthesis in isolated rat kidney glomeruli. *Proc. Natl Acad. Sci. USA*, **76**, 1155–1159

59. Kreisburg, J. I., Karnovsky, M. J. and Levine, L. (1982). Prostaglandin production by homogeneous cultures of rat glomerular epithelial and mesangial cells. *Kidney Int.*, **22**, 355–359

60. Pirotzky, E., Ninio, E., Bidault, J., Pfister, P. and Benveniste, J. (1984). Biosynthesis of platelet activating factor: VI. Precursors of platelets activating factor and acetyl transferase activity in isolated rat kidney cells. *Lab. Invest.*, **51**, 567–572

61. Lovett, D. H., Ryan, J. L. and Sterzyl, R. B. (1983). Stimulation of rat mesangial cell proliferation by macrophage interleukin 1. *J. Immunol.*, **131**, 2830–2836

62. Dubois, C. H., Foidart, J. B., Hautier, M. B., Dechenne, C. A., Lemiere, M. J. and Mahieu, P. R. (1981). Proliferative glomerulonephritis in rats: Evidence that mononuclear phagocytes infiltrating the glomeruli stimulate the proliferation of endothelial and mesangial cells. *Eur. J. Clin. Invest.*, **11**, 91–104

63. Schreiner, G. F., Kiely, J. M. and Cotran, R. S. (1981). Characterization of resident glomerular cells in the rat expressing Ia determinants and manifesting genetically restricted interactions with lymphocytes. *J. Clin. Invest.*, **68**, 290–931

64. Baud, L., Sraer, J., Perez, J., Nivez, M. and Ardaillou, R. (1985). Leukotriene C4 binds to human glomerular epithelial cells and promotes their proliferation in vitro. *J. Clin. Invest.*, **76**, 374–377

65. Kasinath, B. S., Maaba, M. R., Schwartz, M. M. and Lewis, E. J. (1986). Demonstration and characterization of C3 receptors on rat glomerular epithelial cells. *Kidney Int.*, **30**, 852–861

66. Magil, A. B. (1985). Histogenesis of glomerular crescents. Immunohistochemical demonstration of cytokeratin in crescent cells. *Am. J. Pathol.*, **120**, 222–226

67. Hancock, W. W. and Atkins, R. C. (1984). Cellular composition of crescents in human rapidly progressive glomerular nephritis, identified using monoclonal antibodies. *Am. J. Nephrol*, **3**, 177–182

68. Pober, J. S. and Gimbrone, M. A. (1983). Expression of Ia-like antigens by human vascular endothelial cells is inducible in vitro. Demonstration by monoclonal antibody binding and immunoprecipitation. *Proc. Natl Acad. Sci. USA*, **79**, 6641–6643

69. Pober, J. S., Gimbrone, M. A., Cotran, R. S., Riess, C. S., Burakoff, S. J., Fiers, W. and Ault, K. A. (1983). Ia expression by vascular endothelium is inducible by activated T cells and by human T interferon. *J. Exp. Med.*, **157**, 1339–1353

70. Pober, J. S., Collins, T., Gimbrone, M. A., Cotran, R. S., Gitlin, J. D., Fiers, W., Clayberger, C., Krensky, A. M., Burakoff, S. J. and Reiss, C. S. (1983). Lymphocytes recognise human vascular endothelial and dermal fibroblast Ia antigens induced by recombinant immune interferon. *Nature*, **305**, 726–729

71. Bevilacqua, M. P., Pober, J. S., Majeau, G. R., Cotran, R. S. and Gimbrone, M. A. (1984). Interleukin 1 (IL-1) induces biosynthesis and cell surface expression of procoagulant activity in human vascular endothelial cells. *J. Exp. Med.*, **160**, 618–623

72. Naworth, P. P. and Stern, D. M. (1986). Modulation of endothelial cell hemostatic properties by tumor necrosis factor. *J. Exp. Med.*, **163**, 740–745

73. Bevilacqua, M. P., Pober, J. S., Majeau, G. R., Fiers, W., Cotran, R. S. and Gimbrone, M. A. (1986). Recombinant tumor necrosis factor induces procoagulant activity in cultured human vascular endothelium. Characterization and comparison with the actions of interleukin 1. *Proc. Natl. Acad. Sci. USA*, **83**, 4533–4537

74. Emeis, J. J. and Vooistra, T. (1986). Interleukin 1 and lipopolysaccharide induce an inhibitor of tissue type plasminogen activator in vivo and in cultured endothelial cells. *J. Exp. Med.*,

163, 1260–1265
75. Nachman, R. L., Hajjar, K. A., Silverstein, R. L. and Dinarello, C. A. (1986). Interleukin 1 induces endothelial cell expression of plasinmogen activator inhibitor. *J. Exp. Med.*, **163**, 1595–1604
76. Cotran, R. S. (1987). New roles for the endothelium in inflammation and immunity. *Am. J. Pathol.*, **129**, 407–413
77. Pober, J. S., Gimbrone, M. A., Lapierre, L. M., Mendrick, D. L., Fiers, W., Rothlein, R. and Springer, T. A. (1986). Overlapping patterns of activation of human endothelial cells by interleukin 1, tumor necrosis factor and immune interferon. *J. Immunol.*, **137**, 1893–1894
78. Thomson, N. M., Holdsworth, S. R., Glasgow, E. F. and Atkins, R. C. (1979). The macrophage in the development of experimental glomerulonephritis. Studies using tissue culture and electron microscopy. *Am. J. Pathol.*, **94**, 233–240
79. Holdsworth, S. R., Neale, T. J. and Wilson, C. B. (1981). Abrogation of macrophage-dependent injury in experimental glomerulonephritis in the rabbit. Use of an anti-macrophage serum. *J. Clin. Invest.*, **68**, 686–698
80. Tipping, P. G. and Holdsworth, S. R. (1986). The participation of macrophages, glomerular procoagulant activity and Factor VIII in glomerular fibrin deposition. Studies in anti-glomerular basement antibody induced glomerulonephritis in rabbits. *Am. J. Pathol.*, **124**, 10–17
81. Wiggins, R. C., Eldredge, C. and Kunkel, S. (1987). Monokine production by glomeruli at different stages of crescent formation in the rabbit. *Proceedings of the Xth International Congress of Nephrology*, p. 368 (Abstract)
82. Boswell, J. M., Yui, M. A., Burt, D. W. and Kelley, V. E. (1988). Increased tumor necrosis factor and IL-1 β gene in kidneys of mice with lupus nephritis. *J. Immunol.*, **141**, 3050–3054
83. McInnes, A. and Rennick, D. M. (1988). Interleukin 4 induces cultured monocytes/macrophages to form giant multinucleated cells. *J. Exp. Med.*, **167**, 598–611
84. Min, K. W., Györkey, F., Györkey, P., Yium, J. J. and Eknoyan, G. (1974). The morphogenesis of glomerular crescents in rapidly progressive glomerulonephritis. *Kidney Int.*, **5**, 47–56
85. Kalowski, S., MacKay, D. G., Howes, E. L., Csauossy, I. and Wolfson, M. (1976). Multinucleated giant cells in antiglomerular basement membrane antibody induced glomerulonephritis. *Nephron*, **16**, 415–426
86. Cattell, V. and Jamieson, S. W. (1978). The origin of glomerular crescents in experimental nephrotoxic serum nephritis in the rabbit. *Lab. Invest.*, **39**, 584–590
87. Holdsworth, S. R. and Tipping, P. G. (1985). Macrophage induced glomerular fibrin deposition in experimental glomerulonephritis in the rabbit. *J. Clin. Invest.*, **76**, 1367–1374
88. Cochrane, C. G., Unanue, E. R. and Dixon, F. J. (1965). A role of polymorphonuclear leukocytes and complement in nephrotoxic nephritis. *J. Exp. Med.*, **122**, 99–116
89. Simpson, I. J., Amos, N., Evans, F. J., Thomson, N. M. and Peters, D. K. (1975). Guinea pig nephrotoxic nephritis I. The role of complement and polymorphonuclear leukocytes and the effect of antibody subclass and fragments in the heterologous phase. *Clin. Exp. Immunol.*, **19**, 449–551
90. Lavelle, K. J., Durland, B. D. and Yum, M. N. (1981). The effect of antimacrophage antiserum on immune complex glomerulonephritis. *J. Lab. Clin. Med.*, **98**, 195–205
91. Matsumoto, K. and Hatona, M. (1989). Production of interleukin 1 in glomerular cell cultures from rats with nephrotoxic serum nephritis. *Clin. Exp. Immunol.*, **75**, 123–128
92. Tipping, P. G., Lowe, M. G. and Holdsworth, S. R. (1991). Glomerular interleukin 1 production is dependent on macrophage infiltration in anti-GBM glomerulonephritis. *Kidney Int.*, **39**, 103–110
93. Melcion, C., Lachman, L., Killen, P. D., Morel-Maroger, L. and Striker, G. E. (1982). Mesangial cells; effects of monocyte products on proliferation and matrix synthesis. *Transplant. Proc.*, **14**, 559–564
94. MacCarthy, E. P., Hsu, A., Ooi, U. M. and Ooi, B. S. (1985). Modulation of mouse mesangial cell proliferation by macrophage products. *Immunology*, **56**, 695–699
95. Humair, L., Kwann, H. C. and Potter, E. (1979). The role of fibrinogen in renal disease. II. Effect of anticoagulants and urokinase on experimental lesions in mice. *J. Lab. Clin. Med.*, **74**, 72–78
96. Thomson, N. M., Simpson, I. J., Evans, D. S. and Peters, D. K. (1975). Defibrination with ancrod in experimental chronic immune-complex nephritis. *Clin. Exp. Immunol.*, **20**, 527–535

97. Tipping, P. G. and Holdsworth, S. R. (1986). Comparison of fibrinolytic and defibrinating agents in fibrin related experimental glomerulonephritis. *Br. J. Exp. Pathol.*, **67**, 481–491

98. Naish, P. F., Evans, D. J. and Peters, D. K. (1975). The effects of defibrination with Ancrod in experimental allergic glomerular injury. *Clin. Exp. Immunol.*, **20**, 303–309

99. Pollack, V. E., Glueck, H. E., Weiss, M. A., Lebron-Berges, A. and Miller, M. A. (1982). Defibrination with Ancrod in glomerulonephritis. Effect on clinical and histologic findings and on blood coagulation. *Am. J. Pathol.*, **2**, 195–207

100. Nathan, C. F. (1987). Secretory products of macrophages. *J. Clin. Invest.*, **79**, 319–326

101. Tipping, P. G. and Holdsworth, S. R. (1988). Isolation and characterization of glomerular macrophages in experimental glomerulonephritis. *Immunol. Cell. Biol.*, **66**, 147–152

102. Cook, H. T., Smith, J. and Cattell, V. (1987). Isolation and characterization of inflammatory leukocytes from glomeruli in an in situ model of glomerulonephritis in the rat. *Am. J. Pathol.*, **126**, 126–136

103. Boyce, N. W., Tipping, P. G. and Holdsworth, S. R. (1989). Glomerular macrophages produce reactive oxygen species in experimental glomerulonephritis. *Kidney Int.*, **35**, 778–781

104. Cook, H. T., Smith, J., Salmon, J. A. Q. and Cattell, V. (1989). Functional characteristics of macrophages in glomerulonephritis in the rat. O_2^- generation, MHC Class II expression and eicosanoid synthesis. *Am. J. Pathol.*, **134**, 431–437

105. Tipping, P. G., Lowe, M. G. and Holdsworth, S. R. (1988). Glomerular macrophages express augmented procoagulant activity in experimental fibrin-related glomerulonephritis in rabbits. *J. Clin. Invest.*, **82**, 1253–1259

106. Wiggins, R. C. and Eldredge, C. (1987). Monocyte/macrophage heterogeneity and migration into Bowmans space early in crescentic nephritis in the rabbit. *Kidney Int.*, **31**, 333 (Abstract)

107. Rees, A. J., Lockwood, C. M. and Peters, D. K. (1977). Enhanced allergic tissue injury in Goodpasteurs syndrome by intercurrent bacterial infusion. *Br. Med. J.*, **2**, 723–726

108. Boyce, N. W., Tipping, P. G. and Holdsworth, S. R. (1986). Lymphokine (MIF) production by glomerular T-lymphocytes in experimental glomerulonephritis. *Kidney Int.*, **30**, 673–677

109. Neild, G. H., Ivory, K., Hiramatsu, M. and Gwyn-Williams, D. (1983). Cyclosporin A inhibits acute serum sickness nephritis in rabbits. *Clin. Exp. Immunol.*, **52**, 586–594

110. Bolton, W. K., Benton, F. R. and Lobo, P. I. (1978). Requirement of functional T-cells in the production of autoimmune glomerulo-tubular nephropathy in mice. *Clin. Exp. Immunol.*, **33**, 474–477

111. Hagstrom, G. L., Bloom, P. M., Yum, M. N., Sloan, R. S. and Luft, F. C. (1981). Immune complex nephritis in nude mice. *Nephron*, **29**, 95–98

112. Bhan, A. K., Collins, A. B., Schneeberger, E. E. and McCluskey, R. T. (1979). A cell-mediated reaction against glomerular-bound immune complexes. *J. Exp. Med.*, **150**, 1410–1420

113. Bolton, W. K., Chandra, M., Tyson, T. M., Kirkpatrick, P. R., Sadovnic, M. J. and Sturgill, B. C. (1988). Transfer of experimental glomerulonephritis in chickens by mononuclear cells. *Kidney Int.*, **34**, 578–610

114. Dvorak, H. F., Galli, S. J. and Dvorak, A. M. (1986). Cellular and vascular manifestations of cell mediated immunity. *Hum. Pathol.*, **17**, 122–137.

115. Cohen, S. (1986). Physiological and pathologic manifestations of lymphokine action. *Hum. Pathol.*, **17**, 112–121

116. Leonard, E. J., Ruco, L. P. and Meltzar, M. S. (1978). Characterization of macrophage activation factor, a lymphokine that cause macrophages to become cytotoxic for tumor cells. *Cell. Immunol.*, **41**, 347–350

117. Farram, E., Geczy, C. L., Moon, D. K. and Hopper, K. (1983). The ability of lymphokine and lipopolysaccharide to induce procoagulant activity in mouse macrophage cell lines. *J. Immunol.*, **130**, 2750–2756

118. Geczy, C. L., Farram, E., Moon, D. K., Meyer, P. A. and McKenzie, I. F. C. (1983). Macrophage procoagulant activity as a measure of cell-mediated immunity in the mouse. *J. Immunol.*, **130**, 2743–2749

119. Geczy, C. L. and Meyer, P. A. (1982). Leukocyte procoagulant activity in man: an 'in vitro' correlate of delayed type hypersensitivity in man. *J. Immunol.*, **128**, 331–335

120. Colvin, R. B., Mosesson, M. W. and Dvorak, H. F. (1979). Delayed type hypersensitivity skin reactions in congenital afibrinogenaemia lack fibrin deposition and induration. *J. Clin. Invest.*, **635**, 1302–1306

121. Edwards, R. L. and Rickles, F. R. (1978). Delayed hypersensitivity in man effects of systemic anticoagulation. *Science*, **200**, 541–543

122. Tipping, P. G., Dowling, J. P. and Holdsworth, S. R. (1988). Glomerular procoagulant activity in human glomerulonephritis. *J. Clin. Invest.*, **81**, 199–225

123. Tipping, P. G., Worthington, L. A. and Holdsworth, S. R. (1987). The quantitation and characterisation of glomerular procoagulant activity in experimental glomerulonephritis. *Lab. Invest.*, **45**, 77–81

124. Cole, E. H., Sweet, J. and Levy, G. A. (1986). Expression of macrophage procoagulant activity in murine systemic lupus erythematosis. *J. Clin. Invest.*, **78**, 887–893

125. Helin, H. and Edgington, T. S. (1983). Allogenic induction of the human T cell instructed monocyte procoagulant response is rapid and is elicited by HLA-DR. *J. Exp. Med.*, **158**, 962–975

126. Edwards, R. L. and Rickles, F. R. (1980). The role of human T cells (and T cell products) for monocyte tissue factor generation. *J. Immunol.*, **125**, 606–609

127. Gregory, S. A. and Edgington, T. S. (1985). Tissue factor induction in human monocytes. Two distinct mechanisms displayed by different alloantigen-responsive T cell clones. *J. Clin. Invest.*, **76**, 2440–2445

128. Ryan, J. and Geczy, C. L. (1986). Characterization and purification of mouse macrophage procoagulant-inducing factor. *J. Immunol.*, **137**, 2864–2870

129. Henson, P. M. (1972). Pathological mechanisms in neutrophil mediated injury. *Am. J. Pathol.*, **68**, 593–612

130. Cochrane, C. G., Müller-Eberhard, H. J. and Aikin, B. S. (1970). Depletion of plasma complement 'in vivo' by a protein of cobra venom: Its effects on various immunologic reactions. *J. Immunol.*, **105**, 55–69

131. Holdsworth, S. R. (1983). Fc dependence of macrophage accumulation and subsequent injury in experimental glomerulonephritis. *J. Immunol.*, **130**, 735–739

132. Boyce, N. W. and Holdsworth, S. R. (1991). A role for macrophage-Fc-receptor affinity in determining the cellular mediation of antibody initiated glomerulonephritis in the rabbit. *Kidney Int.* (In press)

133. Nolasco, F., Cameron, J. S., Harley, B. and Coelho, R. A. (1987). Changing patterns of glomerular T cells and monocytes according to the timing of biopsy in crescentic nephritis. *Proceedings of the Xth International Congress of Nephrology*, p. 396 (Abstract)

134. Bolton, W. K. and Couser, W. G. (1979). Pulse intravenous methylpredinsolone therapy of acute crescentic rapidly progressive glomerulonephritis. *Am. J. Med.*, **66**, 495–502

135. Couser, W. G. (1982). Idiopathic rapidly progressive glomerulonephritis. *Am. J. Nephrol.*, **2**, 57–69

136. Peters, D. K., Rees, A. J., Lockwood, C. M. *et al.* (1982). Treatment and prognosis in anti-basement membrane antibody mediated nephritis. *Transplant. Proc.*, **14**, 513–519

137. Bendixon, G. (1968)., Organ specific inhibition of the 'in-vitro' migration of leukocytes in human glomerulonephritis. *Acta. Med. Scad.*, **184**, 99–103

138. Rocklin, R. E., Lewis, E. J. and David, J. R. (1970). In vitro evidence for cellular hypersensitivity to glomerular basement membrane antigens in human glomerulonephritis. *N. Engl. J. Med.*, **283**, 497–501

139. Mahieu, P., Dardenne, M. and Bach, J. F. (1972). Detection of humoral and cell mediated immunity to kidney basement membrane in human renal diseases. *Am. J. Med.*, **53**, 185–192

140. Fillit, H. M., Read, S. E., Sherman, R. L., Zabriski, J. B. and van de Rijn, I. (1971). Cellular reactivity to altered basement membrane in glomerulonephritis. *N. Engl. J. Med.*, **298**, 861–868

141. Mallick, N. P., Williams, R. J., McFarlane, H., Orr, W. M., Taylor, G. and Williams, G. (1972). Cell-mediated immunity in nephrotic syndrome. *Lancet*, **1**, 507–509

142. Mallick, N. P. (1977). The pathogenesis of minimal lesion glomerulonephritis. *Clin. Nephrol.*, **7**, 87–95

143. Glassock, R. J., Cohen, A. H., Bennett, C. M. and Martinez-Maldonado, M. (1981). Primary glomerular diseases. In Brenner, B. and Rector, F. C. (eds.) *The Kidney*, pp. 1419–1427. (Philadelphia: W. B. Saunders)

144. LaGrue, G., Branellec, A., Blanc, C., Xhencumont, S., Beaudoux, F., Sobel, A. and Weil, B. (1975). A vascular permeability factor in lymphocyte culture supernatants from patients with nephrotic syndrome. I. Pharmacologic and physicochemical properties. *Biomedicine*, **23**, 73–75

145. Moreau, J. F., Payrat, M. A., Vie, H., Bonneville, M. and Soulillou, J. P. (1985). T cell colony forming frequency of mononucleated cells extracted from rejected human kidney transplants. *Transplantation*, **39**, 649–656

7
Eicosanoids and Cytokines in Glomerular Injury

J. D. WILLIAMS and M. DAVIES

INTRODUCTION

Damage to the renal glomerulus is usually the result of an inflammatory process which is triggered by the deposition of immune reactants. The presence of antibody, either directed against trapped or endogenous glomerular antigens, or in the form of immune complexes, usually results in the activation of complement, the accumulation of inflammatory phagocytes and platelets and the modulation of endogenous glomerular cell function. It is now evident that the development of glomerular injury in most forms of immune-mediated glomerulonephritis involves the interaction of infiltrating leukocytes with intrinsic glomerular cells as well as with extracellular matrices. Evaluation of this cell–cell interaction within the glomerulus has been difficult in man and largely limited to the examination of renal biopsies by immunohistochemistry and, more recently, by *in situ* hybridization with labelled cDNA probes. Functional analysis of the infiltrating cells is also problematic, but some progress has been achieved with animal models and to a limited degree with clinical renal biopsy material. In an attempt to study cell–cell interactions relevant to human glomerular disease, researchers have relied on isolated glomeruli and cultured glomerular cells and their response to co-culture with leukocytes (mainly macrophages) and exposure to soluble mediators. Using this approach, progress has been greatly enhanced by the availability of a wide spectrum of recombinant cytokines, as well as highly purified growth factors and their precipitating antibodies. Together with results from animal models of renal disease and clinical data, such *in vitro* models have indicated that glomerular injury results from inflammatory cell activation coupled with the synthesis and release of a plethora of pro-inflammatory mediators. It is likely that such molecules, either derived from the invading cell or from the intrinsic cells of the glomerulus, play a central role in the initiation and

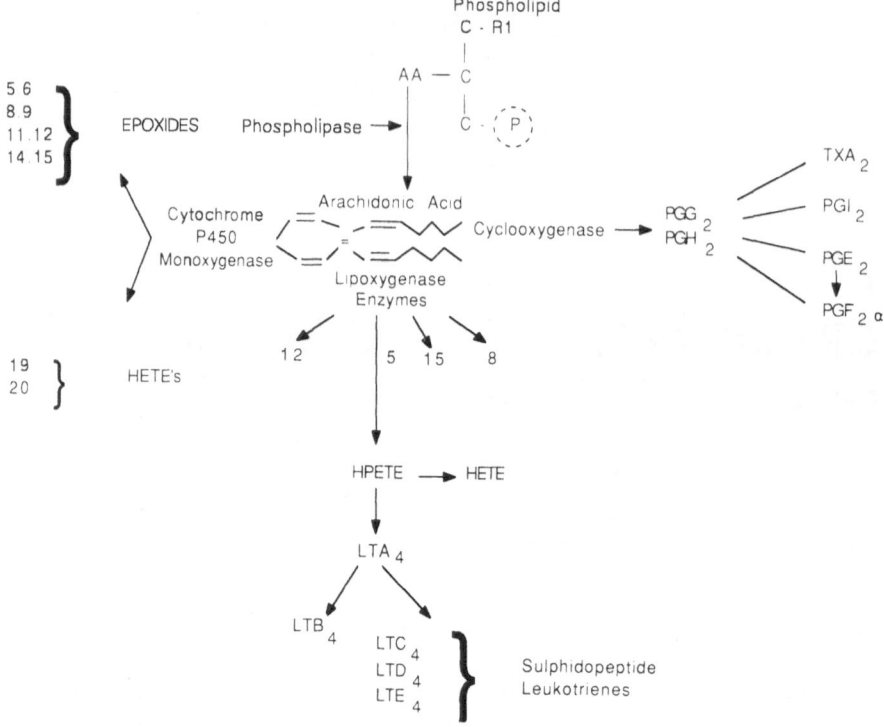

Figure 1 Potential arachidonic acid metabolism within the kidney

progression of glomerular injury. A comprehensive review of all the possible interactions of these compounds is clearly beyond the scope of this chapter, but specific examples of a role for eicosanoids and cytokines in glomerular injury will be emphasized.

GENERAL BACKGROUND TO EICOSANOIDS AND CYTOKINES

Eicosanoids

Eicosanoids are a group of compounds generated as a result of the oxidative metabolism of polyunsaturated fatty acids of 20-carbon-atom chain length (Figure 1). Usually the term is associated with the production of metabolites of arachidonic acid, a 20-carbon-atom fatty acid commonly found in membrane phospholipids. Subsequent to its release, arachidonic acid becomes available to serve as a substrate for one of three enzymatic systems— cyclooxygenase, lipoxygenase, and cytochrome P450 mixed-function oxidases— giving rise to a variety of active products[116,122,197] (Figure 2).

The sites of arachidonic acid metabolism within the kidney are well defined and integrated in that each contributes appropriately to overall renal function. Cyclooxygenase pathway enzymes are located in glomerular cells[95], the collecting tubules[87], and the interstitium[236] as well as in the vascular endothelium[218]. Lipoxygenase pathway enzymes are less well localized and

124

PGE$_2$	Vasodilator
	Mesangial Relaxation
	↓IL-1 production
	↑Renin Secretion
PGI$_2$	↓Platelet Aggregation
	Vasodilator
	Mesangial Relaxation
TXA$_2$	↑Platelet Aggregation
	↑Mesangial Protein Synthesis
	Mesangial Contraction
	Vasoconstriction
	↑PGE$_2$
LTB$_4$	Chemoattractant
	↑Vascular Permeability
LTD$_4$	↓ERPF
	Mesangial Contraction
	↑PGE$_2$

Figure 2 Eicosanoid function

probably arise from resident or invading macrophages[126], or from accumulating polymorphs, although cultured glomerular epithelial cells are reported to possess lipoxygenase activity[101]. The cytochrome P450 monooxygenase system is distributed intermittently around the nephron, being localized mainly to the proximal tubules[75] and to the thick ascending limb of the loop of Henle[197]. Thus it is likely that the products of both cyclooxygenase and lipoxygenase systems play a role in glomerular function during disease, while the products of the cytochrome P450 system, although influenced by glomerular events, will be less likely to have a direct effect during glomerular injury.

Cytokines/growth factors

Cytokine is a collective term used to embrace a number of low-molecular-weight glycosylated polypeptides known variously as lymphokines, monokines, growth factors and mitogens that alone or collectively affect the function of various cells[11,29,61,62,118,199]. In general, cytokines possess the ability to stimulate or augment cell proliferation, initiate protein synthesis, and modify the production of pro-inflammatory molecules such as eicosanoids, platelet-activating factor and procoagulant activity. In addition, this distinct group of polypeptides may act in an autocrine or paracrine manner, are active in the 10^{-12} M range, and interact with target cells via specific cell surface receptors.

To date, the cytokine family consists of eight well-characterized interleukins (IL1–8)[11,91], tumour necrosis factor (TNF)[29,118,199], and interferons α, β

125

and γ. In addition, a number of factors which are usually referred to as growth factors/mitogens must be considered. These include platelet-derived growth factor (PDGF)[92,188], epidermal growth factor (EGF)[39], transforming growth factor (TFG)[185], fibroblast growth factor (FGF)[86], and insulin-like growth factor-1 (somatomedin, ILGF-1)[54]. These molecules are relatively small peptides, many are potent mitogens for glomerular cells, and interact with specific high-affinity cell surface receptors (with the exception of TGF-α, which competes for the same receptor as EGF)[220]. This chapter will concentrate on the inflammatory response to cytokines and focus mainly on IL-1, TNF and PDGF.

Interleukin-1 (IL-1). Interleukin-1 in practice consists of two polypeptides (IL-1α and IL-1β), which exhibit limited homology, yet exert similar if not identical biological activities[61,62]. The alpha form is an acetylated 33 kD membrane-associated protein, whereas IL-1β, the predominant form, is readily secreted from activated cells as a 17 kD non-acetylated polypeptide[36]. The genes for both IL-1α and IL-1β have been cloned and located to chromosome 2[1,129,141]. Interestingly, despite their limited homology, IL-1α and IL-1β both bind to the same receptor molecule, for which they share the same affinity[30,67]. A number of cells exhibit receptors for IL-1, which once occupied are rapidly internalized, probably via receptor-mediated endocytosis[31,138,150]. The post-internalization fate of the IL-1 receptor–ligand complex is still unclear. In certain cells there is evidence for down-regulation of the receptor, which may represent a feedback control mechanism[146,150]. On the other hand, up-regulation has been described for T cells[68,200]. Internalized radiolabelled IL-1 is located in the nucleus; in addition, a significant amount is channelled to the vesicles of the lysosomal system, where it is slowly degraded[138].

Tumour necrosis factor (TNF). TNF, also known as cachectin, is secreted mainly by monocytes and macrophages in response to agonists such as bacterial products[29,199], and opsonized glomerular basement membrane (GBM)[226]. TNF was originally defined by its ability to cause haemorrhagic necrosis and occasionally complete regression of transplanted tumours. In addition, TNF displays a variety of other activities which exhibit remarkable similarities to those of IL-1, in particular the non-immunological properties[29,62,118]. TNF and IL-1, however, do not share any apparent homology, and recognize and bind to separate receptors[28,146]. These two cytokines can also act together in a synergistic manner, resulting in enhanced leukocyte migration[228], the production of prostaglandin E_2 (PGE_2) by both fibroblasts[74] and mesangial cells[222], aggregation of neutrophils, and the synthesis of thromboxane[49].

TNF, as well as IL-1, exerts important regulatory effects on vascular endothelial cells. These effects, which are relevant to the pathophysiology of glomerular disease[52,171], include the induction of the leukocyte adhesion molecules ELAM-1 and ICAM-1, as well as alterations in the synthesis of components of the coagulant/anti-coagulant system in favour of coagulation, and an increase in the production of PGE_2, prostacyclin (PGI_2) and platelet-activating factor. Such findings indicate possible mechanisms whereby the effects of TNF and IL-1 on the endothelium may initiate vascular damage. Furthermore, TNF, unlike IL-1, serves to prime neutrophils for subsequent ligand stimulation and results in an increase in neutrophil phagocytic action, reactive oxygen species production, degranulation and leukotriene B4 synthesis[109,165,211]. This action of TNF on neutrophils further emphasizes the potential role of TNF in vascular damage, since reactive oxygen species and neutrophil neutral proteinases, alone and in combination, kill endothelial cells and degrade basement membrane[55,56,224].

Platelet-derived growth factor (PDGF). PDGF is a growth factor for cells of mesenchymal origin and consists of two closely related peptides (A and B) of similar size and composition but encoded on different chromosomes[92,188]. Independent regulation of expression of each peptide results in the production of at least three different but related molecules, i.e. PDGF-AA, PDGF-BB and PDGF-AB. All three peptides are potent mitogens, bind to specific cell surface receptors, and initiate DNA synthesis[73,152]. In general, higher concentrations of the PDGF-AA dimer are required to elicit the same effect as the PDGF-BB dimer. However, in human fibroblasts and smooth muscle cells it has been shown that IL-1-induced proliferation is mediated by the induction and release of cell-associated PDGF-AA, but not -AB or -BB[181]. In addition to DNA synthesis, PDGF acts as a chemoattractant for fibroblasts and smooth muscle cells, effects phosphatidylinositol turnover and ion transport, and initiates alterations in cytoskeletal elements[92]. Occupancy of PDGF-receptor also influences the status of receptors for other growth factors such as ILGF (up-regulated)[47,181], and EGF (down-regulated)[33].

TISSUE CULTURE STUDIES

Over the last decade the ability to study glomerular cells in culture has greatly contributed to our understanding of normal glomerular physiology, as well as the pathophysiology of glomerular disease. The glomerulus consists of at least four different types of cells and to date methods are available for the successful culture of two of these, namely mesangial and epithelial (probably of visceral origin)[103,111,133,215]. As yet, efforts to establish a reliable and reproducible technique for glomerular endothelial cells have not met with the same success. However, methods have been reported[139,213] and a recent report by Ballerman has documented a novel method for the routine isolation and maintenance of bovine glomerular endothelial cells utilizing fluorescence-activated cell sorting and cloning together with the use of selective culture medium.[13]

While tissue culture of glomerular cells offers a valuable model for the investigation of glomerular function and metabolism at the cellular level, it is important to stress that maintenance of glomerular cells in culture is beset with difficulties. Results have to be interpreted in the context of dedifferentiation as well as the artificial environment of the cultured cells. Indeed, it is likely that glomerular cells in culture represent activated cells since fetal bovine serum, an essential ingredient of most culture medium, contains a number of platelet-derived products. In contrast, glomerular cells *in vivo* are exposed to autologous plasma or its ultrafiltrate. A full discussion of the difficulties involved in the isolation and charcterization of glomerular cells in culture is beyond the scope of this chapter, and the reader is referred to several extensive reviews on the subject[103,111,133,215].

Eicosanoids and glomerular cells

The isolation of intact glomeruli and their stimulation with appropriate ligands has demonstrated production of the vasodilator PGE_2 and to a lesser extent PGI_2, as well as the vasoconstrictor eicosanoids prostaglandin $F_{2\alpha}$ ($PGF_{2\alpha}$) and thromboxane B_2 (TXB_2)[80,95,145,194,205].

Lipoxygenase pathway products appear to be less abundant, although in the isolated rat glomerular preparation a product of the 12-lipoxygenase enzyme (12HETE)[207] can be found, as well as small amounts of leukotriene B_4 (LTB_4) and 5HETE (of the 5-lipoxygenase pathway)[42]. In addition, glomerular epithelial cells have receptors for leukotriene C_4 (LTC_4)[18], and the culture of rat mesangial cells with LTC_4 results not only in the contraction of these cells but also in their proliferation[17]. Whether or not this proliferation is under cyclooxygenase product control, as is the fibroblast response to LTC_4, remains to be determined.

Individually, however, none of the intrinsic glomerular cells appears to possess a 5-lipoxygenase pathway and by inference it is likely that the products of this pathway are the result of activation of the resident macrophage population. Similarly, the 15-lipoxygenase pathway products from human glomeruli also appear to be of macrophage origin[207]. Thus it is essential to appreciate that analysis of the inflammatory reaction within the glomerulus, for either eicosanoids or cytokines, must take into account the respective roles of endogenous and exogenous cells. In addition, the relative importance of individual eicosanoids appears to vary between species. The apparent difference in eicosanoid production between rodent and human glomeruli is reflected by the fact that the major vasodilatory product of rat glomeruli is PGE_2, whereas the human glomerulus, in response to angiotensin II stimulation, secretes mainly PGI_2 [206,209]. These findings are confirmed when the system is dissected further by examining homogeneous cultures of individual glomerular cells. Cultured rat mesangial cells again produce mainly PGE_2 [205], while their human counterparts produce mainly PGI_2 [4]. Despite these differences there are, however, certain common rules that can be applied whatever the species studied. If the glomerulus is exposed to any one of a wide variety of vasoconstrictor hormones or mediators, then the result is the secretion of vasodilator prostaglandins. This appears to occur in all species and serves to create a balance between vasodilatory and vasoconstrictor forces. These findings are confirmed by studies on cultured cells where a variety of compounds which result in mesangial cell contraction, by a mechanism which is dependent on a rise in intracellular calcium, also result in the release of PGE_2 and PGI_2. These eicosanoids are themselves also able to modulate mesangial cell function through the activation of adenylate

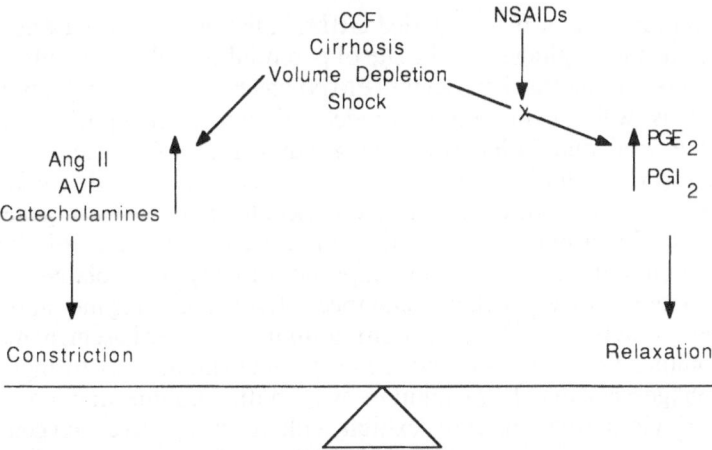

Figure 3 Renal blood flow under conditions of stress is a balance of constrictor and relaxation forces

cyclase, and promote cell relaxation[166]. The mechanism of this relaxation is unclear but may reflect inhibition of myosin light-chain kinase and disaggregation of stress fibres. The importance of this balance between contraction and relaxation is highlighted clinically by the deleterious effect of inhibitors of the cyclooxygenase pathway in patients with impaired renal function (Figure 3).

It is also of interest to note at this point that vasodilator prostanoid synthesis can be modulated by mechanisms which are independent of calcium mobilization. Included here are the capacity of IL-1 and TNFα to increase PGE_2 synthesis in both rodent[20] and human mesangial cells[222]. Similar changes occur by mechanisms which alter the surface charge of the glomerular cell. Glomerular epithelial cells in culture respond significantly to the addition of a variety of polycations, by an increase in the production of both PGE_2 and PGI_2[176]. That this was associated with neutralization of surface charge in these studies was confirmed by the co-incubation of polyanions such as heparin, which reversed the effect. The importance of such mechanisms can be appreciated if one considers that neutrophil degranulation results in the release of a number of polycations, including lactoferrin, and that these may neutralize glomerular and basement membrane charge as well as serving as binding molecules between two anionic cell surfaces.

Cytokine/growth factor interaction with renal glomerular cells

Insight into the contribution of infiltrating leukocytes to glomerular injury has emerged mainly from tissue culture studies. Co-culture studies with rat peritoneal macrophages have demonstrated that phagocytes adhere to isolated glomeruli in a time- and cell-dependent manner[19]. This binding was independent of a requirement for activation of the complement cascade but appeared to be influenced by lipoxygenase products of arachidonic acid, since pretreatment of the glomeruli with nordihydroguaniaretic acid, but not indomethacin, significantly inhibited this phenomenon. Macrophage attachment occurred predominantly to denuded GBM, indicating an intimate association between the macrophage and the site of potential stimulus. A similar location for polymorphonuclear leukocytes (PMN) has been shown in human biopsy material as well as in animal models of glomerulonephritis. Activated monocytes and macrophages secrete a number of soluble factors that are involved in the complex interactions associated with growth, inflammation and fibrosis[59]. Some are constitutive molecules but most are generated in response to direct macrophage activation. Recent observations indicate that these inflammatory cells, when exposed directly to isolated GBM or GBM-coated antigen, exhibit enhanced lysosomal enzyme and neutral proteinase secretion[94,225,232]. In addition, immune-coated basement membrane also promotes TNF and IL-1 production by human monocytes. Intraglomerular macrophages isolated from animals with both immune and non-immune forms of glomerular disease exhibit enhanced reactive oxygen species production, eicosanoid secretion and synthesis of IL-1 compared to control macrophages[51,144], indicating that they are in an activated state. In addition, macrophages adhere to cultured glomerular mesangial cells[69], resulting in an increased synthesis by the mesangial cell of a unique type IV collagenase[142]. These results provide considerable evidence of a pathological role for invading macrophages in immune-mediated glomerulonephritis.

From the above studies it is evident that the interaction of monocytes/macrophages with glomerular cells, or with GBM, generates enzymes and other molecules which have the potential to contribute to cellular and matrix damage. The exact mechanism of interaction of macrophages and mesangial cells is less well defined. Initial studies on the interaction of macrophages with defined glomerular cells described a protein factor in the conditioned medium of rat peritoneal macrophages that potentiated the proliferation of rat mesangial cells[130]. In consequence, the mesangial cells responded by releasing several potent pro-inflammatory mediators, including PGE_2, PGI_2 and TXB_2[135], a thymocyte-activating factor (subsequently shown to be IL-1)[131], and type IV collagenase[132,142]. Further studies indicated that the protein constituents present in macrophage-conditioned medium also induced the release from mesangial cells of reactive oxygen species[178], and a growth factor that had many properties in common with PDGF[2]. Purification of the macrophage-conditioned medium demonstrated that a number of factors were in fact responsible for mesangial activation. These possessed similar biological and physiological properties to PDGF, IL-1 and TNFα. More important, these studies indicated that cultured mesangial cells, when stimulated by macrophage-conditioned medium, themselves respond with the production of growth factors, suggesting a potential amplification of the inflammatory response. Such evidence has recently been presented for IL-6[237]. Rat mesangial cells have been shown to express IL-6 mRNA by northern blot analysis and to secrete a molecule that has been characterized both biochemically and biologically as IL-6. Furthermore, it was clear that as well a possible paracrine role within the glomerulus, mesangial IL-6 may also serve as an autocrine function in relation to mesangial cell proliferation.

Attempts to elucidate the events following macrophage–mesangial cell interaction have largely made use of the availability of highly purified and recombinant cytokines. Mesangial cells exhibit a proliferative response to a number of cytokines and growth factors, including TGFα and β, PDGF, ILGF and EGF. Since the cytokines investigated are derived mainly from monocytes/macrophages, it can be argued that their secretion *in vivo* may form an important contribution to the hypercellularity commonly reported in glomerular inflammation.

In the normal adult kidney, the intrinsic cells of the glomerulus have a very low replicative rate[156]. Mesangial cells in culture have a relatively fast turnover but can be brought into G_0 by holding them for 3–4 days in serum-free medium[223]. When the culture medium is reconstituted with serum, quiescent mesangial cells are rapidly induced to leave G_0, traverse G_1, and enter S phase[170]. Growth factors function at precise stages of the cell cycle and trigger specific biochemical events, which in turn induce quiescent cells to transform from G_0 to a DNA-replicative S phase. Broadly speaking, mitogens are placed into one of two groups: those factors that effect early G_0/G_1 events and which are called competence factors (e.g. PDGF, FGF, thrombin), and those acting on latter cell cycle events and called progression factors (e.g. EGF, IGF)[134,139]. The G_2 phase has no requirements for specific growth factors. Therefore, cells exposed first to a competence factor and then to a progression factor are capable of completing the cell cycle. For example, the addition of PDGF to quiescent (G_0) fibroblasts will produce a rapid increase in DNA synthesis, but the addition of a progression factor, e.g. epidermal growth factor (EGF), is required for full mitogenic activity[170]. In contrast, when added to human mesangial cells, PDGF appears to function as a complete growth factor, since it induces a mitogenic response (i.e. enhanced [³H]thymidine incorporation in association with increased cell numbers[100,201,202,223]) without the requirement fror a competence factor. This response is achieved with all dimers of PDGF, but PDGF-BB and PDGF-AB were considerably more effective than the PDGF-AA dimer[100]. This unique response is not restricted to PDGF alone since EGF, FGF, TGFα and TNFα act in a similar manner.

It has been demonstrated that the above cytokines, as well as exogenous PDGF, also induce increased synthesis and secretion of a PDGF-like factor by mesangial cells. This factor shares biological activity and immunological cross-reactivity with PDGF purified from human platelets. It has also been reported that precipitating antibodies to PDGF are capable of partially neutralizing the mitogenic response of mesangial cells to EGF.

These data are consistent with the possibility that PDGF may have a controlling influence on the proliferation of mesangial cells. Thus, exogenous PDGF might induce proliferation directly. In addition, it might act to stimulate the local release of PDGF and serve to perpetuate and amplify the mitogenic response. Finally, it could be the mediator that in part accounts for the proliferative effect on mesangial cells of other cytokines or growth factors.

However, it is important to stress that not all cytokines enhance PDGF-induced mesangial cell proliferation. Recent studies have shown that TGF-β can cause inhibition of mesangial cell proliferation induced by a plethora of mitogens, including PDGF. IL-1 can also modify the mitogenic response of mesangial cells to PDGF.

Lovett and coworkers have provided convincing evidence that one of the principal mesangial cell mitogens secreted by activated rat peritoneal macrophages is an IL-1-like molecule, and further demonstrated that this cytokine can act as a progression factor[130,131,134]. As with PDGF, IL-1 has also been identified as an autocrine factor secreted by mesangial cells. Cycling, but not quiescent, cells express mRNA which hybridizes with specific probes for IL-1α and β[137]. Significantly, IL-1 mRNA expression in quiescent cells could be induced by the combination of PDGF and EGF, which again underlines the multiple effects of polypeptide mitogens on mesangial cells.

Conflicting results have appeared on the growth response of mesangial cells to TNF. It has been reported that TNF, alone or in combination with competence factors, was effective in the stimulation of cell growth[100,202], again in the absence of other competence factors. However, other reports have demonstrated that TNF inhibits proliferation, including that induced by the PDGF-BB dimer[58,143,223].

In contrast to their putative role in cell proliferation, the co-culture of mesangial cells with IL-1 and TNF, either alone or in combination, directly stimulates *de novo* synthesis of several mesangial cell-derived proteins relevant to the inflammatory response in the glomerular disease. These include a type IV collagenase, a neutral proteinase capable of degrading GBM[57,142], interstitial collagens, which are constituents of sclerotic lesions of renal disease but not normal glomeruli[78,214], proteoglycans[58], and prostaglandin endoperoxide synthetase, together with other distal enzymes responsible for the synthesis of effector prostaglandins[222]. Moreover, it has been demonstrated that phospholipase A$_2$ is translocated and released in increased amounts by cells stimulated with a combination of IL-1 and TNF[167,222]. In addition, the release of oxygen-derived free radicals in response to IL-1 and TNF implies that NADP oxidase synthesis is enhanced[178]. Finally, as intimated above, IL-1-treated mesangial cells synthesize and release an IL-1-like peptide[134]. All these products may play a role as mediators of glomerular inflammation. As yet it is not known whether either macrophage IL-1 or TNF stimulates TNF production by mesangial cells, but the production of this cytokine can be induced by bacterial lipopolysaccharide (LPS)[21,230].

Thus, the principal action of IL-1 and TNF on mesangial cells is to up-regulate cellular metabolism and increase expression of genes coding for biologically active molecules. With respect to TNF, while this cytokine can indeed stimulate catabolic events in glomerular mesangial cells, its major role in glomerular disease is most likely through its ability to up-regulate neutrophil activity and induce changes in endothelial membranes that favour coagulation and neutrophil adhesion.

While much information has been gained from tissue culture studies on the factors that modify mesangial cell function, comparatively little is known about factors that modulate glomerular epithelial and endothelial cells. Glomerular epithelial cells have been reported to proliferate in response to conditioned medium from macrophages[18], and to respond to IL-1 by enhanced type IV collagen synthesis[93]. In contrast, TGF-β inhibited the proliferation of glomerular epithelial (and endothelial) cells[139] induced by EGF, IGF-1 and PDGF, and did not augment collagen production. TGF-β did, however, increase fibronectin production in glomerular epithelial cells.

To date, only two studies have investigated in any detail cytokine-mediated interactions with glomerular endothelial cells[13,139]. In one[139], TGF-β inhibited endothelial proliferation, but in the second[13] FGF-α in the presence of heparin and TGF-β modulated the growth rate of subconfluent cells. In addition, it has been reported that supernatants from mesangial cells in culture can inhibit the growth of endothelial cells. Since medium conditioned by confluent glomerular mesangial cells enhances proliferation of subconfluent endothelial cells, it is apparent that these glomerular cells, as with mesangial cells, are influenced by autocrine and paracine mechanisms. Cotran and Pober[52] have provided an authoritative review of the interaction of cytokines, including TNF, with the endothelium in general, and have indicated consequences relevant to renal diseases.

ELCOSANOIDS IN EXPERIMENTAL GLOMERULAR DISEASE

A potential role for eicosanoids in glomerular injury was initially highlighted by the capacity of cyclooxygenase inhibitors to cause a reduction in proteinuria[6] and a decrease in glomerular filtration[66] in patients with nephrotic syndrome. In addition, studies on obstructive uropathy in rabbits demonstrated that an increase in thromboxane synthesis represented a change in the pattern of eicosanoids released in disease states[151]. More recently, in the early stages of a rat model of immune mediated glomerular disease (nephrotoxic serum nephritis) there was a rapid decrease in glomerular filtration rate and renal plasma flow, which coincided with a significant increase in prostanoid formation. The major product was TXB_2 and not PGE_2 as seen in control animals[123]. An increase in thromboxane production is a common feature of many forms of experimental renal diseases, including SLE nephropathy[107], adriamycin nephropathy[184], endotoxaemia[8], Heymann nephritis[53], glycerol toxicity[22], and diabetic nephropathy[48]. The source of the increased thromboxane production is, however, unidentified and several candidate cells must be considered. While the intrinsic mesangial and epithelial cells have a capacity for thromboxane production, little evidence is available to support their role as a major source of this eicosanoid in disease states, although studies with either cell type suggests that the interaction with the membrane attack complex of complement may result in a significant increase in TXB_2 synthesis[136]. A role for platelets in the pathogenesis of glomerular injury has been suggested by numerous studies, most recently in a model of immune complex nephritis, where their depletion significantly reduced albuminuria[102]. Platelets have also been suggested as a major source of thromboxane in experimental renal disease[177], although the use of a cyclooxygenase inhibitor, ibuprofen, which abolished platelet thromboxane production, did not reduce glomerular thromboxane synthesis or prevent glomerular injury in an autoimmune model of nephritis in mice[105]. In contrast, the isolation of mononuclear phagocytes (macrophages) from the glomeruli of mice with spontaneous lupus erthematosus has demonstrated that these are immunologically active cells in which the synthesis of the various eicosanoids is significantly altered when compared to macrophages from control animals. In animals with active nephritis, isolated cells produced virtually no PGl_2 and showed markedly decreased PGE_2 synthesis. In contrast, thromboxane A_2 (TXA_2) levels were proportionately increased, and further stimulation of these cells with IL-1 resulted in a significant rapid rise only in TXB_2[3]. This finding has been most recently confirmed by the isolation of macrophages from glomeruli of rats with nephrotoxic nephritis, demonstrating a decrease in all eicosanoids with the exception of TXB_2[51]. Thus, it seems that a number of cell types may contribute to the synthesis and excretion of thromboxane, and that the exact source of this eicosanoid will vary with the aetiology of the injury.

In addition to cyclooxygenase pathway products, numerous studies have also identified and characterized lipoxygenase pathway products in both rat[101,207,208] and human[207] glomeruli. In glomeruli isolated from normal rats, both LTB_4[42] and LTC_4[207] have been demonstrated, and it is postulated that the likely source is the resident macrophage population of the glomerulus. These results have more recently been confirmed by the use of gas chromatography and mass spectroscopy[120]. In addition, studies using ^{14}C-labelled arachidonic acid have demonstrated a limited capacity for rat glomeruli to synthesize sulphidopeptide leukotrienes[5]. The isolation of glomeruli from a rat model of anti-GBM nephritis allowed the demonstration of enhanced synthesis of products of the 12-lipoxygenase pathway[124]. Subsequent studies using the same model confirmed the presence of 12 HETE, but also demonstrated an early and significant rise in 5 HETE and LTB_4. The capacity to activate the 5-lipoxygenase pathway appeared to be related to the amount of antibody employed and was dependent on activation of the complement pathway and on the presence of PMN, but not on the presence of platelets[124,125]. This synthesis of LTB_4 by glomeruli from rats with nephrotoxic serum nephritis has also been confirmed by the use of gas chromatography and mass spectrometry to identify and authenticate the LTB_4[231]. In addition, models of nephritis independent of inflammatory cell infiltrates also demonstrated enhanced lipoxygenase products, suggesting a role for intrinsic glomerular cells, perhaps resident macrophages[27,180]. Thus, the synthesis of both lipoxygenase and cyclooxygenase products appears to be increased during experimental glomerular injury, and the relative proportions of the various eicosanoids change in different disease states. Their importance, however, in the pathogenesis of injury can only be evaluated under conditions where either their synthesis is limited or their target organ receptors are blocked.

Inhibition of thromboxane activity in experimental models of nephritis

Studies which have concentrated on the selective modification of thromboxane were prompted by the observation that comprehensive inhibition of prostanoid synthesis in disease states results in a decrease in renal function[25,179,212]. In contrast, the selective inhibition of platelet cyclooxygenase by sulindac with relative sparing of renal eicosanoid synthesis resulted in an amelioration of proteinuria and an improvement in glomerular histology[25], suggesting the involvement of platelets and circulating inflammatory cells. In addition, a number of studies have highlighted a relative increase in glomerular thromboxane concentrations in experimental nephritis, and suggested that selective inhibition of TXA_2 function would leave the cytoprotective and haemodynamic benefits of PGE_2 and PGI_2 intact.

The use of thromboxane synthase inhibition in animal models of glomerular disease has, however, produced conflicting results. In a nephrotoxic nephritis model the functional importance of thromboxane is closely dependent on the stage of the disease. The administration of a thromboxane synthase inhibitor during the first 2–3 hours (the early heterologous phase) protects against the decreased glomerular filtration rate (GFR) seen in the untreated nephrotoxic animal[123]. If the administration of the drug is delayed until the heterologous phase of the disease, it has little effect on proteinuria or GFR despite clear evidence of thromboxane synthase inhibition[212]. Similarly, in a nephritis model triggered by the administration of cationic bovine gamma globulin (immune complex nephritis) there is an increased synthesis of both PGE_2 and TXB_2, and the rise in the latter correlates significantly with proteinuria. Neither the use of a thromboxane synthase inhibitor, nor of a selective thromboxane receptor antagonist, influenced proteinuria or GFR[179]. The administration of indomethacin, however, which results in the comprehensive inhibition of cyclooxygenase product synthesis, caused a significant decrease of GFR, highlighting the beneficial effects of vasodilator prostaglandins in this model.

Thus, it seems that, under conditions where there is reduced glomerular blood flow and reduced GFR, at least part of the vasoconstrictor element is provided in the early stages by TXA_2, generated either by endogenous glomerular cells or by infiltrating cells (platelets or macrophages). The administration of either a thromboxane synthase inhibitor or a thromboxane receptor antagonist may prevent this decrement. This observation is supported by a number of studies using different animal models of glomerular injury—adriamycin nephrosis[184], glycerol nephrosis[157], and endotoxaemia[8]— where a reduced GFR is part of the natural history of the disease process, where there is a relative increase in thromboxane synthesis, and where a functional decrease in thromboxane activity appears, at least in the short term, to be beneficial.

A role for thromboxane in the pathogenesis of proteinuria has also been proposed[53]. In the passive Heymann nephritis model, where glomerular injury is complement-mediated, the use of a thromboxane synthase inhibitor reduced proteinuria by more than 80%. This decrement was identical to that seen when indomethacin was used, but in the presence of selective thromboxane inhibition the changes were independent of a significant alteration in renal haemodynamics. Similarly, in the adriamycin model of nephropathy[184] there was a significant reduction of proteinuria following inhibition of thromboxane production. In contrast, the inhibition of thromboxane in a model of membranous nephropathy[210], and in separate studies on cationic immune complex nephropathy[50,179] failed to influence glomerular protein loss. The reasons behind these differences in effect on proteinuria are unclear. The timing of administration of the drug may be important in haemodynamics, but proteinuria is a relatively late event. The importance of thromboxane is not confined to experimental models where there is cellular infiltration of the glomerulus, since non-infiltrative models also appear to respond to thromboxane inhibition. In any study where modulation of eicosanoid synthesis is attempted it is important not only to establish that there is indeed a modification of product generation but also to distinguish between the role of glomerular cells and infiltrating cells in supplying or generating these eicosanoids. In most studies of experimental nephritis the source of thromboxane appears to be glomerular cells. Confirmation of its adequate inhibition is not always presented and the demonstration of receptor inhibition within the kidney by the use of receptor antagonists is extremely difficult. In addition, the disparity between studies must depend not only on the individual model but also on the characteristics of the pharmacological agents employed.

The efficacy of a synthase inhibitor, e.g. of thromboxane, must be compared not only in terms of platelet enzymes but also in terms of enzymes within endogenous renal cells. This should be taken into consideration when examining the effects of eicosanoid inhibition on progression of disease in models of chronic renal failure. Surgical removal of three-quarters of the renal mass results in proteinuria, hypertension and progressive sclerosis, changes that have been linked to glomerular hyperperfusion and hyperfiltration[34,60,97]. In partially nephrectomized animal studies, a persistent and significant rise in the rate of urine excretion of thromboxane after surgery was demonstrated. Treatment with a thromboxane synthase inhibitor resulted in an increase in single nephron GFR and reduction of progression to the uraemic state, i.e. the thromboxane synthase inhibitor prevented progression of disease despite an increase in renal plasma flow and GFR[177]. The cause of this apparent benefit is difficult to ascertain, since there was both inhibition of thromboxane and also a fall in blood pressure in the treated group. In addition, although a case was made for platelets to have a central role as a source of thromboxane, the effect of the inhibitor on endogenous renal thromboxane synthesis was unclear. In a separate study in the same model using low-dose aspirin, i.e. selective inhibition of platelet cyclooxygenase, progression of disease was not inhibited. In this case there was no change in blood pressure and no inhibition of endogenous renal thromboxane generation[233]. Furthermore, in a model of glomerulosclerosis (the Milan normotensive rat) in which there was no hyperfiltration[175] inhibition of endogenous thromboxane production was accompanied by the amelioration of progressive sclerosis[190]. These studies suggest that in such well-defined models of progression the intraglomerular synthesis of thromboxane contributes to glomerulosclerosis, and that this occurs independently of hypertension and hyperfiltration, possibly through the direct effect of thromboxane on the glomerular cells.

Lipoxygenase products, inhibition and glomerular injury

The contribution of lipoxygenase products to glomerular injury is less well-defined. 12 HETE is increased in animals with nephrotoxic nephritis and this may serve as a chemotactic agent and promote cell infiltration[124].

Leukotriene B_4 has also been isolated from the glomeruli of rats with nephrotoxic serum nephritis[231]. The source of this potent chemotactic agent is unknown, but it seems to be produced only during the early stages of the disease[125]. Neutrophil depletion only partly ameliorated the synthesis of LTB_4 and the most likely candidate cell must therefore be the glomerular macrophage. More recent studies by Cook et al.[51], using a model of acute proliferative nephritis from which glomerular macrophages were isolated, failed to demonstrate any LTB_4 production. Unfortunately, whole glomeruli were not examined for LTB_4 release, and therefore an accurate assessment of glomerular macrophages as a source of LTB_4 cannot be made.

A role for the sulphidopeptide leukotrienes in the kidney was initially postulated by the demonstration of LTC_4 receptors in glomeruli[12,18], and following studies which examined the effect of LTC_4 on renal and systemic vasculature[7]. Following an infusion of LTC_4 in the anaesthetized rat there was a dramatic rise in systemic and renal vascular resistance, followed by an increase in vascular permeability and a subsequent fall in plasma volume. The net result of these effects was a decrease in renal plasma flow and glomerular filtration rate. Interestingly, the vasoactive effect was demonstrated to be mediated directly through a sulphidopeptide receptor, while the change in vascular permeability was blocked not only by a sulphidopeptide receptor antagonist but also by indomethacin, indicating a secondary role for the cyclooxygenase pathway in effecting these functional changes to the vessel wall. This work has more recently been extended by studies using micropuncture techniques in which LTD_4 was shown to increase efferent glomerular arteriolar resistance[9]. A potential role for sulphidopeptide leukotrienes in glomerular injury has been demonstrated in a model of endotoxin-induced glomerular disease[8] as well as in nephrotoxic nephritis. In both studies a sulphidopeptide receptor antagonist prevented the early fall in GFR by maintaining glomerular haemodynamics[10]. A long-term beneficial effect of the inhibition of these vasoactive compounds remains to be established.

The protective effect of prostaglandins

A rationale for the administration of vasodilator eicosanoids in the form of analogues of PGE_2 and PGI_2 is based on the postulated protective effects of these compounds on renal haemodynamics. Indeed, in several models of acute renal failure the infusion of such compounds ameliorated the acute changes and limited the duration of injury. In addition to these findings, however, prostaglandins of the E series may have a direct influence on the immune process[235], and may modify cell function through their capacity to activate adenylate cyclase and increase intracellular cyclic AMP[81]. Other studies have demonstrated not only the capacity of IL-1 to increase PGE_2 synthesis[167] but also the negative feedback effect of PGE_2 at high concentrations on IL-1 and TNF generation and release[110]. Prostaglandins of the E series inhibit mitogenesis[84], decrease antibody production by plasma cells[229], decrease killing by natural killer (NK) cells[35], and reduce degranulation of PMN in response to a variety of stimuli[234]. Thus a decrease in prostaglandin synthesis during the disease process may be detrimental to the immunocompetence of the host and destroy the balance between natural immunity and glomerular damage and sclerosis.

In the murine SLE model the administration of PGE_1 and PGE_2 results in modification of glomerular injury, with a reduction in both glomerular hypercellularity and antibody deposition[104]. Similar results were seen in the NZB/NZW F_1 hybrid lupus mouse, in which the administration of either PGE_1 or iloprost (a synthetic prostaglandin analogue) at a stage of the disease when proteinuria was established resulted in amelioration of the disease[158]. In a model of anti-GBM nephritis the administration of 15(S)-15-methyl-PGE_1 resulted in a reduction in proteinuria and a decrease in glomerular hypercelluarity[114]. More recently this decrease in hypercelluarity has been shown to be linked to the suppression of macrophage infiltration in the glomerulus, with a consequent beneficial effect on glomerular damage[43].

FATTY ACID MANIPULATION AND RENAL DISEASE

The amelioration of glomerular injury by the manipulation of dietary fatty acids has been documented in a number of studies. Two distinct approaches have been employed: (1) diets deficient in essential fatty acids; (2) diets supplemented by polyunsaturated fatty acids. Although encouraging results have been demonstrated in certain disease models where a consistent improvement is seen, the overall picture remains confusing and the underlying mechanisms are unknown.

Essential fatty acid deficiency

In the NZB/NZW F_1 hybrid model of systemic lupus erythematosus (SLE), a diet deficient in essential fatty acids (EFA) prevented the development of glomerulonephritis and significantly improved the survival of the deficient animals[98]. Histologically there was a decrease in glomerular cellularity and a diminution in the deposition of IgG and IgM. More recently, in the nephrotoxic nephritis model, a diet deficient in essential fatty acids resulted in an 80% depletion of resident glomerular macrophages and limited the accumulation of macrophages within the glomerulus following nephrotoxic serum[195]. These changes were not due to an intrinsic defect in macrophage chemotaxis[189], but were possibly related to a decrease in glomerular chemoattractant generation[120,196]. The results in this nephrotoxic nephritis study are somewhat in contrast to earlier studies, where EFA deficiency failed to influence the hypercellularity of rats exposed to nephrotoxic serum[70]. The reason for the differences between these two studies is not clear. The earlier study demonstrated that the EFA deficient diet led to a 50% reduction in glomerular PGE_2 and PGI_2 production as well as a decrease in glomerular cell proliferation. There was, however, no depletion of glomerular macrophages either before or after exposure to nephrotoxic nephritis, nor was there a decrease in proteinuria in the diseased animals as was seen later in Lefkowith's study. One possible explanation for these differing results is the extent of the fatty acid depletion. The Dubois study used coconut oil (which contains mainly saturated fats) as the fatty acid supplement but Lefkowith used a strictly fat-free diet.

The net effect of fatty acid withdrawal is the depletion of arachidonic acid from the cell membrane. This results in a lack of available substrate for both cyclooxygenase and lipoxygenase pathways. Such an effect is clearly seen in fatty acid-deficient animals, since the capacity of isolated cells to synthesize cyclooxygenase products could be restored by supplementation with exogenous arachidonic acid[70,120]. In addition, there is an accumulation of mead acid in the membranes of fatty acid-deficient animals. This compound is unique to the fatty acid-deficient state since it is a poor substrate for either enzymatic pathway and will clearly influence the synthesis of fatty acid products. These studies demonstrate that the net effect of EFA deficiency is a decrease in the resident macrophage population of the glomerulus together with an inability by the animal to mount an adequate inflammatory response.

Polyunsaturated fatty acids

The effect of fish oil, on progressive renal disease has been studied most extensively in murine models of lupus nephritis. Diets supplemented with fish oil, substitute eicosapentaenoic (EPA) and other ω-3 (or N-3) polyunsaturated fatty acids for eicosatetraenoic acid (arachidonic acid) which is an ω-6 (N-6) fatty acid. In both the NZB/NZW F_1 hybrid and in the MRL-1pr mouse dietary supplementation with fish oil instead of safflower oil (linoleic acid and a precursor of arachidonic acid) suppressed the progression of renal injury and prolonged survival[106,173,187]. Indeed, in the NZB/NZW F_1 hybrid the addition of fish oil even after the appearance of proteinuria ameliorated the progression of the disease[174], indicating a therapeutic value of dietary intervention. Similar findings were reported when fish oil was administered in a rat nephrotoxic nephritis model[149], and in the immune complex model of renal disease induced by injections of apoferritin[108].

In models of chronic glomerulosclerosis, however, the benefit is less evident. In the uninephrectomized obese Zucker rat, fish oil supplements instigated at the time of surgery ameliorated the development of progressive renal disease (Wheeler et al., personal communication). Similarly, in the subtotal nephrectomy model[14] supplementation of chow with fish oil shortly after surgery delayed the onset of chronic renal failure. In contrast, the addition of fish oil to the diet of rats subjected to subtotal nephrectomy 6 weeks post-operatively was detrimental and accelerated the decline in renal function[193]. These results indicate that, in such a 'non-immune' model of renal disease, EPA supplementation, although it may have a protective role, does not have the same therapeutic effect as in models of glomerular injury that clearly involve immunological mechanisms.

The theoretical justification for the use of a diet rich in fish oil is that EPA serves as an alternative substrate for both the lipoxygenase and cyclooxygenase pathways (Figure 4). There is an overall reduction in the total amount of product and the resultant molecules are frequently much less active—in particular, LTB_5 is a significantly poorer chemoattractant than LTB_4, and TXA_3 does not aggregate platelets to one-tenth of the potency of TXA_2.

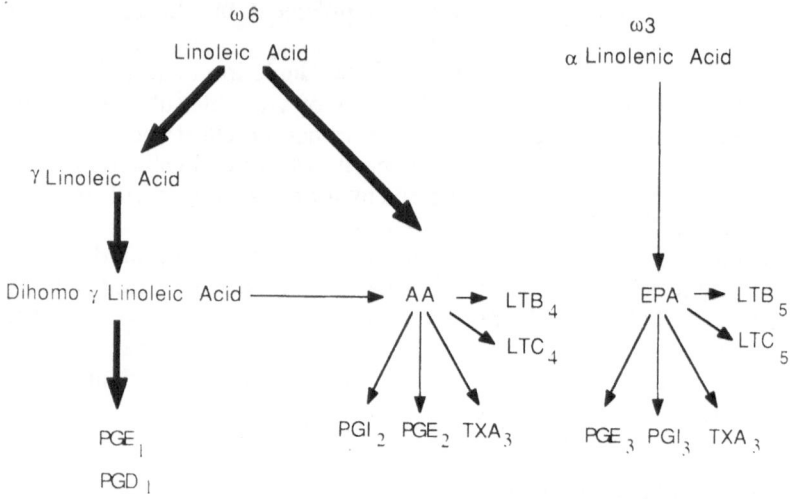

Figure 4 Polyunsaturated fatty acids and their relationships to eicosanoids

These observations would imply that in models of immune injury the decrease of pro-inflammatory mediators such as LTB_4 and TXA_2 is of significant influence in ameliorating the disease. In the established model of glomerulosclerosis, however, the presence of active vasodilatory molecules such as PGE_2 and PGI_2 is essential to maintaining renal function. Although PGE_3 and PGI_3 (products of EPA) are also vasoactive, the net total vasodilatory component is likely to be reduced in the EPA-treated animals, thus impairing the haemodynamic equilibrium of the remaining glomeruli and promoting a decline in renal function. Dietary manipulation of fatty acids is not, however, confined to fish oil supplementation, nor is the modulation of eicosanoid synthesis the only means whereby polyunsaturated fatty acids can exert their effects. Many physiological functions are influenced by polyunsaturated fatty acid supplementation: reduction in serum lipids[99], suppresion of cell proliferation[217], decrease in BP[96], and change in blood rheology[203], although the importance of these remains unexplained.

In the study in which Barcelli et al.[14] demonstrated that fish oil could prevent chronic glomerulosclerosis in the subtotal nephrectomy model, renal function was equally preserved in animals fed a diet rich in linoleic acid (safflower oil) or in linoleic acid plus gamma linolenic acid (evening primrose oil). The control group in this study, who demonstrated a progressive decline of renal function, was fed a diet of beef tallow, which is particularly rich in saturated fatty acids, e.g. oleic acid. Supplementation with linoleic acid was also beneficial in the appoferritin immune complex model[108]. In contrast, it had no effect on either the NZB/NZW F_1 hybrid mouse or the MRL-1pr mouse. The influence of dietary ω-6 fatty acids on glomerulonephritis is partly based on their effects on eicosanoid production. Similarly, linoleic and gamma linolenic acid are converted to dihomo-gamma linolenic acid, which serves as a substrate for the production of PGE_1, as well as being available for conversion to arachidonic acid (Figure 4). The preferential production of such a vasodilator compound in conditions where prostaglandins of the E series have an important role, both haemodynamically and in terms of immunoregulation, may clearly influence the outcome of the disease.

The relative importance of these mediators differs not only between disease models but also at varying times during the course of a single disease. Thus, a role for fatty acids, as either a preventative or a therapeutic manoeuvre, must be defined carefully with respect to the particular disease under consideration.

CYTOKINES IN EXPERIMENTAL NEPHRITIS

In vivo experiments with IL-1 and TNF

While tissue culture studies indicate a potential role for cytokines/growth factors in renal glomerular disease, it is less clear whether they exert a similar role *in vivo*. The gap between tissue culture and the *in vivo* situation has to some extent been bridged by experiments which demonstrated that macrophages isolated from animals with induced glomerular disease were activated to secrete several different types of pro-inflammatory products[51,144]. More pertinent, however, is the finding that homogenates of glomeruli removed from animals with immune-complex glomerulonephritis showed increased IL-1 gene expression[230], as did glomeruli from animals pretreated with non-toxic doses of TNF[40]. These increases in expression of the IL-1 gene must be seen in the light of the finding that quiescent human mesangial cells do not express IL-1 mRNA[137].

Some evidence that cytokines can initiate renal damage is now emerging from animal studies. In one study, the direct perfusion of TNF (8000 U/kg/h) over 5 hours induced a rise in serum creatinine[27]. The principal morphological changes observed were endothelial cell damage and the accumulation of neutrophils, together with some evidence of fibrin deposition. There was no significant proteinuria, and 24 hours after cessation of the infusion glomerular morphology had returned to normal. In a model of glomerular disease induced by anti-glomerular basement membrane antibody[221], LPS, IL-1 and TNF all enhanced the antibody-mediated injury, as demonstrated by a significant increase in albuminuria and the deposition of thrombi within the capillary wall. Anti-rat TNF antibodies significantly reduced the cytokine-induced proteinuria in animals treated with LPS, suggesting that TNF was involved in LPS-induced enhancement of glomerular injury in nephrotoxic nephritis in rats. The above animal model may explain the clinical observation that microbial infection in patients with established anti-GBM nephritis is associated with a deterioration in renal function in the absence of detectable circulating anti-GBM antibodies.

On the basis of the tissue culture studies described above and the limited data available to date from animal models of renal disease, it is apparent that the growth status of mesangial cells, and to a lesser extent of glomerular epithelial and endothelial cells, is influenced by a wide variety of cytokines. Furthermore, the same factors also control the production of the extracellular matrix, which in turn can promote growth of glomerular cells[79]. Initiation

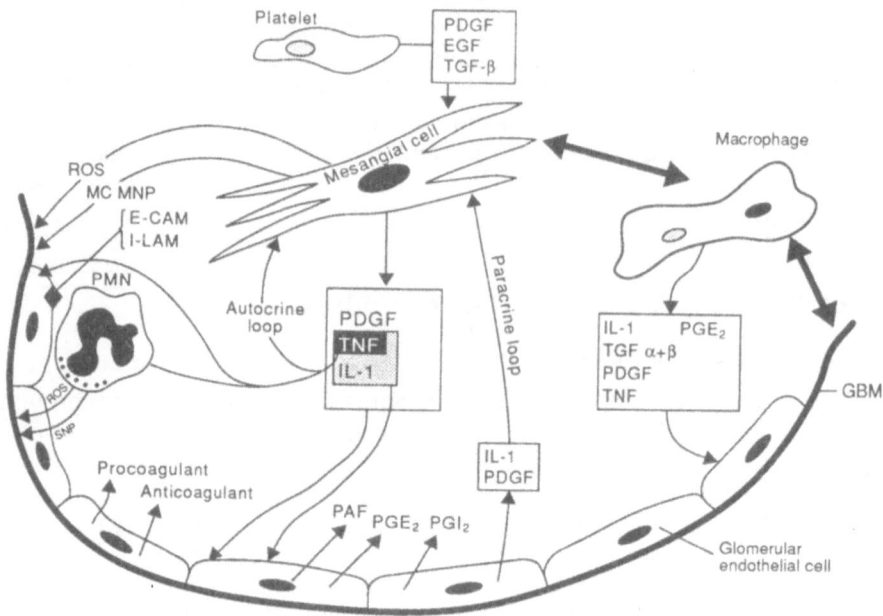

Figure 5 Cell–cell interaction relevant to glomerular vascular injury. In addition to abbreviations used in the text: ROS = reactive oxygen species; MC-MNP = mesangial cell metallo neutral proteinase; PMN = polymorphonuclear leukocytes; SNP = serine neutral proteinase (PMN-derived); PAF = platelet-activating factor; I-LAM = intracellular adhesion molecule-1; E-LAM = endothelium leukocyte adhesion molecule; ↔ denotes possible cell activation through direct contact of mesangial cell-MO and MO-GBM

of the events that control proliferation and matrix production by glomerular cells would appear to be a complex process requiring cell–cell interaction between the growth factor and specific cell surface receptors. A common feature of glomerular disease is the infiltration of extrinsic inflammatory cells. Platelets accumulate in some forms of renal disease[15] and platelet-related antigens have been localized within the glomerulus[38]. Activated platelets release PDGF, EGF and TGF-β and these could directly induce cell proliferation and matrix turnover. The involvement of macrophages is well established in acute and proliferative forms of nephritis, and their ability to respond to immune complexes, C5b-9 membrane attack complex, and bacterial products by the release of cytokines (TNF, IL-1, PDGF) could be important in the pathophysiology of kidney disease.

Although not discussed in detail in this review, the secretion of cytokines by macrophages may in addition be influenced by lymphokines derived from T lymphocytes. Since T lymphocytes have been recognized in certain forms of glomerulonephritis, a role for cell-mediated immunity in the release of mitogens is implicated.

Thus, activated glomerular cells produce growth factors that may have autocrine activity or act in a paracrine manner to stimulate the other cells of the glomerulus. A scheme to embrace most of these events and interactions is shown in Figure 5. Most, but not all, of the cell–cell interactions represented in the scheme and discussed in the text are up-regulatory and result in enhanced cell proliferation and/or the secretion of pro-inflammatory products. In contrast, TGF-β[139], and in one report IL-1[223], have a down-regulatory action. This suggests a role for cytokines in both positive and negative feedback mechanisms in glomerular cells. In addition, secretory products from glomerular epithelial cells (probably a heparan sulphate) can modulate the proliferative response of mesangial cells[41]. In other cell systems, cytokine-induced synthesis of proteins appears to be regulated by PGE$_2$ and cAMP[115,121,182]. Furthermore, in mouse macrophages the consumption of arginine and the production of ornithine, a metabolic pathway important for the induction of T cell-mediated immune response *in vivo*, is regulated by an autoregulatory loop which involves the PGE$_2$-dependent elevation of cAMP[121].

EICOSANOIDS AND HUMAN STUDIES

Elevation of urinary prostaglandins and thromboxane in patients with glomerular disease, as well as studies using non-steroidal anti-inflammatory agents, have provided evidence that eicosanoids have a role in human renal disease. The exact contribution of these molecules to the pathogenesis of individual diseases, however, requires careful analysis in any clinical study. The identification of a renal, as opposed to a systemic, origin for urinary prostaglandins is dependent on the recovery of unmetabolized molecules from the urine[82]. In addition, the PGE$_2$ content of seminal fluid confines precise studies of prostanoid synthesis and turnover to women[160]. The need for accuracy is emphasized by studies using the selective inhibition of extrarenal cyclooxygenase activity by sulindac or low-dose aspirin[162], which did not influence urinary secretion of either 6-keto-PGF$_{1\alpha}$ (the stable metabolite or prostacyclin) or TXB$_2$[44,161] but abolished the synthesis and excretion of 2,3-dinor-6-keto-PGF$_{1\alpha}$ and 2,3-dinor-TXB$_2$ — metabolites which therefore reflected systemic generation of PGI$_2$ and TXA$_2$ respectively.

The role for prostaglandins in the maintenance of glomerular function in normal fasting individuals is contentious. In an individual with a replete intravascular volume, prostaglandin inhibition does not influence either GFR or renal plasma flow[77]. A decrease in plasma volume or the depletion of total body sodium will, however, markedly increase the sensitivity of the kidneys to cyclooxygenase inhibitors, emphasizing the dependence of the stressed kidney on vasodilatory prostaglandins (Figure 3). In addition, under circumstances where there is diminished renal perfusion, e.g. in cardiac or hepatic failure, renal homeostasis depends on a balance between vasodilatory prostaglandins and vasoconstrictor molecules, including catecholamines, angiotensin II and vasopressin[71].

A role for prostaglandins in the maintenance of glomerular function in patients with renal impairment was initially proposed following the observation that indomethacin caused a significant decrease in renal function in patients with chronic renal disease[65]. More recently, a comparison of the non-steroidal anti-inflammatory drugs ibuprofen and sulindac in patients with chronic glomerulonephritis confirmed the dependence of glomerular function on an intact intrarenal cyclooxygenase system[44]. In particular, the inhibition of renal PGI_2 synthesis by ibuprofen correlated with a significant fall in both glomerular filtration rate and renal plasma flow. Furthermore, exposure of the same patients to sulindac, which spared the glomerular cyclooxygenase system, did not influence glomerular haemodynamics. The majority of non-steroidal anti-inflammatory drugs have been examined for their effect on urinary prostaglandin excretion and, with the exception of sulindac, renal cyclooxygenase is reduced by between 50 and 80% by all drugs of this class[164]. Of particular importance is the fact that sulindac does not influence cortical cyclooxygenase activity in the kidney, although it may reduce medullary PGE_2 synthesis[44,45,186,198]. The mechanisms of this renal sparing effect of sulindac are poorly understood but are possibly related to its redox pro-drug nature.

Renal selecivity is also exhibited by low-dose aspirin[159], and this is thought to be due to the different aspirin sensitivity of renal cyclooxygenase and to the irreversible nature of platelet cyclooxygenase inhibition compared to the relatively rapid turnover of glomerular cyclooxygenase.

The ability of cyclooxygenase inhibitors to reduce proteinuria in patients with the nephrotic syndrome has been known for some time[148]. The administration of indomethacin to patients with the nephrotic syndrome resulted in the simultaneous fall in glomerular filtration rate and in urinary protein excretion[66], and the mechanism of this event was attributed to the inhibition of prostaglandins[6]. The decrement in proteinuria, although accompanied by a fall in GFR, was not directly proportional to GFR and studies on the clearance of polyvinyl pyrole particles demonstrated a selectivity in their filtration. Particles of size greater than 4 nm units showed a decrease in fractional clearance, whereas the clearance of molecules of less than 4 nm was unaffected[219].

In a more recent study[83], the effect of indomethacin on dextran clearance was studied in 20 patients with the nephrotic syndrome. Although the fractional clearances of albumin and IgG were reduced by equal amounts, the clearance of neutral dextran followed a pattern seen earlier with polyvinyl pyrole. Indomethacin decreased the clearance of dextrans of radius 55–66 nm while it increased the fractional clearance of molecules of radius 2.8–3.8 nm. In the light of this observation, two mechanisms were proposed to explain the ability of cyclooxygenase inhibitors to reduce proteinuria in patients with nephrotic syndrome:

(1) Reduction in glomerular ultrafiltration pressure, being a combination of an increase in plasma osmotic pressure and a reduction in glomerular capillary hydraulic pressure;
(2) A change in the size selectivity of the filtration barrier.

Whether this is accomplished by a change within each nephron, or by the shunting of blood away from nephrons with a higher permeability for macromolecules, remains to be established. It does seem, however, that such changes are closely linked to cyclooxygenase inhibition, since they are common to all non-steroidal anti-inflammatory agents (other than sulindac), occur rapidly after drug administration, and are reversible when the agent is withdrawn.

A role for platelets?

The changes in glomerular function which occur in glomerulonephritis are not infrequently accompanied by the deposition of platelets and fibrin within the glomerular vasculature. Although it has been argued that intraglomerular coagulation is merely the result rather than the cause of glomerular damage[32], a role for the platelet in the progression of glomerular disease has been proposed[37,46].

In their consideration of glomerular injury, the scheme proposed by Purkerson[177] (Figure 6) demonstrates how platelets might be involved in the pathogenesis of glomerular sclerosis. While the validity of this hypothesis in relation to the specific model used has been questioned[233], platelet endothelial interaction may play an important role in the progression of renal disease. It would therefore seem logical to examine the role of platelets in a disease where secretion of urinary thromboxane is known to be increased. In patients with SLE, urinary thromboxane levels are indeed elevated, and on careful examination this increase appears to be due to intrarenal synthesis of the eicosanoid. The urinary excretion of 2,3-dinor-TXB$_2$ is unchanged[163],

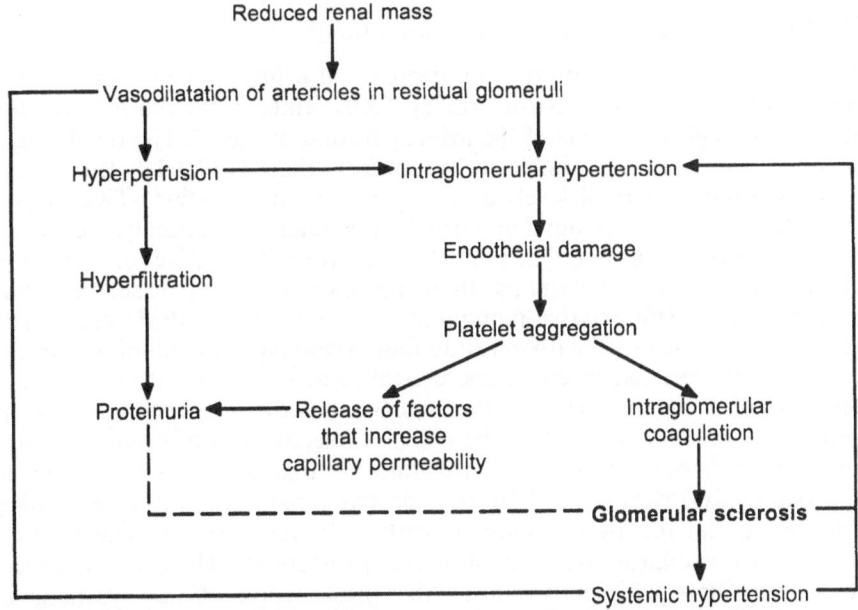

Figure 6 Proposed scheme for pathogenesis of the progressive glomerulosclerosis that occurs in rats with subtotal renal ablation and postulated sites of different interventions known to ameliorate the progression of the renal disease. (Reproduced with permission from Purkerson et al.[177])

indicating that systemic production of thromboxane is not elevated in this disease. In addition, the selective inhibition of platelet cyclooxygenase by low-dose aspirin in patients with SLE over a 4-week period, although causing a significant change in haemostasis, did not influence glomerular haemodynamics nor did it reduce the output of renal TXB_2 [168]. These results suggest that platelets do not play an active role in glomerular haemodynamics in this group of patients. Nevertheless, since glomerular thrombi occur in more than 50% of patients with severe lupus nephritis, and as platelets may serve as a source of growth factors such as PDGF and EGF as well as mediators such as platelet-activating factor, their potential role in chronic glomerular damage cannot be discounted[26].

Indeed, anti-platelet therapy in a group of patients with mesangial proliferative glomerulonephritis significantly slowed the deterioration of renal function[63]. Forty patients were treated for one year in a randomized double-blind placebo-controlled study with dipyramidole (225 mg/day). Patients receiving anti-platelet therapy showed a significant decrease in the rate of decline of function, although proteinuria remained unchanged. Furthermore, a 7-year follow-up demonstrated a significantly greater number of placebo-treated patients reaching end-stage therapy than patients who received anti-platelet drugs. Although the effect of aspirin on glomerular cyclooxygenase was not reviewed in this group, and further studies are required to support these findings, long-term inhibition of platelet function may have a role in the treatment of progressive renal disease.

Role of thromboxane in glomerular injury

Patients with SLE, in addition to a decrease in urinary 6-keto-$PGF_{1\alpha}$, also exhibit a significant increase in urinary TXB_2. Indeed, the more active the disease, the higher the level of the urinary thromboxane[163]. The renal origin of this thromboxane is confirmed by the facts that (1) platelets from these patients produce normal levels of TXB_2; (2) urinary 2,3-dinor-TXB_2 levels are no higher than those found in normal individuals. Interestingly, the kidney seems to depend for haemodynamic balance more on the relative concentration of vasodilatory prostaglandins than on high levels of vasoconstrictor prostaglandins. This relative functional preponderance of PGI_2 and PGE_2 has been confirmed by the observation that cyclooxygenase inhibition results in an overall decrease in creatinine clearance as well as renal plasma flow. The role of TXB_2 in this condition cannot, however, be ignored since its importance was highlighted by the use of a selective thromboxane receptor antagonist[169]. Short-term administration of this antagonist resulted in approximately 25% rise in GFR and effective renal plasma flow, indicating that glomerular function in patients with SLE was partly dependent on a balance of vasodilator and vasoconstrictor prostanoids. Thus, it would seem that in patients with active lupus the preservation of the synthesis of vasodilatory prostaglandins is essential, but that the inhibition of thromboxane synthesis may, at least in the short term, be beneficial in terms of improving glomerular haemodynamics. Any possible long-term benefits of the inhibition of thromboxane function require further investigation.

146

A role for thromboxane in the pathogenesis of proteinuria has also received some attention. A recent study in patients with nephrotic syndrome using a selective TXA_2 inhibitor showed a mean 50% decrease in urinary protein excretion and a concomitant rise in plasma albumin[153]. These results were complementary to a previous study in a small group of diabetic patients, where a thromboxane synthase inhibitor significantly reduced urinary albumin excretion rates[16]. In neither study was the inhibition of thromboxane accompanied by any change in glomerular haemodynamics.

It would at this point seem appropriate to examine the possible mechanisms whereby the activity of thromboxane might be modulated, and to compare the relative merits of synthase inhibition and receptor blockade[155]. The inhibition of thromboxane through the use of thromboxane synthase inhibitor results in the accumulation of endoperoxides both intra- and extracellularly. Although these are unstable compounds with relatively short half-lives, they increase the substrate pool for other eicosanoids. Thus in a cell such as the macrophage, which has more than one cyclooxygenase end product, there may be an increase in the synthesis of PGE_2 and PGI_2. In the platelet, in contrast, the excess endoperoxide may be released into the extracellular space and be taken up by the vascular endothelium, increasing the output of PGI_2 from this cell[192]. Thus, in addition to an inhibition of TXA_2 synthesis there is a shift in the balance towards vasodilatory and anti-aggregatory molecules[154]. It has also been suggested that the accumulation of endoperoxide may partly negate the effects of an inhibitor, since endoperoxides cross-react with the thromboxane receptor, resulting in partial end organ activation[140].

The use of a specific receptor antagonist, on the other hand, clearly overcomes the problem of endoperoxide accumulation, but does not have the advantage of supplementing the vasodilatory prostanoids. As a result of this, such receptor antagonists would not increase thromboxane-independent anti-inflammatory molecules and would have limited use in platelet-dependent injury. It has therefore been proposed that use of a synthetase inhibitor together with a receptor blocker would represent a more rational approach to treatment. To this end, synergistic effects on platelet function of using such a combination have been demonstrated in normal volunteers[88].

DIETARY FATTY ACID MANIPULATION AND HUMAN RENAL DISEASE

Epidemiological studies have demonstrated that diets rich in ω-3 polyunsaturated fatty acids correlate with a low incidence of cardiovascular disease, asthma, rheumatoid arthritis and diabetes mellitus[112,113]. In addition, supplementation of a normal diet of fish oil results in a modification of plasma lipids and a reduction in resting blood pressure[85,90,204]. The mechanism of such changes is poorly understood, but in those conditions characterized by a tissue inflammatory response the modification of eicosanoids by a change in the fatty acid substrate is thought to play an important role. In normal individuals, ω-3 fatty acid supplementation results in a decrease in neutrophil chemotaxis and impairment of synthesis of products of 5-lipoxygenase[119]. In addition, the incorporation of such fatty acids into cell membranes is

147

accompanied by a significant fall in PGE_2 production and in the capacity of monocytes to synthesize IL-1 and TNF in response to endotoxin[76]. This alteration in cytokine synthesis is as yet unexplained; but may relate to a modification in eicosanoid production since exogenous LTB_4 can enhance endotoxin-stimulated IL-1 production. The concomitant reduction of LTB_4 in individuals on a fish oil diet may reduce the ability of the monocyte to respond to endotoxin.

Thus, the capacity of fish oil to modulate cytokine production as well as eicosanoid synthesis would indicate its potential value in the treatment of renal disease. Indeed, the addition of fish oil to the diet of 10 healthy volunteers resulted in a significant increase in both renal plasma flow and glomerular filtration rate in the absence of a change in blood pressure. In view of the lack of effect of cyclooxygenase inhibitors on normal renal function, it is unlikely that the changes in response to fish oil can be accounted for by changes in eicosanoids alone, although a change in the balance of dilator versus constrictor eicosanoids may potentiate such an effect[72]. The same authors also examined the effect of fish oil on the renal response to a high-protein meal in patients with impaired renal function, and demonstrated an increase in GFR and effective renal plasma flow as well as a decrease in the total renal vascular resistance[191].

Few studies have been conducted in patients with defined glomerulopathies. A small study in patients with active lupus nephritis demonstrated that EPA supplementation resulted in a decrease in quantitative urinary red cell casts and this was taken as an improvement of renal histological activity. Interestingly, in this group of patients there was also a significant fall in GFR during the course of EPA therapy which was reversed when the fish oil was withdrawn[117]. Conflicting studies have been reported in patients with IgA nephropathy, where EPA apparently slowed the progression of the disease in one group of patients[89] but made no difference to a similar group in a separate study[24]. More recently, a pilot study in 11 patients with mesangial IgA nephropathy demonstrated a decrease in proteinuria and improved renal fucntion[64]. It is worth noting that in the second of these studies EPA did not appear to have an adverse effect on renal haemodynamics.

Thus, the results of fish oil supplementation remain far from conclusive. Further studies are required in both the acute and the chronic stages of particular diseases.

CYTOKINES AND HUMAN DISEASE

A defined role for cytokines in the pathogenesis of human disease remains speculative. An increased capacity for cytokine production is often seen in monocytes isolated from patients with sepsis[23,227], whereas decreased levels are reported from patients with SLE and other systemic immunological conditions[128]. There is accumulating evidence of increased circulating levels of these molecules in defined diseases, for example raised TNF, IL-1 and IL-2 levels in renal allograft rejection, raised IL-6 in burns patients, and raised TNF in *Neisseria* meningitis. Most recently, the examination of a group of patients with nephrotic syndrome revealed a 5-fold increase in circulating levels of TNF compared with normals, but no change in IL-1, IL-2, interferon-α and interferon-γ[216]. More recently a role for IL-6 in renal disease has been suggested[238]. Transgenic mice carrying the human IL-6 gene fused with a human immunoglobulin heavy chain not only developed myeloma, but also mesangial proliferative glomerulonephritis. It has also been recently shown that patients with mesangial proliferative glomerulonephritis secrete significantly raised levels of urinary IL-6[239]. In a separate study[240] there was a selective increase in urinary IL-6 in patients with mesangial proliferative and focal segmental glomerulosclerosis but not in individuals with membranous nephropathy or minimal change disease, suggesting a selective role for this particular molecule. A fundamental role for cytokines in the initial pathogenic events of glomerulonephritis remains unproven.

The exacerbation of immunologically mediated renal disease during episodes of superadded infection is well established[172,183]. This may be partly explained by the observation that circulating TNF levels are elevated in human volunteers injected with endotoxin[147]. Such a phenomenon is well documented in patients with glomerulonephritis, in which intercurrent infection results in a marked deterioration in renal function. The direct cause-and-effect link, however, will require studies into either specific inhibitors or receptor antagonists to the cytokines in question.

CONCLUSION

There is little doubt that products of the cyclooxygenase pathway become involved in preserving the 'status quo' of glomerular function during periods of stress. Their importance is increased during disease states where significant inhibition of vasodilatory molecules may contribute to a loss of glomerular filtration. A role for thromboxane and products of the 5-lipoxygenase pathway remains hypothetical, although the availability of specific enzyme inhibitors and receptor antagonists will shortly allow a more critical approach and permit a better understanding of the role of such molecules in disease states.

Similarly, a role for TNF and IL-1 in clinical disease continues to gain support. There is ample evidence that cytokines and growth factors have the potential to be involved in the control of glomerular cell turnover, matrix production and protein synthesis, as well as in modulating the pathogenesis of established diseases. What is less certain is whether the documented changes are due to direct effects of cytokines or whether they represent the cumulative effect of a number of mediators acting synergistically to augment the underlying disease process.

References

1. Aaron, P. E., Webb, A. C., Rosenwasse, L. J., Mucci, S. F., Rich, A., Wolff, S. M. and Dinarello, C. A. (1984). Nucleotide sequence of human monocyte interleukin-1 precursor cDNA. *Proc. Natl Acad. Sci. USA*, **81**, 7907–7911
2. Abboud, H. E., Poptic, E. and Dicorleto, P. (1987). Production of platelet-derived growth factor-like protein by rat mesangial cells in culture. *J. Clin. Invest.*, **80**, 675–683

3. Altboum, I., Boswell, J. and Kelley, V. E. (1987). Thromboxane production by activated renal cortical macrophages. *Kidney Int.*, **31**, 257 (A)

4. Ardaillou, N., Hagege, J., Nivez, M. P., Ardaillou, R. and Schlöndorff, D. (1985). Vasoconstrictor evoked prostaglandin synthesis in cultured human mesangial cells. *Am. J. Physiol.*, **248**, F240–F246

5. Ardaillou, R., Baud, L. and Sraer, J. (1988). Leukotrienes and reactive oxygen species as mediators of glomerular injury. *Am. J. Nephrol.*, **9** (suppl. 1), 17–22

6. Arisz, L., Donker, A. J. M., Brentjend, J. R. H. and van der Hem, G. K. (1976). The effect of indomethacin on proteinuria and kidney function in the nephrotic syndrome. *Acta Med. Scand.*, **199**, 121–125

7. Badr, K. F., Bayliuss, C., Pfeffer, J. M., Pfeffer, M. A., Soberman, R. J., Lewis, R. A., Austen, K. F., Corey, E. J. and Brenner, B. M. (1984). Renal and systemic haemodynamic responses to intravenous infusion of leukotriene C_4 in the rat. *Circ. Res.*, **54**, 492–499

8. Badr, K. F., Kelley, V. E., Rennke, H. G. and Brenner, B. M. (1986). Roles of thromboxane A_2 and leukotrienes in endotoxin-induced acute renal failure. *Kidney Int.*, **30**, 474–480

9. Badr, K. F., Brenner, B. M., Wasserman, M. and Ighikawa, I. (1986). Evidence for local glomerular actions of LTD_4. *Kidney Int.*, **29**, 328(A)

10. Badr, K. F., Schreiner, G. F., Wasserman, M. and Ighikawa, I. (1986). Preservation of the glomerular capillary ultrafiltration coefficient during rat nephrotoxic serum nephritis by a specific leukotriene D_4 receptor antagonist. *J. Clin. Invest.*, **81**, 1702–1709

11. Balkwill, F. R. and Burke, FR. (1989). The cytokine network. *Immunol. Today*, **10**, 299–304

12. Ballerman, B. J., Lewis, R. A., Corey, E. J., Austen, K. F. and Brenner, B. M. (1985). Identification and characterisation of leukotriene C_4 receptor in isolated rat renal glomeruli. *Circulation Res.*, **56**, 324–330

13. Ballermann, B. J. (1989). Regulation of bovine glomerular endothelial cell growth *in vitro*. *Am. J. Physiol.*, **256**, C182–C189

14. Barcelli, U., Miyata, J., Ito, Y., Gallon, L., Laskarzewski, P., Weiss, M., Hitzemann, R. and Pollack, V. E. (1986). Beneficial effects of polyunsaturated fatty acids in partially nephrectomized rats. *Prostaglandins*, **32**, 211–219

15. Barnes, J. C. and Venkatchalam, M. A. (1985). The role of platelets and polycationic mediators in glomerular vascular injury. *Semin. Nephrol.*, **5**, 57–68

16. Barnett, A. H., Leatherdale, B. A., Polak, A., Toop, M., Wakelin, K., Britton, J. R., Bennett, J., Rowe, D. and Dallinger, R. (1984). Specific thromboxane synthase inhibition and AER in insulin dependent diabetics. *Lancet*, **1**, 1322–1324

17. Barnett, R., Goldwasser, P., Scharschmidt, C. A. and Schlöndorff, D. (1986). Effects of luekotrienes on isolated rat glomeruli and cultured mesangial cells. *Am. J. Physiol.*, **250**, 838–844

18. Baud, L., Sraer, J., Perez, J., Nivez, M. P. and Ardaillou, R. (1985). Leukotriene C4 binds to human glomerular epithelial cells and promotes their proliferation in vitro. *J. Clin. Invest.*, **76**, 374–377

19. Baud, L., Sraer, J., Delarue, F., Bens, M., Balavoine, F., Schlondorff, D., Ardaillou, R. and Sraer, J-D. (1985). Lipoxygenase products mediate attachment of rat macrophages to glomeruli *in vitro*. *Kidney Int.*, **27**, 855–863

20. Baud, L., Perez, J., Friedlander, G. and Ardaillou, R. (1988). Tumour necrosis factor stimulates prostaglandin production and cyclic AMP levels in rat cultured mesangial cells. *FEBS*, **239**, 50–54

21. Baud, L., Oudinet, J-P., Bens, M., Noe, L., Peraldi, M-N., Rondeau, E., Etienne, J. and Ardaillou, R. (1989). Production of tumour necrosis factor by rat mesangial cells in response to bacterial lipopolysaccharide. *Kidney Int.*, **35**, 1111–1118

22. Benabe, J. E., Klahr, S., Hoffmann, M. K. and Mamsai, A. R. (1980). Production of thromboxane A_2 by the kidney in glycerol-induced acute renal failure in the rabbit. *Prostaglandins*, **19**, 333–347

23. Bendtzen, K., Baek, J., Berild, D., Haselbach, H., Dinarello, C. A. and Wolff, S. M. (1984). Demonstration of circulating leucocyte pyrogen/interleukin-1 during fever. *N. Engl J. Med.*, **310**, 596

24. Bennett, W. M., Walker, R. G. and Kincaid-Smith, P. (1989). Treatment of IgA nephropathy with eicosapentaenoic acid: a two-year prospective trial. *Clin. Nephrol.*, **31**, 128–131

25. Bertani, T., Benigni, A., Cutillo, F., Rocchi, G., Morelli, C., Carminatti, C., Verroust, P. and Remuzzi, G. (1986). Effect of aspirin and sulindac in rabbit nephrotoxic nephritis. *J.*

Lab. Clin. Med., **107**, 261–268

26. Bertani, T., Livio, M., Macconi, D., Morigi, M., Bisogno, G., Patrono, C. and Remuzzi, G. (1987). Platelet activating factor as a mediator of injury in nephrotoxic nephritis. *Kidney Int.*, **31**, 1248–1256

27. Bertani, T., Abbate, M., Zoja, C., Corna, D., Perico, N., Ghezzi, P. and Remuzzi, G. (1989). Tumour necrosis factor induces glomerular damage in the rabbit. *Am. J. Pathol.*, **134**, 419–430

28. Beutler, B. and Cerami, A. (1985). Recombinant interleukin-1 suppresses lipoprotein lipase activity in 3T3 cells. *J. Immunol.*, **135**, 3969–3971

29. Beutler, B. and Cerami, A. (1988). Tumour necrosis, cachexia, shock, and inflammation: a common mediator. *Ann. Rev. Biochem.*, **57**, 505–518

30. Bird, T. A. and Saklatvala, J. (1986). Identification of a common class of high affinity receptors for both types of porcine interferon-1 on connective tissue cells. *Nature*, **324**, 263–266

31. Bird, T. A. and Saklatvala, J. (1987). Studies on the fate of receptor-bound ^{125}I-interleukin β in procine synovial fibroblasts. *J. Immunol.*, **139**, 92–97

32. Border, W. A. (1984). Anticoagulants are of little value in the treatment of renal disease. *Am. J. Kidney Dis.*, **3**, 308–312

33. Bowen-Pope, D. F., Dicorleto, P. E. and Ross, R. (1983). Interaction between the receptors for platelet-derived growth factor and epidermal growth factor. *J. Cell. Biol.*, **96**, 679–683

34. Brenner, B. M., Meyer, T. W. and Hostetter, T. H. (1982). Dietary protein intake and the progressive nature of kidney disease: the role of haemodynamically mediated injury in the pathogenesis of progressive glomerular sclerosis in ageing, renal ablation and intrinsic renal disease. *N. Engl J. Med.*, **307**, 652–659

35. Brunda, M. J., Heberman, R. B. and Holden, H. T. (1980). Inhibition of murine natural killer cell activity by prostaglandins. *J. Immunol.*, **124**, 2682–2687

36. Burstein, S. L., Locksley, R. M., Ryan, J. L. and Lovett, D. H. (1988). Acylation of monocytic and glomerular mesangial cell proteins. *J. Clin. Invest.*, **82**, 1479–1488

37. Cameron, J. S. (1984). Platelets in glomerular disease. *Ann. Rev. Med.*, **35**, 175–180

38. Camussi, G., Tetta, G., Mazzucco, G., Monga, G., Roffinello, C., Alberton, M., Dellabona, P., Malavasi, F. and Vercellone, A. (1986). Platelet cationic proteins are present in glomeruli of lupus nephritis patients. *Kidney Int.*, **30**, 555–565

39. Carpenter, G. and Cohen, S. (1979). Epidermal growth factor. *Annu. Rev. Biochem.*, **48**, 193–216

40. Cashman, S. J., Koshino, Y., Tomosgui, N. and Rees, A. J. (1989). Induction of glomerular interleukin-1β gene expression after liposaccharide (LPS) or tumour necrosis factor. *7th International Congress on Immunology*, Berlin.

41. Castellot, J. J., Hoover, R. L., Harper, P. A. and Karnovsky, M. J. (1985). Heparin and glomerular epithelial cell-secreted heparin like species inhibit mesangial cell proliferation. *Am. J. Pathol.*, **120**, 427–435

42. Cattell, V., Cook, H. T., Smith, J., Salmon, J. A. and Moncada, S. (1987). Leukotriene B$_4$ production in normal rat glomeruli. *Nephrol. Dial. Transplant.*, **2**, 154–157

43. Cattell, V., Smith, J. and Cook, H. T. (1989). Prostaglandin E$_1$ (PGE$_1$) suppresses macrophage infiltration and ameliorates injury in accelerated nephrotoxic nephritis. *Abstracts of the Renal Association*, Spring 1989

44. Ciabattoni, G., Cinotti, G. A., Pierucci, A., Simonetti, B. M., Manzi, M., Pugliese, F., Barsotti, P., Pecci, G., Taggi, F. and Patrono, C. (1984). Effects of sulindac and ibuprofen in patients with chronic glomerular disease. Evidence for the dependence of renal function on prostacyclin. *N. Engl. J. Med.*, **310**, 279–283

45. Ciabattoni, G., Boss, A. H., Patrignani, P., Catella, F., Simonetti, B. M., Pierucci, A., Pugliese, F., Filabozzi, P. and Patrono, C. (1987). Effects of sulindac on renal and extrarenal eicosanoid synthesis. *Clin. Pharmacol. Ther.*, **41**, 380–383

46. Clarke, W. F., Friesen, M., Linton, A. L. and Lindsay, R. M. (1976). The platelet as a mediator of tissue damage in immune complex nephritis. *Clin. Nephrol.*, **6**, 287–289

47. Clemmons, D. R., Van Wyk, J. J. and Pledger, W. J. (1980). Sequential addition of platelet factor and plasma to BA1B/3T3 fibroblasts in cultures stimulates somatomedin C-binding early in the cycle. *Proc. Natl Acad. Sci. USA*, **77**, 6644–6648

48. Collins, D. M., Coffman, T. M., Ruiz, P. and Klotman, P. (1989). High protein feeding stimulates renal thromboxane production in the diabetic rat. *Kidney Int.*, **35**, 425(A)

49. Conti, P., Cifone, M. G., Alesse, E., Reale, M., Fieschi, C. and Dinarello, C. A. (1986). *In vitro* enhanced thromboxane B$_2$ release by polymorphonuclear leukocytes and macrophages

after treatment with human recombinant interleukin-1 and tumour necrosis factor. *Prostaglandins*, **32**, 111–115

50. Cook, H. T., Cattell, V., Smith, J., Salmon, J. A. and Moncada, S. (1986). Effect of a thromboxane synthetase inhibitor on eicosanoid synthesis and glomerular injury during acute unilateral glomerulronephritis in the rat. *Clin. Nephrol.*, **26**, 195–202

51. Cook, H. T., Smith, J., Salmon, J. A. and Cattell, V. (1989). Functional characteristics of macrophages in glomerulonephritis in the rat. *Am. J. Pathol.*, **134**, 431–437

52. Cotran, R. S. and Pober, J. S. (1989). Effects of cytokines on vascular endothelium: Their role in vascular and immune injury. *Kidney Int.*, **35**, 967–975

53. Cybulsky, A. V., Lieberthal, W., Quigg, R. J., Renke, H. G. and Salant, D. J. (1987). A role for thromboxane in complement-mediated glomerular injury. *Am. J. Pathol.*, **128**, 45–51

54. D'Ercole, A. J. (1987). Somatomedins/insulin-like growth factors and foetal growth. *J. Dev,. Physiol.*, **9**, 481–495

55. Davies, M., Barrett, A. J., Travis, I., Sanders, E. and Coles, G. A. (1978). The degradation of human glomerular basement membrane with purified lysosomal proteinases. *Clin. Sci. Mol. Med.*, **54**, 233–240

56. Davies, M., Coles, G. A. and Harber, M. J. (1984). Effect of glomerular basement membrane on the initation of chemiluminescence and lysosomal enzyme release in human polynuclear leucotyes: an *in vitro* model of glomerular disease. *Immunology*, **52**, 151–159

57. Davies, M., Thomas, G. J., Martin, J. and Lovett, D. H. (1988). The purification and characterization of a glomerular basement membrane degrading neutral proteinase from rat mesangial cells. *Biochem. J.*, **251**, 419–425

58. Davies, M., Shewring, L., Thomas, G. and Jenner, L. (1989). Stimulation of proteoglycan synthesis in rat mesangial cells in response to tumour necrosis factor. *Clin. Sci.*, **76**, (suppl. 20), 25(A)

59. Davies, P., Bonney, R. J., Humes, J. L. and Kuehl, F. A. (1981). Secretory function of macrophages participating in inflammatory reactionary responses. In Dingle, J. T. and Gordon, J. L. (eds.) *Cellular International*, pp. 32–42. (Amsterdam: Elsevier–North Holland)

60. Deen, W. M., Maddox, D. A., Robertson, C. R. and Brenner, B. M. (1974). Dynamics of glomerular ultrafiltration in the rat: VII. Response to reduced renal mass. *Am. J. Physiol.*, **227**, 556–562

61. Dinarello, C. A. (1988). Biology of interleukin-1. *FASEB J.*, **2**, 108–115

62. Dinarello, C. A. (1988). Interleukin-1 and its biologically related cytokines. *Ann. Rev. Immunol.*, **44**, 153–205

63. Donadio, J. V., Anderson, C. F., Mitchell, J. C., Holley, K. E., Ilstrup, D. M., Fuster, V. and Chesibro, J. H. (1984). Membranoproliferative glomerulonephritis. A prospective clinical trial of platelet-inhibitory therapy. *N. Engl. J. Med.*, **310**, 1421–1426

64. Donadio, J. V., Holman, R. T., Holub, B. J. and Bergstrain, E. J. (1990). Effects of omega (ω)-3 polyunsaturated fatty acids (PUFA) in mesangial IgA nephropathy. *Kidney Int.*, **37**, 255(A)

65. Donker, A. J. M., Arisz, L., Brentjens, J. R. H., Hem, G. K. van der and Hollemans, H. J. G. (1976). The effect of indomethacin on kidney function and plasma renin activity in man. *Nephron*, **17**, 288–296

66. Donker, A. J. M., Brentjens, J. R. H., Hem, G. K. van der and Arisz, L. (1978). Treatment of the nephrotic syndrome with indomethacin. *Nephron*, **22**, 374–381

67. Dower, S. K., Kronheim, S. R., Hepp, T. P., Contrell, M., Deeley, M., Gillis, S., Henney, C. S. and Urdal, D. L. (1986). The cell surface receptors for interleukin-1α and β are identical. *Nature*, **324**, 266–268

68. Dower, S. K. and Urdal, D. L. (1987). The interleukin-1 receptor. *Immunol. Today*, **8**, 46–51

69. Dubois, C. H., Goffinet, G., Foidart, J. B., Dechenne, C. A., Foidart, J. M. and Mathieu, P. R. (1982). Evidence for a particular binding capacity of rat peritoneal macrophages to rat glomerular mesangial cells *in vitro*. *Eur. J. Clin. Invest.*, **12**, 239–246

70. Dubois, C. H., Foidart, J. B., Dechenne, C. A. and Mahieu, P. R. (1982). Effects of a diet deficient in essential fatty acids on the glomerular hypercellularity occurring in the course of nephrotoxic serum nephritis in rats. *Kidney Int.*, **21**, 539–545

71. Dunn, M. J. and Zambraski, E. J. (1980). Renal effects of drugs that inhibit prostacyclin synthesis. *Kidney Int.*, **18**, 609–622

72. Dusing, R., Struck, A., Scherf, H., Pietsch, R. and Kramer, H. J. (1987). Dietary fish oil supplements: Effect on renal hemodynamic and renal excretory function in healthy

volunteers. *Kidney Int.*, **31**, 268(A)

73. Ek, B. and Heldin, C. H. (1983). Characterization of a tyrosine-specific kinase activity in human fibroblast membranes stimulated by platelet-derived growth factor. *J. Biol. Chem.*, **257**, 10486–10492

74. Elias, J. A., Gustilio, K., Baeder, W. and Freundlich, B. (1987). Synergistic stimulation of fibroblast prostaglandin production by recombinant interleukin-1 and tumour necrosis factor. *J. Immunol.*, **138**, 3812–3816

75. Endou, H. (1983). Cytochrome P450 monoxygenase system in the rabbit kidney; its intranephron localisation and its induction. *Jpn J. Pharmacol.*, **33**, 423–433

76. Endres, S., Ghorbani, R., Kelley, V. E., Georgilis, K., Lonneman, G., Meer, J. W. M. van der, Cannon, J. G., Rogers, T. S., Klemper, M. S., Weber, P. C., Schaefer, E. J., Wolff, S. M. and Dinarello, C. A. (1989). The effects of dietary supplementation with n-3 polyunsaturated fatty acids on the synthesis of interleukin-1 and tumour necrosis factor by mononuclear cells. *N. Engl J. Med.*, **320**, 265–271

77. Epstein, M. and Lifshiftz, M. D. (1980). Volume status as a determinant of the influence of renal PGE on renal function. *Nephron*, **25**, 157–159

78. Foellmer, H. G., Sterzel, R. B. and Kashgarian, M. (1986). Progressive glomerulosclerosis in experimental anti-glomerular basement membrane glomerulonephritis. *Am. J. Kidney Dis.*, **7**, 5–11

79. Foellmer, H. G., Perfetto, M., Kashgarian, M. and Sterzel, R. B. (1987). Matrix constituents promote adhesion and proliferation in glomerular mesangial cells in culture. *Kidney Int.*, **31**, 318(A)

80 Folkart, V. W. and Schlöndorff, D. (1979). Prostaglandic synthesis in isolated glomeruli. *Prostaglandins*, **17**, 79–86

81. Friedlander, G., Chansel, D., Sraer, J., Bens, M. and Ardaillou, R. (1983). PGE_2 binding sites and PG-stimulated cyclic AMP accumulation in rat isolated glomeruli and glomerular cultured cells. *Mol. Cell. Endocrinol.*, **30**, 201–214

82. Frolich, J. C., Wilson, T. W., Sweetman, B. J., Smigel, M., Nies, A. S., Carr, K., Watson, J. T. and Oates, J. A. (1975). Urinary prostaglandins; identification and origin. *J. Clin. Invest.*, **55**, 763–770

83. Golbetz, H., Black, V., Shemesh, O. and Myers, B. D. (1989). Mechanism of the antiproteinuria effect of indomethacin in nephrotic humans. *Am. J. Physiol.*, **255**, F44–F51

84. Goodwin, J. S. and Cuppens, J. (1983). Regulation of the immune response by prostaglandins. *J. Clin. Immunol.*, **3**, 295–315

85. Gorlin, R. (1988). The biological actions and potential clinical significance of dietary ω-3 fatty acids. *Arch. Intern. Med.*, **148**, 2034–2048

86. Gospodarowicz, D., Neufeld, G. and Schweiggerer, L. (1987). Fibroblast growth factor: structural and biological properties. *J. Cell. Physiol.*, *Supplement 5*, 15–26

87. Grenier, F. C., Rollins, T. E. and Smith, W. L. (1981). Kinin induced prostaglandin synthesis by renal papillary collecting tubule cells in culture. *Am. J. Physiol.*, **241**, 94–104

88. Gresele, P., Arnout, J., Deckmyn, H., Huybrechts, E., Pieters, G. and Vermyhan, J. (1987). Role of pro-aggregatory and anti-aggregatory prostaglandins in hemostasis studies with combine thromboxane synthase inhibition and thromboxane receptor antagnoism. *J. Clin. Invest.*, **80**, 1435–1445

89. Hamazaki, T., Tateno, S. and Shishido, H. (1984). Eicosapentaenoic acid and IgA nephropathy. *Lancet*, **1**, 1017–1018

90. Hamazaki, T., Nakazawa, R., Tateno, S., Shishido, H., Isoda, K., Kattori, Y., Yoshida, T., Fujita, T., Yano, S. and Kumagai, A. (1984). Effects of fish oil rich in eicosapentaenoic acid on serum in hyperlipidemic hemodialysis patients. *Kidney Int.*, **26**, 81–84

91. Hamblin, A. S. (1988). Lymphokines and interleukins. *Immunology*, *Supplement 1*, 39–41

92. Hannink, M. and Donoghue, D. J. (1989). Structure and function of platelet-derived growth factor (PDGF) and related proteins. *Biochim. Biophys. Acta*, **989**, 1–10

93. Hänsch, G-M., Torbohm, I., Kempis, J. and Rother, K. (1988). Modulation of collagen synthesis in glomerular epithelial cells by interleukin-1 and the supernatants of mesangial cells. *Kidney Int.*, **33**, 317(A)

94. Harry, T. R., Hughes, K. T. and Davies, M. (1980). The secretion of neutral proteinases from rat peritoneal macrophages. In Richards, R. J. and Rajan, K. I. (eds.), *Tissue Culture in Medical Research (II)*, pp. 109–111. (Oxford: Pergamon Press)

95. Hassid, A., Konieczkowski, M. and Dunn, M. J. (1979). Prostaglandin synthesis in isolated rat kidney glomeruli. *Proc. Natl. Acad. Sci. USA*, **76**, 1155–1159

96. Heifets, M., Purkerson, M. and Klahr, S. (1985). A diet rich in linoleic acid improves renal function and decreases blood pressure in rats with a remnant kidney. *Kidney Int.*, **27**, 244(A)

97. Hostetter, T. H., Olson, J. L., Rennke, H. G., Venkatachalam, M. A. and Brenner, B. M. (1981). Hyperfiltration in remnant nephrons: a potentially adverse response. *Am. J. Physiol.*, **241**, 85–93

98. Hurd, E. R., Johnson, J. M., Okita, J. R., Macdonald, P. C., Ziff, M. and Gillian, J. N. (1981). Prevention of glomerulonephritis and prolonged survival in New Zealand Black/New Zealand White P_1 hybrid mice fed an essential fatty acid deficient diet. *J. Clin. Invest.*, **67**, 476–485

99. Ito, Y., Barcelli, U., Yamashita, W., Weiss, M., Glas-Greenwalt, P. and Pollack, V. E. (1988). Fish oil has beneficial effects on lipids and renal disease of nephrotic rats. *Metabolism*, **37**, 352–357

100. Jaffer, F., Saunders, C., Shultz, P., Throckmorton, D., Weinshell, E. and Abboud, H. E. (1989). Regulation of mesangial cell growth by polypeptide mitogens. Inhibitory role of transforming growth factor beta. *Am. J. Pathol.*, **135**, 261–269

101. Jim, K., Hassid, A., Sun, F. and Dunn, M. J. (1982). Lipoxygenase activity in rat kidney glomeruli, glomerular epithelial cells and cortical tubules. *J. Biol. Chem.*, **257**, 10294–10299

102. Johnson, R. J., Alpers, C. E., Pritzl, P., Schulze, M., Baker, P., Pruchno, C. and Couser, W. G. (1988). Platelets mediate neutrophil dependent immune complex nephritis in the rat. *J. Clin. Invest.*, **82**, 1225–1235

103. Karnovsky, M. J. (1984). Improved method for culturing rat glomerular cells. *Kidney Int.*, **26**, 875–880

104. Kelley, V. E., Winklestein, A., Izui, S. and Dixon, F. J. (1981). Prostaglandin E_1 inhibits T-cell proliferation and renal disease in MRL/1 mice. *Clin. Immunol. Immunopathol.*, **21**, 190–203

105. Kelley, V. E., Izui, S. and Halushka, P. V. (1982). Effect of ibuprofen, a fatty acid cyclooxygenase inhibitor on murine lupus. *Clin. Immunol. Immunopathol.*, **25**, 223–231

106. Kelley, V. E., Ferretti, A., Izui, S. and Strom, T. B. (1985). A fish oil diet rich in eicosapentaenoic acid reduces cyclooxygenase metabolites and suppresses lupus in MRL-1pr mice. *J. Immunol.*, **134**, 1914–1919

107. Kelley, V. E., Sneve, S. and Musinski, S. (1986). Increased renal thromboxane production in murine lupus nephritis. *J. Clin. Invest.*, **77**, 252–259

108. Kher, V., Barcelli, U., Weiss, M., Gallon, L., Pajel, P., Laskarzewski, P. and Pollack, V. E. (1986). Protective effect of polyunsaturated fatty acid supplementation in apoferritin induced murine glomerulonephritis. *Prostaglandins, Leukotrienes and Medicine*, **22**, 323–334

109. Klebanoff, S. J., Vadas, M. A., Harlan, J. M., Sparks, L. H., Gamble, J. R., Agosti, J. M. and Waltersdorph, A. M. (1986). Stimulation of neutrophils by tumor necrosis factor. *J. Immunol.*, **136**, 4222–4225

110. Knudsen, P. J., Dinarello, C. A. and Strom, T. B. (1986). Prostaglandins post-transcriptionally inhibit monocyte expression of interleukin-1 activity by increasing cyclic adenosine monophosphate. *J. Immunol.*, **137**, 3189–3194

111. Kreisberg, J. I. and Karnovsky, M. J. (1983). Glomerular cells in culture. *Kidney Int.*, **23**, 439–447

112. Kromann, N. and Green, A. (1980). Epidemiological studies in the Upernavik district, Greenland: incidence of some chronic diseases 1950–1974. *Acta Med. Scand.*, **208**, 401–406

113. Kromhout, D., Bosschieter, E. B. and de Lezenne Coulander, C. (1985). The inverse relation between fish consumption and 20-year mortality from coronary heart disease. *N. Engl. J. Med.*, **312**, 1205–1209

114. Kunkel, S. L., Zanetti, M. and Sapin, C. (1982). Suppression of nephrotoxic serum nephritis in rats by prostaglandin E_1. *Am. J. Pathol.*, **108**, 240–245

115. Kunkel, S. L., Spengler, M., May, M. A., Spengler, R., Larrick, J. and Remick, D. (1988). Prostaglandin E_2 regulates macrophage-derived tumour necrosis factor gene expression. *J. Biol. Chem.*, **263**, 5380–5384

116. Lands, W. E. M. (1979). The biosynthesis and metabolism of prostaglandins. *Annu. Rev. Physiol.*, **41**, 633–642

117. Leaker, B., Salehi, P. and Kincaid-Smith, P. (1986). The effect of eicosaentanoic acid on active lupus nephritis. *Kidney Int.*, **30**, 629(A)

118. Le, J. and Vilcek, J. (1987). Tumour necrosis factor and interleukin-1: cytokines with

multiple overlapping biological activities. *Lab. Invest.*, **56**, 234–248

119. Lee, T. H., Hoover, R. L., Williams, J. D., Sperling, R. J., Ravalese, J., Spur, B. W., Robinson, D. R., Corey, E. J., Lewis, R. A. and Austen, K. F. (1985). Effect of dietary enrichment with eicosapentaenoic and docosahexaenoic acids on in vitro neutrophil and monocyte leukotriene generation and neutrophil function. *N. Engl. J. Med.*, **312**, 1217–1224

120. Lefkowith, J. B., Morrison, A. R. and Schreiner, G. F. (1988). Murine glomerular leukotriene B_4 synthesis: Manipulation by (n-6) fatty acid deprivation and cellular origin. *J. Clin. Invest.*, **82**, 1655–1660

121. Lehmmann, V., Benninghoff, B. and Dröge, W. (1988). Tumour necrosis factor-induced activation of peritoneal macrophages is regulated by prostaglandin E_2 and cAMP. *J. Immunol.*, **141**, 587–591

122. Lewis, R. A. and Austen, K. F. (1984). The biologically active leukotrienes. Biosynthesis, metabolism, receptors, functions and pharmacology. *J. Clin. Invest.*, **73**, 889–897

123. Lianos, E. A., Andres, G. A. and Dunn, M. J. (1983). Glomerular prostaglandin and thromboxane synthesis in rat nephrotoxic nephritis: Effects on renal haemodynamics. *J. Clin. Invest.*, **72**, 1439–1448

124. Lianos, E. A., Rahman, M. A. and Dunn, M. J. (1985). Glomerular arachidonate lipoxygenation in rat nephrotoxic serum nephritis. *J. Clin. Invest.*, **76**, 1355–1359

125. Lianos, E. A. (1988). Synthesis of hydroxyeicosatetraenoic acids and leukotrienes in rat nephrotoxic serum glomerulonephritis. Role of anti-GBM antibody dose, complement and neutrophils. *J. Clin. Invest.*, **82**, 427–435

126. Lianos, E. A. (1989). Leukotriene synthesis in experimental membranous nephropathy — Potential role of the glomerular macrophage. *Kidney Int.*, **35**, 295(A)

127. Lianos, E. A. and Noble, B. (1989). Glomerular leukotriene synthesis in Heyman nephritis. *Kidney Int.*, **36**, 998–1002

128. Linker-Israeli, M., Bakke, A. C., Kitridon, R. C., Gendler, S. and Horowitz, D. A. (1983). Defective production of interleukin-1 and interleukin-2 in patients with systemic lupus erythematosis. *J. Immunol.*, **130**, 2651–2655

129. Lomedico, P. T., Gubler, U., Hellman, C. P., Dukovich, M., Giri, J. G., Pan, Y. E., Collier, K., Seminonow, R., Chua, A. O. and Mizel, S. B. (1984). Cloning and expression of murine interleukin-1 in *Escherichia coli*. *Nature*, **312**, 458–462

130. Lovett, D. H., Ryan, J. L. and Sterzel, R. B. (1983). Stimulation of rat mesangial cell proliferation by macrophage interleukin-1. *J. Immunol.*, **131**, 2830–2836

131. Lovett, D. H., Ryan, J. L. and Sterzel, R. B. (1983). A thymocyte activating factor derived from glomerular mesangial cells. *J. Immunol.*, **130**, 1796–1801

132. Lovett, D. H., Sterzel, R. B., Kashgarian, M. and Ryan, J. L. (1983). Neutral proteinase activity produced *in vitro* by cells of the glomerular mesangium. *Kidney Int.*, **23**, 342–349

133. Lovett, D. H. and Sterzel, R. B. (1986). Cell culture approaches to the analysis of glomerular inflammation. *Kidney Int.*, **30**, 246–254

134. Lovett, D. H., Szamel, M., Ryan, J. L., Sterzel, R. B., Gemsa, D. and Resch, K. (1986). Interleukin-1 and the glomerular mesangium. I. Purification and characterization of a mesangial cell-derived autogrowth factor. *J. Immunol.*, **136**, 3700–3705

135. Lovett, D. H., Resch, K. and Gemsa, D. (1987). Interleukin-1 and the glomerular mesangium. II. Monokine stimulation of mesangial cell prostanoid secretion. *Am. J. Pathol.*, **129**, 543–551

136. Lovett, D. H., Hänsch, G. M., Goppelt, M., Resch, K. and Gemsa, D. (1987). Activation of glomerular mesangial cells by the terminal membrane attack complex of complement. *J. Immunol.*, **138**, 2473–2480

137. Lovett, D. H. and Larsen, A. (1988). Cell cycle-dependent interleukin-1 gene expression by cultured glomerular mesangial cells. *J. Clin. Invest.*, **82**, 115–122

138. Lowenthal, J. W. and MacDonald, H. R. (1986). Binding and internalization of interleukin-1 by T cells: direct evidence of high and low affinity classes of interleukin-1 receptor. *J. Exp. Med.*, **164**, 1060–1074

139. MacKay, K., Striker, L. J., Stauffer, J. W., Dol, T., Agodao, L. Y. and Striker, G. E. (1989). Transforming growth factor-β. Murine glomerular receptors and responses of isolated glomerular cells. *J. Clin. Invest.*, **83**, 1160–1167

140. Mais, D. E., Burch, R. M., Saussy, D. L. Jr., Kochel, P. J. and Halushka, P. V. (1985). Binding of a thromboxane A_2/prostaglandin H_2 receptor antagonist to washed human platelets. *J. Pharmacol. Exp. Ther.*, **235**, 729–734

141. March, C. H., Mosley, B., Larsen, A., Cerretti, D. P., Braedt, G., Price, V., Gillis, S., Henney, C. S., Kronheim, S. R., Grabstein, K., Conlon, P. J., Hopp, T. P. and Cosman, D. (1985). Cloning sequence and expression of two distinct human interleukin-1 complementary DNA's. *Nature*, **315**, 641–646

142. Martin, J., Lovett, D. H., Gemsa, D., Sterzel, R. B. and Davies, M. (1986). Enhancement of glomerular mesangial cell neutral proteinase secretion by macrophages: role of interleukin-1. *J. Immunol.*, **137**, 525–529

143. Martin, M., Schwinzer, R., Schellekens, H. and Resch, K. (1989). Glomerular mesangial cells in local inflammation: Induction of the expression of MHC Class II antigens by IFN-γ. *J. Immunol.*, **142**, 1887–1894

144. Matsumoto, K. and Atkins, R. C. (1989). Glomerular cells and macrophages in the progression of experimental focal and segmental glomerulonephritis. *Am. J. Pathol.*, **134**, 933–945

145. Matsumura, Y., Ozawa, Y., Suzuki, H. and Saruta, I. (1986). Synergistic action of angiotensin II on norepinephrine induced prostaglandin release from rat glomeruli. *Am. J. Physiol.*, **250**, 811–816

146. Matsushima, K., Yodoi, J., Tagaya, Y. and Oppenheim, J. J. (1986). Down regulation of interleukin-1 receptor expression by IL-1 and fate of internalized ^{125}I-labelled IL-1 beta in a human large granular lymphocyte cell line. *J. Immunol.*, **137**, 3183–3188

147. Michie, H. R., Manogue, K. R., Springs, D. R., Revhaug, A., O'Dwyer, S., Dinarello, G. A., Cerami, A., Wolff, S. M. and Wilmore, D. W. (1988). Detection of circulating tumour necrosis factor after endotoxin administration. *N. Engl. J. Med.*, **318**, 1481–1486

148. Michielsen, P., Verberckmoes, R., Desmel, V. and Hemeruckx, W. (1967). Evolution histologique des gloméulonéphrites proliferatives diffuses traitées par l'indométhacine. *J. Urol. Nephrol.*, **75**, 315

149. Miller, M., Holthoffer, H., Sinha, A., Gibbons, N., Santiago, A. and Scharschmidt, L. (1988). A fish oil diet is protective against accelerated nephrotoxic serum nephritis. *Kidney Int.*, **33**, 322(A)

150. Mizel, S. B., Kilian, P. L., Lewis, J. C., Paganelli, K. A. and Chizzonite, R. A. (1987). The interleukin-1 receptor. Dynamics of interleukin-1 binding and internalization in T cells and fibroblasts. *J. Immunol.*, **138**, 2906–2912

151. Morrison, A. R., Nishikana, A. and Needleman, P. (1977). Unmasking of thromboxane A_2 synthesis by ureteral obstruction in the rabbit kidney. *Nature*, **267** 259–260

152. Nishimura, J., Huang, J. S. and Deuel, T. F. (1982). Platelet-derived growth factor stimulates tyrosine-specific protein kinase activity in Swiss mouse 3T3 cell membranes. *Proc. Natl Acad. Sci. USA*, **79**, 4303–4307

153. Niwa, T., Maeda, K., Shibata, M. and Yamada, K. (1988). Clinical effects of selective thromboxane A_2 synthetase inhibitor in patients with nephrotic syndrome. *Clin. Nephrol.*, **30**, 276–281

154. Nowak, N. and Fitzgerald, G. A. (1989). Redirection of prostaglandin endoperoxide metabolism at the platelet-vascular interface in man. *J. Clin. Invest.*, **83**(2), 380–385

155. Oates, J. A., Fitzgerald, G. A., Branch, R. A., Jackson, E. K., Knapp, H. R. and Roberts, L. J. (1988). Clinical implications of prostaglandin and thromboxane A_2 formation. *New Engl J. Med.*, **319**, 689–698

156. Pabst, R. and Sterzel, R. B. (1983). Cell renewal of glomerular cell types in normal rats. An autoradiographic analysis. *Kidney Int.*, **24**, 626–631

157. Papanicoleau, N., Hatziatoniou, C. and Bariety, J. (1986). Selective inhibition of thromboxane synthesis partially protected while inhibition of angiotensin II formation did not protect rats against acute renal failure induced with glycerol. *Prostaglandins, Leukotrienes and Medicine*, **1**, 29–35

158. Parbtani, A., Clark, W. F. and McDonald, J. W. C. (1988). Reversal of proteinuria and reduction of fatality in MZB/W F_1 lupus mice by prostaglandin E_2, iloprost and a thromboxane synthase inhibitor. *Kidney Int.*, **33**, 321(A)

159. Patrignani, P., Filabozzi, P. and Patrono, C. (1982). Selective cumulative inhibition of platelet thromboxane production by low-dose aspirin in healthy subjects. *J. Clin. Invest.*, **69**, 1366–1372

160. Patrono, C., Wennmalm, A., Ciabattoni, G., Nowak, J., Pugliese, F. and Cinotti, G. A. (1979). Evidence for an extrarenal origin of urinary prostaglandin E_2 in healthy men.

Prostaglandins, **18**, 623–629

161. Patrono, C., Ciabattoni, G., Patrignani, P., Filabozzi, P., Pinca, E., Satta, M. A., Van Dorne, D., Cinotti, G. A., Pugliese, F., Pierucci, A. and Simonetti, B. M. (1983). Evidence for a renal origin of urinary thromboxane B$_2$ in health and disease. In Samuelsson, B., Paoletti, R. and Ramwell, P. (eds.) *Advances in Prostaglandin, Thromboxane and Leukotriene Research*, Vol. II, pp. 493–498. (New York: Raven Press)

162. Patrono, C. (1984). Tissue-selective inhibition of prostaglandin and thromboxane synthesis in man: Investigative and therapeutic implications. *Clin. Physiol.*, **4**, 443–447

163. Patrono, C., Ciabattoni, G., Remuzzi, G. and Galti, E. (1985). Functional significance of renal prostacyclin and thromboxane A$_2$ production in patients with SLE. *J. Clin. Invest.*, **76**, 1011–1018

164. Patrono, C. and Dunn, M. J. (1987). The clinical significance of inhibition of renal prostaglandin synthesis. *Kidney Int.*, **32**, 1–12

165. Petersen, M., Steadman, R., Hallet, M. B., Matthews, N. and Williams, J. D. (1990). Zymosan induced leukotriene B4 generation by human neutrophils is augmented by rhTNFα but not chemotactic peptide. *Immunology*, **70**, 75–81

166. Pfeilschifter, J. (1989). Cross-talk between transmembrane signalling systems: A prerequisite for the delicate regulation of glomerular haemodynamics by mesangial cells. *Eur. J. Clin. Invest.*, **19**, 347–361

167. Pfeilschifter, J., Pignat, W., Vosbeck, K. and Märki, F. (1989). Interleukin-1 and tumour necrosis factor synergistically stimulate prostaglandin synthesis and phospholipase A$_2$ release from rat renal mesangial cells. *Biochem. Biophys. Res. Commun.*, **159**, 385–394

168. Pierucci, A., Simonetti, B. M., Pecci, G., Feriozzi, S., Mavrikakis, G., Cinotti, G. A., Patrignani, P., Patrono, C. (1988). Low dose aspirin in patients with lupus nephritis. *Kidney Int.*, **33**, 281(A)

169. Pierucci, A., Simonetti, B. M., Pecci, G., Mavrikakis, G., Feriozzi, S., Cinotti, G. A., Patrignani, P., Ciabattoni, G. and Patrono, C. (1989). Thromboxane antagonism improves renal function in lupus nephritis. *N. Engl. J. Med.*, **320**, 421–425

170. Pledger, W. J., Stiles, C. D., Antoniades, H. N. and Scher, C. D. (1978). An ordered sequence of events is required before BA1B c3TC cells become committed to DNA synthesis. *Proc. Natl Acad. Sci. USA*, **75**, 2839–2843

171. Pober, J. S. (1987). In *Tumour Necrosis Factor and Related Cytokines*, Ciba Foundation 131, pp. 170–184

172. Praga, M., Gutierrez-Millet, V., Navas, J. J., Ruilope, L. M., Morrales, J. M., Alcazar, J. M., Bello, I. and Rodicio, J. L. (1985). Acute worsening of renal function during episodes of macroscopic hematuria in IgA nephropathy. *Kidney Int.*, **28**, 69

173. Prickett, J. D., Robinson, D. R. and Steinberg, A. D. (1981). Dietary enrichment with the polyunsaturated fatty acid eicosapentaenoic acid prevents proteinuria and prolongs survival in NZB/×NZW/F$_1$ mice. *J. Clin. Invest.*, **68**, 556–559

174. Prickett, J. D., Robinson, D. R. and Steinberg, A. D. (1983). Effects of dietary enrichment with eicosapentaenoic acid upon autoimmune nephritis in female NZB×NZW/F$_1$ mice. *Arthritis Rheum.*, **26**, 133–139

175. Pugliese, F., Mene, P. and Cinotti, G. A. (1984). Glomerular prostaglandin and thromboxane synthesis in normotensive and hypertensive rats of the Milan strain before and after development of hypertension. *J. Hypertens.*, **4** (suppl. 3), S391–S393

176. Pugliese, F., Singh, A. K., Kasinath, B. S., Kreisberg, J. I. and Lewis, E. J. (1987). Glomerular epithelial cell, polyanion neutralization is associated with enhanced prostanoid production. *Kidney Int.*, **32**, 57–61

177. Purkerson, M. L., Jolst, J. H., Yates, J., Valdes, A., Morrison, A. and Klahr, S. (1985). Inhibition of thromboxane synthesis ameliorates the progressive kidney disease of rats with subtotal renal ablation. *Proc. Natl Acad. Sci. USA*, **82**, 193–197

178. Radeke, H. H., Meier, B., Topley, N., Floege, J., Habermehl, G. G. and Resch, K. (1990). Interleukin-1α and tumour necrosis factor-α induce oxygen radical production in mesangial cells. *Kidney Int.*, **37**, 767–775

179. Rahman, M. A., Emancipator, S. N. and Dunn, M. J. (1987). Immune complex effects on glomerular eicosanoid production and renal haemodynamics. *Kidney Int.*, **31**, 1317–1326

180. Rahman, M. A., Nakazawa, M., Emancipator, M. J. and Dunn, M. J. (1988). Increased leukotriene B$_4$ synthesis in immune injured rat glomeruli. *J. Clin. Invest.*, **81**, 1945–1952

181. Raines, E. L., Dower, S. K. and Ross, R. (1989). Interleukin-1 mitogenic activity for fibroblasts and smooth muscle cells is due to PDGF-AA. *Science*, **243**, 393–396
182. Raz, A., Wyche, A., Siegel, N. and Needleman, P. (1988). Regulation of fibroblast cyclooxygenase synthesis by interleukin-1. *J. Biol. Chem.*, **263**, 3022–3028
183. Rees, A. J., Lockwood, C. M. and Peters, D. K. (1977). Enhanced allergic tissue injury in Goodpasture's syndrome by intercurrent bacterial infection. *Br. Med. J.*, **2**, 723
184. Remuzzi, G., Imberti, L., Ressini, M., Marelli, C., Carminati, G., Cattanes, M. and Bertani, T. (1985). Increased glomerular thromboxane synthesis as a possible cause of proteinuria in experimental nephrosis. *J. Clin. Invest.*, **75**, 94–101
185. Roberts, A. B. and Sporn, M. B. (1985). Transforming growth factors. *Cancer Surv.*, **4**, 683–705
186. Roberts, D. G., Gerber, J. G., Barnes, J. S., Zerbe, G. O. and Nies, A. S. (1985). Sulindac is not renal sparing in man. *Clin. Pharmacol. Ther.*, **41**, 380–383
187. Robinson, D. R., Prickett, J. D., Polisson, R.l, Steinberg, A. D. and Levine, L. (1985). The protective effect of dietary fish oil on murine lupus. *Prostaglandins*, **30**, 51–75
188. Ross, R., Raines, W. and Bowen-Pope, D. R. (1986). The biology of platelet derived growth factor. *Cell.*, **46**, 155–169
189. Rovin, B. H., Lefkowith, J. B. and Schreiner, G. F. (1988). Macrophage (M0) chemotaxis in the essential fatty acid deficient (EFAD) rat. *Kidney Int.*, **33**, 323(A)
190. Salvati, P., Ferti, C., Duzzi, L., Ferrario, R., Perico, N., Remuzzi G. and Bianchi, G. (1987). Effect of thromboxane synthetase inhibitor on age dependent glomerulosclerosis in Milan normotensive rat. *Abstracts of the Xth International Congress on Nephrology*, p. 517
191. Schaap, G. H., Bilo, H. J. G., Popp-Snijders, C., Oe, P. L., Mulder, C. and Donker, A. J. M. (1987). Effects of protein intake variation and ω-3 polyunsaturated fatty acids on renal function in chronic progressive renal disease. *Life Sci.*, **32**, 211–219
192. Schafer, A. I., Crawford, D. D. and Gimbrone, M. A. (1984). Unidirectional transfer of prostaglandin endoperoxides between platelets and endothelial cells. *J. Clin. Inv.*, **73**, 1105–1112
193. Scharschmidt, L. A., Gibbons, N. A., McGarry, L., Berger, P., Axelrod, M., Janis, R. and Ko, Y. H. (1987). Effects of dietary fish oil on renal insufficiency in rats with subtotal nephrectomy. *Kidney Int.*, **32**, 700–709
194. Schlöndorff, D., Rocniak, J., Satriano, J. A. and Folkart, V. W. (1980). Prostaglandin synthesis by isolated rat glomeruli, effect of angiotensin II. *Am. J. Physiol.*, **239**, 486–495
195. Schreiner, G. F. and Lefkowith, J. B. (1987). Essential fatty acid (EFA) deficiency in rats regulates the localisation of macrophages to the glomerular mesangium. *Kidney Int.*, **31**, 328(A)
196. Schreiner, G. F., Rovin, B. H. and Lefkowith, J. B. (1989). Essential fatty acid deficiency inhibits monocyte migration in glomerulonephritis (GN). *Kidney Int.*, **35**, 362(A)
197. Schwartzman, M., Carroll, M. A., Ibraham, N. G., Ferreri, N. R., Songu-Mize, E. and McGiff, J. C. (1985). Renal arachidonic acid metabolism. The third pathway. *Hypertension*, **7** (suppl. 1), 136–144
198. Sedor, J. R., Williams, S. L., Chremos, A. N., Johnson, C. L. and Dunn, M. J. (1984). Effects of sulindac and indomethacin on renal prostaglandin synthesis. *Clin. Pharmacol. Ther.*, **36**, 85–91
199. Sherry, B. and Cerami, A. (1988). Cachectin/tumour necrosis factor exerts endocrine, paracrine, autocrine control of inflammatory response. *J. Cell. Biol.*, **107**, 1269–1277
200. Shirakawa, F., Tanaka, Y., Ota, T., Suzuki, H., Eto, S. and Yamashita, U. (1987). Expression of interleukin-1 receptors on human peripheral T cell. *J. Immunol.*, **138**, 4243–4249
201. Shultz, P. J., Dicorleto, P., Silver, B. J. and Abboud, H. E. (1988). Mesangial cells express PDGF mRNAs and proliferate in response to PDGF. *Am. J. Physiol.*, **255**, F674–F684
202. Silver, B. J., Jaffer, E. E. and Abbound, H. E. (1988). Platelet-derived growth factor synthesis in mesangial cells: Induction by multiple peptide mitogens. *Proc. Natl Acad. Sci. USA*, **86**, 1056–1060
203. Simpson, L. O. (1986). Renal disease, polyunsaturated fatty acids and blood rheology. *Nephron*, **44**, 256–258
204. Singer, P., Wirth, M. and Voigt, S. (1985). Blood pressure and lipid-lowering effect of mackerel and herring diet in patients with mild essential hypertension. *Atherosclerosis*, **56**, 223–225
205. Sraer, J., Foidart, J., Chansel, D., Mahieu, P., Kruznetzova, B. and Ardaillou, R. (1979). Prostaglandin synthesis by mesangial and epithelial glomerular cultured cells. *FEBS Lett.*, **15**, 420–424
206. Sraer, J., Ardaillou, N., Sraer, J. D. and Ardaillou, R. (1982). In vitro prostaglandin synthesis

by human glomeruli and papillae. *Prostaglandins*, **23**, 855–864

207. Sraer, J., Rigaud, M., Bens, M., Rubinovitch, H. and Ardaillou, R. (1983). Metabolism of ararchidonic acid via the lipoxygenase pathway in human and murine glomeruli. *J. Biol. Chem.*, **258**, 4325–4330

208. Sraer, J., Bens, M., Oudinet, J. P. and Aradaillou, R. (1986). Biconversion of leukotrienes C by rat glomeruli and papillae. *Prostaglandins*, **31**, 909–921

209. Stahl, R. A. K., Paravicini, M. and Schollmeyer, P. (1984). Angiotensin II stimulation of Prostaglandin E_2 and 6-keto F_1 formation by isolated human glomeruli. *Kid. Int.*, **26**, 30–34

210. Stahl, R. A. K., Adler, S., Baker, P. J., Chen, Y. P., Pritzl, P. M. and Couser, W. G. (1987). Enhanced glomerular prostaglandin formation in experimental membranous nephropathy. *Kidney Int.*, **31**, 1126–1131

211. Steadman, R., Petersen, M., Topley, N., Williams, D., Matthews, N., Spur, B. and Williams, J. D. (1990). Differential augmentation by recombinant human tumour necrosis factor α of neutrophil responses to particulate zymosan and glucan. *J. Immunol.*, **144**, 2712–2718

212. Stork, J. E. and Dunn, M. J. (1985). Haemodynamic roles of thromboxane A_2 and prostaglandin E_2 in glomerulonephritis. *J. Pharmacol. Exp. Ther.*, **233**, 672–678

213. Striker, G. E., Soderland, C., Bowen-Pope, D. F., Gown, A. M., Schmer, G., Johnson, A., Luchtel, D., Ross, R. and Striker, L. J. (1984). Isolation, characterisation and propagation *in vitro* of human glomerular endothelial cells. *J. Exp. Med.*, **160**, 3233–3238

214. Striker, L. M-M., Killen, P. D., Chi, E. and Striker, G. E. (1984). The composition of glomerulosclerosis. I. Studies on focal sclerosis, crescentic glomerulonephritis, and membrano-proliferative glomerulonephritis. *Lab. Invest.*, **51**, 181–191

215. Striker, G. E. and Striker, L. J. (1985). Glomerular cell culture. *Lab. Invest.*, **53**, 122–131

216. Suranyi, M. G., Quiza, C., Gausch, A., Newton, L., Myers, B. D. and Hall, B. M. (1990). Cytokine levels in patients with the nephrotic syndrome. *Kidney Int.*, **37**, 445(A)

217. Tashjian, A. H., Voelkel, E. F., Robinson, D. R. and Levine, L. (1984). Dietary menhaden oil lowers plasma prostaglandins and calcium in mice bearing the prostaglandin-producing HSDM, fibrosarcoma. *J. Clin. Invest.*, **74**, 2042–2048

218. Terragno, N. A., McGiff, J. C. and Terragno, D. A. (1979). Synthesis of prostaglandins by vascular and non-vascular renal tissues and the presence of an endogenous prostaglandin synthesis inhibitor in the cortex. In Vargraftig, B. B. (ed.) *Advances in Pharmacology and Therapeutics*, Vol. 4, pp. 39–46. (Oxford: Pergamon Press)

219. Tiggeler, R. G., Hulme, B. and Wijdeveld, P. G. (1979). Effect of indomethacin on glomerular permeability in the nephrotic syndrome. *Kidney Int.*, **16**, 312–321

220. Todaro, G-J., DeLarco, J. E. and Cohen, S. (1976). Transformation by murine and feline sarcoma viruses specifically block binding of epidermal growth factor to cells. *Nature*, **264**, 26–31

221. Tomosgui, N., Cashman, S. J., Hay, H., Pusey, C. D., Evans, D. J., Shaw, A. and Rees, A. J. (1989). Modulation of antibody mediated glomerular injury *in vivo* by bacterial lipopolysaccharide, tumour necrosis factor, and IL-1. *J. Immunol.*, **142**, 3083–3090

222. Topley, N., Floegge, J., Wessel, K., Hass, R., Radeke, H. H., Kaever, V. and Resch, K. (1989). Prostaglandin E_2 production is synergistically increased in cultured human glomerular mesangial cells by combination of IL-1 and tumour necrosis factor. *J. Immunol.*, **143**, 1989–1995

223. Topley, N., Floege, J., Hoppe, J., Kishimoto, T. and Resch, K. (1990). Lymphokines modulate rather than induce proliferation in cultured human mesangial cells. *Kidney Int.*, **37**, 204

224. Varani, J., Ginsburg, I., Schuger, L., Gibbs, D. F., Bromberg, J., Johnson, K. J., Ryan, S. and Ward, P. A. (1989). Endothelial cell killing by neutrophils. Synergistic interaction of oxygen products and proteases. *Am. J. Pathol.*, **135**, 435–438

225. Vissers, M. C. M., Wiggins, R. and Fantone, J. C. (1989). Comparative ability of human monocytes and neutrophils to degrade glomerular basement membrane *in vitro*. *Lab. Invest.*, **60**, 831–838

226. Vissers, M. C., Fantone, J. C., Wiggins, R. and Kunkel, S. L. (1989). Glomerular basement membrane-containing immune complexes stimulate tumour necrosis factor and interleukin-1 production by human monocytes. *Am. J. Pathol.*, **134**, 1–6

227. Waage, A., Espevik, T. and Lamvik, J. (1986). Detection of tumour necrosis factor-like cytotoxicity in serum from patients with septicaemia but not from untreated cancer patients. *Scand. J. Immunol.*, **24**, 739–743

228. Wankowitz, Z., Mecyeri, P. and Isselkutz, A. (1988). Synergy between tumour necrosis

factor α and interleukin-1 in the induction of polymorphonuclear leukocytes migration during inflammation. *J. Leuk. Biol.*, **43**, 349–356

229. Webb, D. R. and Oscheroff, P. L. (1976). Antigen stimulation of prostaglandin synthesis and control of immune responses. *Proc. Natl Acad. Sci. USA*, **73**, 1300–1304

230. Werber, H. I., Emancipator, S. N., Tykocinski, M. L. and Sedor, J. R. (1987). The interleukin-1 gene is expressed by rat glomerular mesangial cells and is augmented in immune complex glomerulonephritis. *J. Immunol.*, **138**, 3207–3212

231. Wiemeyer, A., Fauler, J., Marx, K. H., Kuhn, K., Koch, K. M. and Frolich, J. C. (1987). LTB$_4$ in nephrotoxic serum nephritis in rats. *Abstracts Xth International Congress on Nephrology*, pp. 236(A)

232. Williams, J. D., Abrahamson, D. R., Davies, M., Harry, T. and Coles, G. A. (1987). Activation of the complement and of phagocytic cells by isolated glomerular basement membrane. In Price, R. G. and Hudson, B. G. (eds.) *Renal Basement Membranes in Health and Disease*, pp. 375–388. (London: Academic Press)

233. Zoja, C., Benigni, A., Livio, M., Beiganelli, A., Onisio, S., Abbate, M., Bertani, T. and Remmuzzi, G. (1989). Selective inhibition of platelet thromboxane generation with low dose aspirin does not protect rats with reduced renal mass from the development of progressive disease. *Am. J. Pathol.*, **134**, 1027–1038

234. Zurier, R. B., Weissmann, G., Hoffstein, S., Kammerman, S. and Tai, H. H. (1974). Mechanism of lysosomal enzyme release from human leukocytes. II. Effects of cAMP and cGMP, autonomic agonists and agents which effect microtubule function. *J. Clin. Invest.*, **53**, 297–309

235. Zurier, R. B. (1979). Modulation of inflammation and immune responses by prostaglandins. In Ryan, A. (ed.) *Actions of Non-steroidal Agents in the Alteration of Prostaglandin Synthesis*, pp. 46–49. (Minneapolis: Postgraduate Medical Communications)

236. Zusman, R. M. and Keiser, H. R. (1977). Prostaglandin biosynthesis by rabbit renomedullary interstitial cells in tissue culture. *J. Clin. Invest.*, **60**, 215–223

237. Ruef, C., Budde, K., Lacy, J., Northemann, W., Baumann, M., Sterzel, B. R. and Coleman, D. L. (1990). Interleukin 6 is an autocrine growth factor for mesangial cells. *Kidney Int.*, **38**, 249–257

238. Suematsu, S., Matsuda, T., Aozasa, K., Akira, S., Nakano, N., Ohno, S., Miyazaki, J. I., Yamamura, K. I., Hirano, T. and Kishimoto, T. (1989). IgG1 plasmacytosis in interleukin 6 transgenic mice. *Proc. Natl. Acad. Sci. USA*, **186**, 7547–7551

239. Horii, Y., Muraguchi, A., Iwano, M., Matsuda, T., Hirayama, T., Yamada, H., Fujii, Y., Dohi, K., Ishikawa, H., Ohmoto, Y., Yoshizaki, K., Hirano, T. and Kishimoto, T. (1989). Involvement of IL-6 in mesangial proliferative glomerulonephritis. *J. Immunol.*, **143**, 3949–3955

240. Richards, N. T., Gordon, C., Richardson, K., Emery, P., Howie, A. J., Adu, D. and Michael, J. (1990). Urinary IL-6: A marker for mesangial proliferation? *JASN*, **1**, 566A

8
Immunology of Minimal-change Nephropathy

G. CLARK and D. G. WILLIAMS

INTRODUCTION

Despite many advances in our understanding of the immune response, inflammation, and glomerular structure and physiology over the last fifteen years there has been very little progress in solving the aetiology and pathogenesis of minimal-change nephropathy (MCN). The central observation of a disorder characterized by an absence of inflammatory changes and immune reactions in the diseased organ, but with a high response rate to drugs which profoundly alter the immune response and inflammation, continues to pose a problem rich in apparent paradox.

The hypothesis that MCN is a disorder caused by abnormal function of T lymphocytes has been neither proved nor disproved, and still commands attention. Although an abnormal lymphocyte population, or a lymphokine abnormal in quantity or quality, has escaped definition in MCN, there has been an increase in the circumstantial evidence pointing in that direction. More importantly, immunogenetic studies have defined HLA associations which strongly indicate that MCN can be related to T cell function/dysfunction.

Definition of minimal-change nephropathy

This review will include cases described histologically as 'minimal change nephropathy' and the clinically defined 'steroid-responsive nephrotic syndrome (SRNS)'. Because paediatric nephrologists do not routinely perform renal biopsy in children with a nephrotic syndrome which responds to empirical treatment with steroids, many patients with MCN have not had the diagnosis confirmed by histology. At the same time, it must be recognized that the category SRNS can include some patients with focal glomerulosclerosis and membranous nephropathy, as the nephrotic syndrome associated with these conditions may respond to steroids. Furthermore, some patients with a histological diagnosis of MCN may in fact have focal glomerulosclerosis, the correct diagnosis not being made because of sampling error.

Histology

By definition, in the majority of cases there are no abnormalities on light microscopy. A slight increase in numbers of mesangial cells is seen in some cases; these are not lymphocytes or macrophages. The much-quoted fusion or loss of foot processes of the epithelial cells seen on electron microscopy is not peculiar to MCN. Small electron-dense deposits have been noted in the mesangial and subendothelial areas, but they are not associated with immune reactants. Immunohistology in a minority of cases shows mesangial deposits of IgM, and rarely of IgA or IgG, but there is little evidence to suggest that these are different from other cases of MCN. There is no convincing evidence that IgE is deposited.

The general absence of conventionally accepted markers of inflammation and/or immune reactants in the glomeruli seems to exclude the familiar forms of damage caused by immune complexes, antibody deposition, or cell-mediated immunity. None the less, the minor positive findings noted above should not be disregarded, as they may indicate transient or subtle glomerular inflammation.

GENETICS

Familial history

Familial cases of MCN account for 3.3% of the known prevalence of idiopathic nephrotic syndrome in European children[1]. While these data support the hypothesis that genetic factors play a role in the aetiology of the disease, most index cases had affected siblings, thus not excluding environmental factors, with only a few incidences of the nephrotic syndrome occurring in different generations. However, the age at onset, renal morphology on biopsy, and response to treatment were very consistent within the families.

Immunogenetics

In man the important genetic elements that control an individual's immune response to foreign antigens reside within the major histocompatibility complex (MHC) region of chromosome 6. Much research has been undertaken to elucidate the structure and function of these genes[2], which are considered in more detail in Chapter 1.

Combinations of alleles present on chromosomes are called haplotypes. They are inherited together unless, for example, a genetic recombination event takes place within the MHC. Haplotypes which have commonly been described in MCN are HLA-A1-B8-SC01-DR3-DQw2 and HLA-B12-FC31-DR7-DQW2[3]. The nomenclature used in these haplotypes also describes

Table 1 Summary of the major histocompatibility complex alleles associated with minimal-change nephropathy

Histocompatibility antigen associated with MCN	Number of patients	Relative risk	Reference	Comments
MHC Class I antigens				
HLA-B12	104	6.3	[4, 5, 10]	Caucasoid children
HLA-B8; B13	45	2.8; 4.65	[6]	Caucasoid population B8, B13
A1/B8 haplotype		5.24		linked to DR7
HLA-B44	77	5.8	[9]	Asian caucasoids
None	72	–	[7]	
	33	–	[98]	
MHC Class II antigens				
HLA-DR7	45	5.9	[10, 11]	Caucasoid children
	50	4.5		
HLA-DR3, DR7	72	9.3	[8]	Ref. 16 is a family study;
	32		[3]	describes two haplotypes; B8-SC01-DR3, B44-FC31-DR7
DR8, DQw3			[99]	Japanese population
DR2	50	0.23	[11]	Negative association in caucasoids
None	33	–	[98]	
MHC Class III antigens				
C4A*Q0	37		[12]	Occurs commonly in the B8/DR3 haplotype. Increased C4 turnover?

the alleles for the three complement components Bf, C2 and C4 which are present in the MHC region. They are arbitrarily written in the order Bf, C2, C4A and C4B—Bf typing being either fast (F) or slow (S) on plasma electrophoresis, C2 typing being the 'C' variant, C4A having six common variants (1–6) or a null allele (Q0), and C4B having three variants (1–3) and a null allele (Q0). Therefore, SC01 and FC31 are complement phenotypes for the Bf, C2 and C4 loci, as determined by electrophoresis according to the nomenclature described by Alper.

The first report of an HLA association with steroid-responsive nephrotic syndrome was in British children[4]. Thomson found that the frequency of HLA-B12 in 104 children was significantly raised out of the 21 Class I histocompatibility antigens tested. Although atopy was more common in the HLA-B12 patients, a later study by the same group showed that the raised frequency of HLA-B12 was independent of atopy. This report also stated that HLA-B12 patients relapsed earlier after cyclophosphamide than non-B12 patients[5]. Not all studies have found the same MHC Class I antigens to be more prevalent in minimal-change/SRNS patients within a given ethnic population. European serological studies showed that HLA-B8 and B13 were raised, as well as the combination HLA-A1/B8 (probably as a haplotype)[6], whereas others found no associations with MHC Class I antigens in their series, each of which contained 72 steroid-sensitive nephrotic children[7,8]. In a South African study, Adhikari[9] found HLA-B44 (a subtype of B12) to be more prevalent in 33 Indian children with SRNS compared to normal Indian children. By contrast, black African children with membranous nephropathy had a raised frequency of HLA-Bw21, and of these 82% were HBsAg positive. This raises the possibility that if HLA-Bw21 is the Class I histocompatibility antigen used to present a peptide antigen derived from the hepatitis B virus to T lymphocytes, then HLA-B44 or a closely linked molecule, may have a similar function in presenting an undefined protein antigen in MCN.

More recent studies have shown associations with MHC Class II alleles, which are linked to the Class I alleles described above. In 1980, Alfiler et al. showed that MHC Class II antigens defined susceptibility to SRNS, as HLA-DR7 was found to be increased in Australian caucasoid children. Thirty of 42 patients tested had the DR7 antigen compared to 36 of 121 controls giving relative risk of 5.9[10]. No association between this marker and atopy was observed. Comparisons of the frequencies of DR7 and B12 alleles in these patients showed that the prevalence was not due solely to the haplotype carrying B12 and DR7, suggesting that the raised frequency of DR7 was the more important marker of susceptibility. The association between DR7 and SRNS has been confirmed in studies of European populations[8,11], one of which also indicated that HLA-DR2 might protect against the development of the disease. Cambon-Thomsen et al.[8] reported that DR3 and DR7 occurred together significantly more frequently in steroid-sensitive and resistant patients than normal subjects. Recently, in a North American caucasoid family study of frequently relapsing MCN[3], a DR7 and DR3 haplotype were observed in increased frequency.

Research into the immunogenetic background of MCN patients using restriction fragment length polymorphism (RFLP) analysis in our laboratory has confirmed the DR7 association with the disease. This technique allows specific assignment of an individual's MHC genotype for the majority of alleles of the DR, DQ and DP loci, including many subtypes of MHC alleles defined serologically. An increased prevalence of patients typed as DR3,7 was also confirmed, and a significantly increased frequency of DQw2 was observed in 45 MCN patients compared to 60 controls. Both DR7 and DR3 are in linkage disequilibrium with DQw2, so this result is not surprising. Nevertheless, the importance of DQw2, as well as DR7, in determining genetic susceptibility to MCN is shown by the unexpected finding that 30% of the DR7 patients had the DR7-DQw9 haplotype. However, all were also phenotypically DQw2, because the other 6th chromosome carried either a DR3-DQw2 haplotype (22%) or a DR7-DQw2 haplotype (8%). It therefore appears that at least two genes, DRB1 of the DR7 allele and DQB1 of the DQw2 allele (which code for the beta chains of the respective MHC Class II molecules), define the immunogenetic disease susceptibility for minimal-change nephropathy (Figure 1).

Investigation of the class III (complement) allele and phenotype frequencies in MCN have shown the presence of weak associations. Certain alleles of this region, called null alleles, fail to produce a functional complement protein. These null alleles, denoted by C4A*Q0 and C4B*Q0, are found in association

THE MHC REGION

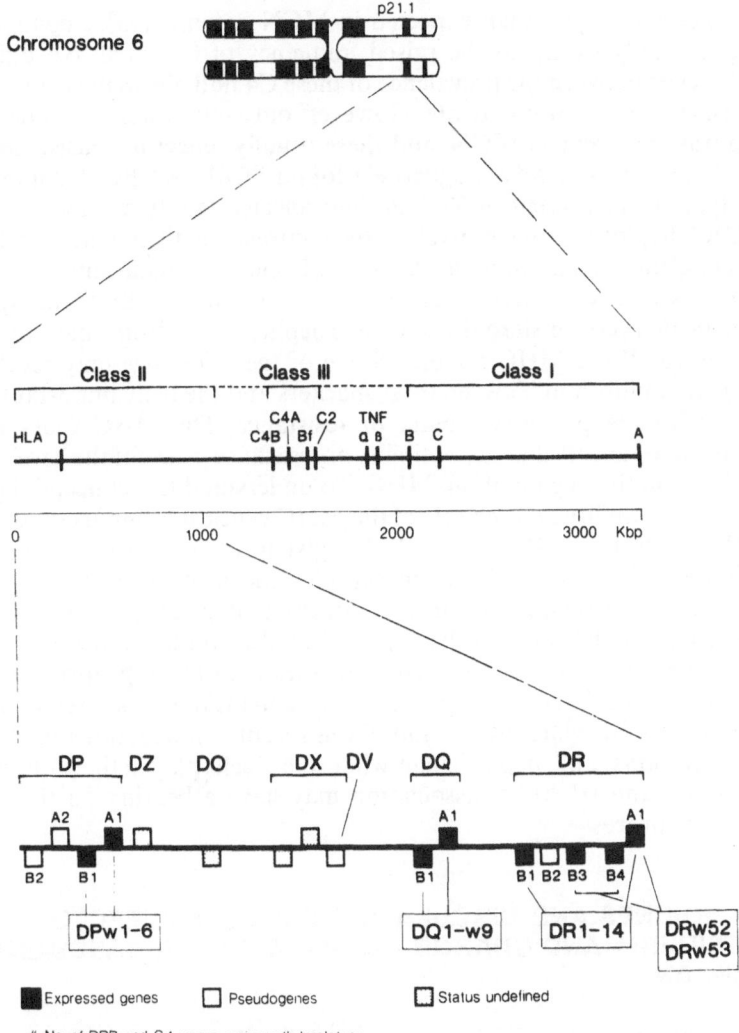

Figure 1 The structure of the major histocompatibility complex. The region on chromosome 6p is subdivided into three areas: the MHC Class I region containing the HLA-A, -B and -C loci; the MHC Class II region with the HLA-D locus comprising DR, DQ and DP loci; and the MHC Class III region containing the genes for Bf, C2 and C4 complement components as well as those for 21-hydroxylase and tumour necrosis factor. The detailed structure of the MHC Class II region (lower diagram) shows the A and B genes which encode the alpha and beta polypeptide chains of the histocompatibility molecules respectively. Some are expressed whilst other genes within the region act as pseudogenes and are known not to produce a protein product. The alleles of the DR, DQ and DP genes give rise to the histocompatibility specificities as shown in the boxes. MHC antigen associations with MCN have been described for the HLA-B locus (B12, B44, B8, B13) and for the DR locus (DR7 and the combination DR3, DR7 in caucasians, and DR8 in orientals). As the genetic and physical distances between the loci in the MHC are small, certain DQ and DP alleles have been linked to these DR associations (authors' unpublished findings).

with certain MHC haplotypes, notably HLA-B8-DR3-DQw2. McClean *et al.*[12] showed that the combined gene frequency of C4A*Q0 and/or C4B*Q0 null alleles was higher than expected in MCN patients (43%) compared to normals, mainly owing to the raised frequency of C4A*Q0. No difference was observed between the prevalence of these C4 null alleles in corticosteroid responsive or resistance patients. However, only minor abnormalities in C4 concentrations occur in MCN, and these usually reflect increased clearance at the kidney[13]. Similarly, Lagueruela found SC01 and FC31 complement phenotypes to be present in 50% of their affected family members, on DR3 and DR7 haplotypes respectively[3]. By contrast, in their study of French children, Cambon-Thomsen *et al.*[8] did not find any significant association, in steroid-sensitive or steroid-resistant patients, with the Bf phenotype.

Genetic markers for steroid-responsive nephrotic syndrome have now been described in all the MHC regions. Some of these findings may result from linkage disequilibrium between these markers and the truly important alleles which define disease susceptibility or resistance. The MHC Class II data most strongly indicate that susceptibility or resistance genes for the development of MCN lie in this region of the MHC. To understand this concept of genetic disease susceptibility and the role of the MHC genes, it is important to realize that the Class I and II genes code for glycoprotein antigens whose main function is to bind self and foreign peptides and to present them to T cells. T-lymphocyte recognition of these antigens is dependent upon the T cell receptor binding not only to the peptide but also to the self MHC molecule. T cell activation may then proceed, which leads to the appropriate immune response, as considered in Chapter 1. What remains to be discovered in MCN are the means by which MHC and T cell receptor interactions mediate the immune response and, in particular, what role T cells play in the pathogenesis. The Class I and III MHC association may have a bearing on this part of the disease process.

LYMPHOKINES AND CIRCULATING FACTORS AFFECTING PROTEINURIA AND CHARGE ON GLOMERULAR BASEMENT MEMBRANE

The hypothesis that MCN is a disorder of T cells led to several attempts to define a product of lymphocytes which caused proteinuria. Other experiments have expanded this approach by examining vascular permeability and alteration in charge on the glomerular basement membrane (GBM) produced not only by lymphocyte products but also by serum or plasma from nephrotic subjects. A summary of these findings is shown in Table 2, and general comments may be made as follows. First, no factor(s) has yet been identified chemically, so no conclusions can be made as to whether or not any of them are identical. Second, the reported effects are not peculiar to MCN, so until the structures of the factors concerned are known we have to conclude that the nephrotic syndrome due to membranous nephropathy and focal glomerulosclerosis are characterized by circulating factor(s) similar to those in MCN. Third, very few experiments have been done to demonstrate whether

Table 2 Investigations of effects of human plasma, serum and lymphocyte culture supernatant on vascular permeability, protein excretion and charge of glomerular basement membrane

Nature of observation	Method and species	Test system	Reference
Vascular permeability	Guinea pig skin and Evans blue	Con A plus lymphocytes (T)	Heslan [100]
	Guinea pig skin and Evans blue	T lymphocytes	Tomizawa [101]
	Guinea pig skin and Evans blue		Bakker [102]
	Guinea pig skin and Evans blue	Lymphocytes	Jones [103]
Proteinuria	Perfusion	Lymphocytes	Lagrue [104]
	Perfusion in vivo of rat kidney	Plasma	Zimmerman [105]
	Perfusion in vivo of rabbit kidney	Plasma	Wilkinson [106]
	Perfusion in vivo of rat kidney via tail vein	Con A plus lymphocytes	Yoshizawa [107]
GBM anions	Rat kidney in vivo	Serum and lymphocytes	Jones [108]
	Rabbit kidney in vivo	Plasma	Wilkinson [106]
	Rat kidney	Con A plus lymphocytes	Bakker [109]

identical samples have more than one action. Finally, leukocytes—T cells or monocytes—have been found to be the source of factors affecting glomerular polyanions and vascular permeability, a finding of considerable importance relating to Shalhoub's hypothesis. Other workers examining these factors have made two interesting obsevations: (i) inhibitory activity in plasma has been found for the factor(s) causing increased vascular permeability[14]; and (ii) factors causing increased vascular permeability have been detected in normal human plasma that are of identical molecular weight to those in nephrotic plasma[15]. Taken together, these observations suggest that there are normally occurring factors in human plasma/serum which can cause proteinuria and reduction in anionic charge on the GBM, and which can inhibit these effects. Thus, MCN may be due to altered control of normally occurring substances rather than to the production of new factors. An interesting approach to examining more accessible factors in MCN was promised by a report of reduction of the negative charge in circulating erythrocytes in patients in relapse[16]. Subsequent workers, however, have failed to confirm this finding, and have also pointed out problems with the methodology[17-19].

Although the most obvious lymphocyte product to be sought in MCN is one causing glomerular permeability, a considerable amount of work has been expended on the demonstration of circulating factors in this disorder that affect lymphocyte function, so accumulating circumstantial evidence that lymphokines are being produced. While there is no doubt that MCN plasma/serum can reduce lymphocyte responses to mitogens, and alter T cell suppressor activity, these findings do not advance our understanding of MCN itself, as the abnormalities are found in other histological forms of nephrotic syndrome and in other hypoproteinaemic conditions. Moreover, factors affecting lymphocyte function have not been identified, so they cannot be unequivocally labelled as lymphokines.

The lymphocyte function most commonly studied has been the response of normal lymphocytes to mitogens in the presence of nephrotic plasma. In summary, there is a decreased response to Con A and PHA of normal lymphocytes in sera from patients with MCN, membranous nephropathy and focal glomerulosclerosis[20-27]. This effect is related to the severity of the nephrotic syndrome as measured by plasma albumin concentration, and, not surprisingly, disappears in MCN with remission. When the results are compared allowing for the severity of nephrotic syndrome, there are no differences between MCN and the other diseases studied, with the exception of one report on the effect of sera on mixed lymphocyte culture in which MCN was found to have a greater effect[21]. The factors suppressing lymphocyte transformation have not been fully identified, but are associated with alpha-2 macroglobulin, lipoproteins, and other undefined substances of low molecular weight. Both alpha-2 macroglobulin and lipoproteins are constituents of normal plasma, the concentrations of which rise in nephrotic syndrome. That these inhibitors are not qualitatively peculiar to MCN is further supported by the demonstration of an inhibitor of lymphocyte blastogenesis (with a molecular weight of 60 to 160 kD) in sera from normal subjects as well as from patients with membranous nephropathy, focal glomerulosclerosis, mesangiocapillary glomerulonephritis, IgA nephropathy, polyarteritis, systemic lupus erythematosus and diabetes mellitus[15]. These authors also found that normal human serum contains a 'counter factor' inhibiting the inhibitor of blastogenesis, again suggesting that the effect of serum/plasma from nephrotic patients may be the result of a disturbance in a normally occurring and balanced system.

Further work along these lines, although promising greater understanding of abnormalities in the nephrotic state and the immune system, will not help to define the pathogenesis of MCN itself unless the factor(s) concerned are shown to be specific for MCN. The evidence to date suggests that this phenomenon is secondary to hypoproteinaemia, which therefore includes nephrotic syndrome of any cause.

PATIENTS' LYMPHOCYTE FUNCTION

Other attempts to define an abnortmality of lymphocyte function in MCN have centred on demonstrating disturbances in patients' lymphocyte response to mitogens, T-suppressor cell function, immunoglobulin production, and phenotypes of circulating lymphocytes. In general, as with the effect of nephrotic plasma/serum on normal lymphocytes, there are clear abnormalities but these are not restricted to MCN.

Table 3 Clinical studies identifying allergens that produce significant proteinuria in minimal-change nephrotic patients and the results obtained upon withdrawal of the allergen or hyposensitization of the patient

Allergen	No.	Positive challenge; influence on proteinuria	Withdrawal of stimulus; hyposensitization	Reference
Tree and grass pollen	2	Seasonal	Successful	[55, 56]
Alternaria, Hormo-dendrums, Helmintho-sporium moulds	1	–	–	[56]
Ragweed pollen	1	Seasonal	Successful	[56]
Cow's milk	6	Proteinuria in 4 patients	Successful	[57]
Pork	1	Proteinuria	Successful	[58]
Wheat flour, egg, cow's milk	17	Proteinuria in 4 patients	Successful	[59]

Lymphocyte transformation by mitogens

Studies using Con A and PHA have demonstrated that patients' lymphocytes show reduced proliferation in MCN in relapse, as well as in membranous nephropathy, focal glomerulosclerosis and mesangiocapillary glomerulonephritis[20,26,28,29]. In MCN in remission, transformation becomes normal, although one group found that impaired transformation persisted into remission in patients with steroid-resistant or frequently relapsing MCN who had been treated with cyclophosphamide[30]. The cause of the persisting hyporesponsiveness in these patients could therefore have been either the treatment or the severity of the nephrotic syndrome.

T-suppressor cell function

Varying results have produced a confusing picture depending on the method used, whether or not the patients were currently receiving steroid treatment, and the stage of disease during which the patients were studied. This extends to other causes of nephrotic syndrome, such as focal glomerulosclerosis and membranous nephropathy, in which both increased and decreased T cell suppressor activity have been found.

Conflicting results have also been presented for MCN in remission. One group reported impaired suppressor cell function in patients previously treated with cyclophosphamide, and also related a greater degree of suppressor cell impairment to an increased incidence of relapses[31]. In another study, which differed in methodology and population (in respect of age and a smaller dose of cyclosphosphamide), these findings were not confirmed[32].

No doubt these discrepant findings represent the rather unsatisfactory situation of inferring *in vivo* lymphocyte function from prolonged *in vitro* experiments.

Lymphocyte phenotyes

Studies employing monoclonal antibodies to identify surface antigens thought to indicate T-suppressor and T-helper cells have shown no difference in relapse or remission in MCN compared to normal controls[33,34].

Interrelationship between monocytes and lymphocytes

Circulating monocytes are intimately related to the immune response and are capable of secreting a large number of lymphokines. Few studies have dissected their role in MCN. Co-culture of rat glomeruli with peripheral blood cells from patients with MCN results in increased sulphate uptake by the glomerular basement membrane; this effect requires both monocytes and lymphocytes[35]. Measurement of IL-1 production *in vitro* by monocytes from patients with MCN showed reduced amounts, which increased in the presence of indomethacin, an inhibitor of prostaglandin production[36].

Apart from demonstrating the extent of the immune disturbance in MCN, these disparate observations point only to the need for more definitive studies on the role of monocytes, especially whether their dysfunction is directly related to the abnormalities of T and B cells found in MCN.

B-cells

Disturbances of B cell function have been examined in MCN by measuring concentrations of total immunoglobulin isotypes and subclasses in serum, specific antibody titres to known antigens (both in the resting state and following immunization), and the surface immunoglobulins on B cells. Overall, while unequivocal abnormalities have been demonstrated, they are not confined to MCN.

Raised serum concentrations of IgM and IgE are found in relapse, and are accompanied by low concentrations of IgG[37-44]. An apparent inverse relationship between IgM and IgG concentrations suggests that the normal immunoglobulin heavy-chain switch mechanism is disturbed, but reports of an increased number of lymphocytes with surface IgG do not support this, and suggest a hold-up at the stage of Ig secretion[45,46]. One report demonstrated that steroids neutralized *in vitro* this secretory impairment[47], and cell culture experiments have confirmed reduced production of IgG[48]. These findings, the abnormal distribution of IgG subclasses in the serum[49], and the well-known selectivity of proteinuria in MCN, are against the explanation that urinary loss causes the low serum IgG. IgA concentrations and IgA-bearing lymphocytes are unchanged in MCN, whereas IgE is increased. The latter finding has been related to the reduced IgG, which in normal individuals suppresses IgE synthesis. The increased serum concentrations of IgE may be related to the Type I reactions which are overtly associated with a minority of cases of MCN. This is discussed later in this chapter.

In MCN in relapse, antibody titres to defined antigens derived from pneumococci and streptococci are reduced in patients without overt infection[40,50,51], whereas studies in which patients have been immunized with a known antigen have mainly shown normal responses, the exception being a reduced response in steroid-resistant patients[51-53]. The humoral immune response in MCN therefore seems generally normal, suggesting that whatever mechanisms are causing hypogammalobulinaemia in the resting state can be overcome.

The occurrence of an increased frequency of autoantibodies against antigens derived from kidney basement membrane, kidney microsomes, smooth muscle and gastric cells is likely to reflect derangement of the mechanisms controlling the formation of what are now known to be normal products of B cell clones[54]. There is no evidence that these autoantibodies play a pathogenetic role in MCN.

When remission of the MCN occurs, IgG levels may return to normal or may remain reduced, but IgM and IgE levels continue to be raised in many cases. Similar changes have been described in other types of nephrotic syndrome, emphasizing once more that the findings are not unique for MCN but are secondary to the nephrotic syndrome.

Serum IgE concentrations have been reported to be high or normal in patients with ongoing relapses or in remission[39]. This is not a specific finding to MCN but probably reflects the derangements of serum Ig concentration which have been observed in nephrotic syndrome of various aetiologies. The early reports that IgE may be found in the glomeruli of MCN patients have not been confirmed, and immunoglobulin deposition, apart from small amounts of IgM, is not a feature of MCN.

ATOPY

Atopy frequently occurs in patients with minimal-change nephrotic syndrome. It has been reported by several authors[4,5,7,42,55] to occur in up to 34% of patients, yet its relationship to MCN in terms of pathogenesis or aetiology remains obscure. Certainly, a small number of patients with well-defined MCN relapse when provoked with specific allergens. Pollen, cow's milk, bee stings, poison ivy and pork have all been implicated as causes of relapse (Table 3)[55-59]. In some instances proteinuria has decreased markedly with the exclusion of the allergic stimulus and rapidly returned upon its reintroduction; for example, the reports on cow's milk and pork challenges[57,59]. However, the weight of clinical evidence indicates that Type I hypersensitivity reactions do not play a significant role in the majority of patients. Not surprisingly, drugs which inhibit the allergic response are generally ineffective in reducing either the frequency or severity of nephrotic relapses.

The association between atopy and minimal-change nephrotic syndrome may reflect a common inheritance of susceptibility, as both have been reported to be more common in HLA-DR7 individuals[8]. Alternatively, stimuli such as allergens or infections may activate common immune processes which subsequently cause proteinuria in the MCN patient; it may be relevant that a patient who relapses with Type I reactions can also relapse with an infection.

Immune complexes

Immune complexes are detectable in the serum of MCN during relapse, with diminution during remission[60-62]. The lack of any of the typical features of immune complex disease in the glomeruli suggests that these complexes are not pathogenetic in MCN, although a cautionary note should be deduced from the report that the complexes in MCN do not bind C1q[61]. The antigenic component of these complexes has been defined only in the study describing autoantibodies, in which it was shown that immunoglobulin isolated from the complexes were reactive with autoantigens[54].

DISEASES ASSOCIATED WITH ONSET OF MCN

Infections

Before the discovery and clinical use of antibiotics, patients with minimal-change nephrotic syndrome often died from sepsis. The common occurrence of less serious infection, particularly by encapsulated bacteria such as pneumococci[63], strongly suggested that these patients had an increased susceptibility to infection due to immune deficiencies. Abnormalities of the immune response in MCN patients lend support to this hypothesis. The first line of protection against invading organisms is the phagocytic system, comprising the monocyte–macrophage lineage and granulocytes. The spleen plays an important function in this system by clearing the blood of foreign antigens. Nephrotic patients were shown to have splenic hypofunction, as measured by the uptake of ^{99m}Tc-labelled, heat-damaged autologous red blood cells[64]. The important observation was made that the patients with defective splenic uptake had developed sepsis following the diagnosis of nephrotic syndrome, compared with none of the patients with normal splenic uptake. Splenic B cell function may also be compromised, as B lymphocyte plaque-forming colony (PFC) counts following antigen stimulation are impaired by a circulating soluble immune response suppressor (SIRS). This is produced by suppressor T cells and activated by macrophages[65]. The plasma concentration of SIRS is elevated during relapse and conversely decreases in remission of the nephrotic syndrome, so antibody responses to invading pathogens may be reduced for this reason[66].

Complement abnormalities in MCN, which affect both classical and alternative pathways, may also increase susceptibility to infections, particularly E. coli peritonitis and urinary tract infection[67]. The alternative pathway factors B and I are low in one-third of patients[13]. Forty per cent of children with MCN have low C1q and 20% low C2 concentrations during relapse, which may be explained by their molecular size in relation to clearance by the glomeruli. Opsonization and granulocyte chemotaxis are diminished during nephrotic relapses[68], reflecting the effect that altered plasma concentrations of complement components may have on opsonization and phagocytosis.

In addition to increased bacterial sepsis in these patients, respiratory viral infections frequently precipitate relapses[69]. Despite identification of the virus in 55% of infections causing relapse, no single agent appeared responsible for the majority of relapses. This suggests that it is the host reaction which triggers the relapse rather than a specific viral antigen.

Other viral infections may have the opposite effect on disease activity. There are several reports that measles produces clinical remission, and it has been postulated that it is the marked impairment of cell-mediated immunity, as assayed by the tuberculin skin test, that prolongs remission[70-73]. Certainly, T lymphocytes possess receptors for the measles virus and it has been demonstrated that a small subpopulation of both T and B cells can produce infectious measles particles. In a description of measles causing several months' remission in two related children with untreated nephrotic syndrome, decreased counts of CD4+ and CD8+ T cells, and B cells, were observed in the peripheral blood[74]. *In vitro* tests of the patients' leukocyte migration in the presence of measles antigen, and of proliferation to lectins, suggested that the lymphocyte response was markedly depressed during the remission period.

It is worth noting that, in common with other cell-mediated immune phenomena, the remission produced by measles has also been noted in forms of nephrotic syndrome other than MCN. Overall, the experimental and clinical evidence demonstrates that abnormal cellular immune reactions and reduced concentrations of antibodies favour increased susceptibility to bacterial and viral pathogens. Some of these abnormalities may be accounted for by the loss of humoral factors in the urine, and by malnutrition in severely affected individuals. Most other findings support the concept that the host immune response alone is responsible for triggering relapses and causing the observed cellular, immunoglobulin and complement anomalies in MCN.

Lymphomas

The occurrence of a nephrotic syndrome histologically identical to MCN in some cases of lymphoma has led to much interest and speculation[75]. An important difference from idiopathic MCN is its steroid resistance, suggesting that the two should not be equated. The most relevant observation concerning lymphoma-related MCN is its abrogation by removal of tumour load even by surgery, i.e. without antimitotic drugs or radiotherapy which might affect the immune system. An attractive supposition in terms of the pathogenesis of MCN is that a lymphokine(s) directly or indirectly responsible for proteinuria has been removed. The fact that only a minority of patients with lymphoma develop MCN is suggestive, once more, that the host response is playing a crucial role in the development of the nephrotic syndrome.

Drug-induced MCN

A drug-induced nephrotic syndrome caused by non-steroidal anti-inflammatory drugs has been labelled as MCN[76]. While it is clear that the glomeruli are normal in this condition (by all criteria used to diagnose MCN), and that the proteinuria responds to steroid therapy as well as withdrawal of the drug, caution is necessary before assuming that this is indeed MCN. The main caveat is that the majority of cases also have an interstitial infiltrate, which is not consistent with idiopathic MCN. It is interesting to speculate whether these drugs induce proteinuria by altering the normal balance of lymphokine production by effects on prostanoid metabolism. An intriguing case report of an MCN-like nephrotic syndrome, again with interstitial infiltrates, clearly related to interferon-α administration, suggests even more strongly that lymphocyte perturbation can cause proteinuria[77].

TREATMENT

Several drugs are currently prescribed to promote remission of the nephrotic state. All, with one exception, have immunosuppressive activity although several have many other actions. By studying their mechanisms of action and clinical efficacy we may glean further insight into the immune system's role in MCN.

Steroids

Glucocorticosteroids remain the major primary treatment in MCN[78-80]. They have several actions on the immune system in man, including: (1) inhibition of IL-1 gene transcription by monocytes, thereby restricting IL-1-dependent T cell activation; (2) reduced IL-2 production by lymphocytes, which decreases lymphocyte proliferation; (3) reduction of total mRNA levels in circulating lymphocytes; and (4) reduced interferon-γ production[81]. Although lymphocytolysis does not occur appreciably in man, steroids do cause lymphocytes to be trapped in the peripheral immune organs such as lymph nodes and Peyer's patches. The fact that steroids regularly induce remission in MCN, in the absence of inflammatory changes, suggests that these mechanisms are operative.

Alkylating agents

Cyclophosphamide and chlorambucil have been used successfully to produce prolonged remission in frequently relapsing steroid-responsive, and steroid-dependent, nephrotic syndrome[82,83]. Cyclophosphamide and chlorambucil are powerful inhibitors of dividing cells by their interference with DNA replication. Consequently, actively dividing cells, such as bone marrow cells or lymphocytes, are held in a state of arrested growth. Lymphopenia occurs during cyclophosphamide therapy, being more marked in CD4+ than CD8+ cells. Consequently, the CD4/CD8 cell ratio falls significantly. Azathioprine given to adults with steroid-resistant nephrotic syndrome over long periods (3–15 years) also produced complete remission in all 13 patients reported by Cade et al.[84]. Again, the known effects of these drugs on lymphocytes points to these cells as operating in the pathogenesis of MCN.

Cyclosporin A

Use of cyclosporin A in nephrotic patients has become widespread following the report of effective immunosuppression in renal transplant patients[85]. Clinically, cyclosporin A has been efficacious in producing and maintaining remission in frequently relapsing and steroid-dependent nephrotic syndrome, often allowing total withdrawal of steroid therapy[86-88]. Little success has also be reported with its use in steroid-resistant MCN and focal glomerular sclerosis[89,90]. Its main immunosuppressive action is the specific inhibition of IL-2 and IL-1 production by activated T cells, whereby further clonal T cell proliferation is suppressed. Consequently IL-2-dependent macrophage function is inhibited. The cyclosporin A binding protein, cyclophylin, has recently been identified as peptidyl-prolyl isomerase, which catalyses the folding of polypeptides at proline residues[91,92].

The low dosage of cyclosporin A required to maintain patients in remission suggests that it specifically inhibits the T cell dysfunction responsible for the pathogenesis of MCN. Other actions of the drug that may have some bearing in MCN include increased vascular wall tone, decreased glomerular filtration rate, increased MHC Class II expression on activated vascular endothelium, and alterations in prostanoid metabolism.

Levamisole

The common therapeutic effect of steroids and alkylating agents is generalized immunosuppression, whereas cyclosporin A has specific immunosuppressive actions on T-helper and T cytotoxic cells, but usually spares T cell suppression. Levamisole differs in having immunostimulant effects, as it may cause increased T cell numbers[93] and restore cell-mediated immunity[94]. Levamisole may achieve immunostimulation by specifically inhibiting T cell suppression and therefore enhancing other T cell functions, although little effect is seen on normal T cells[95].

Aune has reported that levamisole inhibited the release of the lymphokine SIRS from suppressor T cells *in vitro*[96]. This inhibition of T cell suppression by levamisole has led to clinical studies being performed in patients with MCN, as the disease has many features suggestive of disordered T cell regulation.

Mehta reported that of 14 children with otherwise untreated nephrotic syndrome, 6 achieved complete remission, 6 had partial remission and 2 failed to respond to levamisole therapy (2.5 mg/kg per day on alternate days)[94]. Tanphaichitr *et al.* and Niaudet *et al.* had previously reported similar clinical results, with 53% and 100% of patients respectively achieving complete or partial remission[93,97].

AETIOLOGY AND PATHOGENESIS

No evidence has yet confirmed Shalhoub's original hypothesis that T lymphocyte dysfunction underlies the aetiology of MCN. The consistent immunogenetic abnormalities described in well-characterized SRNS/MCN patients strongly suggest T cell involvement during an early and crucial stage of the disease. That the expansion of one or several T cell clones may be important is demonstrated by the effectiveness of cyclosporin A and cytotoxic drugs. Derangements in B cell function may follow early immunological dysfunction as a consequence of the abnormal production of lymphokines by T cells. However, no evidence exists as yet that a primary T cell abnormality or abnormal lymphokine production occurs in MCN.

What T cell dysfunction has been demonstrated in MCN? The disease has many features of an underlying immunosuppressive disorder, with T cell suppression occurring during relapses precipitated by an immune stimulus. Furthermore, this immunosuppressive function of T lymphocytes appears to be under control of CD4+ cells, which are involved in the early stages of the immune response. This may explain: (1) the consistent MHC Class II antigen associations: (2) the observation that production of lymphokines such as SIRS may be blocked by inhibition with CD4+ specific antibody; and (3) the effectiveness of the above therapeutic agents. It is important to distinguish between primary and secondary effects, as most experimental evidence describing the profound immunological abnormalities observed in these patients suggests that they are secondary to changes in nephrotic plasma. It is also probable that abnormalities described in MCN, such as the lymphocyte-derived factors which cause increased vascular permeability, may represent a derangement of normal, rather than solely pathological, processes. To overcome these very significant problems in experimental design and interpretation, current research using modern molecular biological techniques should perhaps re-examine the function of lymphocyte subpopulations in this disease, particularly the role that any lymphokine may play in producing proteinuria.

The selective proteinuria of MCN arises from alterations in the charge-permeability characteristics of the glomerular basement membrane. To understand the pathogenesis of this process, more knowledge about the synthetic pathways of the glomerular basement membrane, including factors which affect the turnover of its constituents, are required. No obvious immune process is apparent from histological evidence, but experimental evidence shows that glomerular permeability to serum proteins may be increased by perfusion of human nephrotic plasma into the kidney of experimental animals. Whether this property of nephrotic plasma, which occurs not only in MCN, has an immunological aetiology can only be speculated upon. It is perhaps in this sphere of knowledge that least is known about the disease. This area of investigation contains the greatest paradox—what specific pathological events in the glomerular basement membrane of these patients produce proteinuria yet show no known underlying immune processes? Only when this pathological enigma is solved can the proposed primary role of the immune system in the aetiology of MCN be better defined.

References

1. White, R. H. R. (1973). The familial nephrotic syndrome: 1. A European survey. *Clin. Nephrol.*, **1**, 215–219
2. Korman, A. J., Boss, J. M., Sorrentino, R., Okada, K. and Strominger, J. L. (1985). Genetic complexity and expression of human class II histocompatibility antigens. *Immunol. Rev.*, **85**, 45–86
3. Langueruela, C., Buettner, T. L., Robson, A. M., Kissane, J. M. and Cole, B. R. (1989). Steroid sensitive nephrotic syndrome of childhood: evidence for genetic susceptibility. *Kidney Int.*, **35**, 57A
4. Thompson, P. D., Barrett, T. M., Stokes, C. R., Turner, M. W. and Soothill, J. F. (1976). HLA antigens and atopic features in steroid-responsive nephrotic syndrome of childhood. *Lancet*, **2**, 765–768
5. Trompeter, R. S., Barrett, T. M., Kay, R., Turner, M. W. and Soothill, J. F. (1980). HLA, atopy and cyclophosphamide in steroid-responsive childhood nephrotic syndrome. *Kidney Int.*, **17**, 113–117
6. Noss, G., Bachmann, H. J. and Obling, H. (1981). Association of minimal change nephrotic syndrome (MCNS) with HLA-B8 and B13. *Clin. Nephrol.*, **15**, 172–174
7. Meadows, S. R., Sarsfield, J. K., Scott, D. G. and Rajah, S. M. (1981). Steroid-responsive nephrotic syndrome and allergy: immunological studies. *Arch. Dis. Child.*, **56**, 517–524
8. Cambon-Thomsen, A., Bouissou, F., Abbal, M., Duprat, M-P., Barthe, Ph., Calot, M. and Ohayon, E. (1986). HLA et Bf dans le syndrome nephrotique idiopathique de l'enfant: différences entre les formes corticosensibles et corticoresistantes. *Pathol. Biol.*, **34**, 725–730
9. Adhikari, M., Coovadia, H. M. and Hammond, M. G. (1985). Associations between HLA antigens and nephrotic syndrome in African and Indian children in South Africa. *Nephron*, **41**, 289–292
10. Alfiler, C. A., Roy, L. P., Doran, T., Sheldon, A. and Bashir, H. (1980). HLA-DR7 and steroid-responsive nephrotic syndrome of childhood. *Clin. Nephrol.*, **14**, 71–74
11. Nunex-Roldan, A., Villechenous, E., Fernandez-Andrade, C. and Martin-Govantes, J. (1982). Increased HLA-DR7 and decreased DR2 in steroid-responsive nephrotic syndrome. *N. Engl. J. Med.*, **306**, 366–367
12. McClean, R. H., Ruley, E. J., Tina, L. and Medani, C. (1988). Increased frequency of silent C4A allele (C4A*Q0) of the fourth component of complement in the idiopathic nephrotic syndrome. *Kidney Int.*, **33**, 165A
13. Strife, C. F., Jackson, E. C., Forristal, J. and West, C. D. (1986). Effect of the nephrotic syndrome on the concentration of serum complement components. *Am. J. Kidney Dis.*, **8**, 37–42
14. Tomizawa, S., Mariiyama, K., Nagasawa, N., Suzuki, S. and Kuroumet, T. (1985). Studies of vascular permeability factor derived from T lymphocytes and inhibitory effect of plasma on its production in minimal change nephrotic syndrome. *Nephron*, **41**, 157–160
15. Thomson, N. M. and Kraft, N. (1987). Normal human serum also contains the lymphotoxin found in minimal change nephropathy. *Kidney Int.*, **31**, 1186–1193
16. Levin, M., Smith, C., Walters, M. D. S. and Gascoine, P. (1985). Steroid responsive nephrotic syndrome: a generalized disorder of membrane charge. *Lancet*, **2**, 239–242
17. Sewell, R. F. and Brenchley, P. E. C. (1986). Red cell surface charge in glomerular disease. *Lancet*, **2**, 635
18. Feehally, J., Samanta, A., Kinghorn, H., Barden, A. C. and Walls, J. (1986). Red cell charge in glomerular disease. *Lancet*, **2**, 635–636
19. Cohen, H. T., Singh, A. K., Kaswith, B. S. and Lewis, E. J. (1988). Red cell surface charge in patients with nephrotic syndrome. *Lancet*, **1**, 1459
20. Moorthy, A. V., Zimmerman, S. W. and Burthholder, P. M. (1976). Inhibition of lymphocyte blastogenesis by plasma of patients with minimal change nephrotic syndrome. *Lancet*, **1**, 1160–1162
21. Iitaka, K. and West, C. D. (1979). A serum inhibitor of blastogenesis in idiopathic nephrotic syndrome transferred by lymphocytes. *Clin. Immunol. Immunopathol.*, **12**, 62
22. Beale, M. G., Hoffsten, P. R., Robson, A. M. and MacDermot, R. P. (1980). Inhibitory factors of lymphocyte transformation in sera from patients with minimal change nephrotic syndrome. *Clin. Nephrol.*, **13**, 271–276
23. Sasdelli, M., Cagnoli, L., Candi, P., Mandreoli, M., Bettrandi, E. and Zuchelli, P. (1981).

Cell mediated immunity in idiopathic glomerulonephritis. *Clin. Exp. Immunol.*, **46**, 27–34

24. Martini, A., Vitiello, M. A., Siena, S., Capelli, V. and Ugazio, A. G. (1981). Multiple serum inhibitors of lectin-induced lymphocyte proliferation in nephrotic syndrome. *Clin. Exp. Immunol.*, **45**, 178–184

25. Minchin, M. A., Turner, K. J. and Bower, G. D. (1980). Lymphocyte blastogenesis in nephrotic syndrome. *Clin. Exp. Immunol.*, **42**, 241–246

26. Taube, D., Chapman, S., Brown, Z. and Williams, D. G. (1981). Depression of normal lymphocyte transformation by sera of patients with minimal change nephropathy and other forms of nephrotic syndrome. *Clin. Nephrol.*, **15**, 286–290

27. Tomizawa, S., Suzuki, S., Oguri, M. and Kuroume, T. (1979). Studies of T lymphocyte function and inhibitory factors in minimal change nephrotic syndrome. *Nephron*, **24**, 179–182

28. Schulte-Visserman, H., Straub, E. and Funke, P. J. (1977). Nephrotic syndrome of childhood and disorders of T cell function. *Eur. J. Pediatr.*, **124**, 121–128

29. Sasdelli, M., Rovinetti, C., Cagnoli, L., Beltrandi, E., Barboni, F. and Zuchelli, P. (1980). Lymphocyte subpopulations in minimal change nephropathy. *Nephron*, **25**, 72–76

30. Chapman, S., Taube, D., Brown, Z. and Williams, D. G. (1982). Impaired lymphocyte transformation in minimal change nephropathy in remission. *Clin. Nephrol.*, **18**, 34–38

31. Taube, D., Brown, Z. and Williams, D. G. (1981). Long-term impairment of suppressor-cell function by cyclophosphamide in minimal change nephropathy and its association with therapeutic response. *Lancet*, **1**, 325–338

32. Feehally, J., Beattie, T. J., Brenchley, P. E. C., Coupes, B. M., Houston, I. B., Mallick, N. P. and Postlethewaite, R. J. (1984). Modulation of cellular immune function by cyclophosphamide in children with minimal change nephropathy. *N. Engl. J. Med.*, **310**, 415–420

33. Herrod, H. G., Stapleton, F. B., Trouy, R. L. and Roy, S. (1983). Evaluation of T lymphocyte subpopulations in children with nephrotic syndrome. *Clin. Exp. Immunol.*, **52**, 581–585

34. Feehally, J., Beattie, T. J., Brenchley, P., Coupes, B., Postlethwaite, R. J., Houston, I. B. and Mallick, N. P. (1983). T lymphocyte subpopulations and lymphocyte function in minimal change nephropathy during long-term remission. *Eur. J. Pediatr.*, **130**, 158

35. Garin, E. H. and Boggs, K. P. (1987). Synergy of monocytes and lymphocytes from idiopathic minimal lesion nephrotic patients in relapse in the population of the supernatant factor that increases rat glomerular basement membrane sulphate uptake. *Int. J. Pediatr. Nephrol.*, **8**, 187–192

36. Matsumoto, K. (1989). Decreased production of interleukin 1 by monocytes from patients with lipoid nephrosis. *Clin. Nephrol.*, **31**, 292–296

37. Giangiacomo, J., Clearly, T. G., Cole, B. R., Hoffsten, P. and Robson, A. M. (1975). Serum immunoglobulins in the nephrotic syndrome. *N. Engl. J. Med.*, **293**, 8–12

38. Mansfield, L. E., Trygstad, C. W., Ajugwo, R. E. and Hewer, D. C. (1980). Serum concentrations of immunoglobulins E and G and alpha-2 macroglobulin in childhood renal disease. *J. Allergy Clin. Immunol.*, **66**, 227

39. Groshong, T., Mendelson, L. and Mendoza, S. (1973). Serum IgE in patients with minimal change nephrotic syndrome. *J. Pediatr.*, **83**, 767–771

40. Baliah, T., Park, B. H. and Neter, E. (1977). Low ASO titre and abnormal immunoglobulin levels in minimal lesion nephrotic syndrome in children. *Fed. Proc.*, **36**, 1055

41. Brouhard, B. H., Goldblum, R. M., Bunce, H. and Cunningham, R. J. (1981). Immunoglobulin synthesis and urinary IgG excretion in the idiopathic nephrotic syndrome of children. *Int. J. Pediatr. Nephrol.*, **2**, 163–169

42. Meadow, S. R. and Sarsfield, J. K. (1981). Steroid-responsive nephrotic syndrome and allergy: clinical studies. *Arch. Dis. Child.*, **56**, 509–516

43. Sobel, A. T., Intrator, L. and Lagrue, G. (1976). Serum immunoglobulins in idiopathic minimal change nephrotic syndrome. *N. Engl. J. Med.*, **294**, 50

44. Chan, M. K., Chan, K. W. and Jones, B. (1987). Immunoglobulins (IgG, IgA, IgM, IgE) and complement components (C3, C4) in nephrotic syndrome due to minimal change and other forms of glomerulonephritis, a clue for steroid therapy? *Nephron*, **47**, 125–130

45. Dall'Aglio, P., Meroni, P. L., Barcellini, P. W., Brigati, C., Chizzoloni, C., De Bartolon, G., Migone, L. and Zanussi, C. (1984). Altered expression of B lymphocyte surface immunoglobulins in minimal change nephrotic syndrome and focal glomerulosclerosis. *Nephron*, **37**, 224–228

46. Yokoyama, H., Kida, H., Tani, Y., Abe, N., Tomosugi, N., Koshimo, Y. and Hattori, N.

(1985). Immunodynamics of minimal change nephrotic syndrome in adults, T and B lymphocyte subsets and serum immunoglobulin levels. *Clin. Exp. Immunol.*, **61**, 601–607

47. Yokoyama, H., Kida, H., Abe, N., Koshimo, Y., Yoshimura, M. and Hattori, N. (1987). Impaired immunoglobulin G production in minimal change nephrotic syndrome in adults. *Clin. Exp. Immunol.*, **70**, 110–115

48. Heslan, J. M., Lautie, J. P., Intrator, L., Blanc, C., Lagrue, G. and Sobel, A. T. (1982). Impaired IgG synthesis in patients with the nephrotic syndrome. *Clin. Nephrol.*, **18**, 144–147

49. Shakir, F., Hardwicke, J., Stanworth, D. R. and White, R. H. R. (1977). Asymmetric depression in the serum level of IgG subclasses in patients with nephrotic syndrome. *Clin. Exp. Immunol.*, **28**, 506–511

50. Lange, K., Ahmed, H., Seligson, G. and Grover, A. (1981). Depression of endostreptosin, streptolysin O and streptozyme antibodies in patients with idiopathic nephrosis with and without a nephrotic syndrome. *Clin. Nephrol.*, **15**, 279–285

51. Spika, J. S., Halsey, N. A., Fish, A. J., Lum, G. M., Lauer, B. A., Schiffman, G. and Giebink, G. S. (1982). Serum antibody response to pneumococcal vaccine in children with nephrotic syndrome. *Pediatrics*, **69**, 219–223

52. Fikrig, S. M., Schiffman, G., Phillipp, J. C. and Moel, D. I. (1978). Antibody response to capsular polysaccharide vaccine of *Streptococcus pneumoniae* in patients with nephrotic syndrome. *J. Infect. Dis.*, **137**, 818–821

53. Wilkes, J. C., Nelson, J. D., Worthen, H. G. and Hogg, R. J. (1979). Pneumococcal vaccination in nephrotic syndrome. *Kidney Int.*, **16**, 914

54. Tina, L. U., Phillips, T. M. and Gilcagno, P. L. (1984). Autoantibodies in minimal change nephrotic syndrome. *Int. J. Pediatr. Nephrol.*, **5**, 63–66

55. Hardewicke, J., Soothill, J. F., Squire, J. R. and Holti, G. (1959). Nephrotic syndrome and pollen hypersensitivity. *Lancet*, **1**, 500–502

56. Wittig, H. J. and Goldman, A. S. (1970). Nephrotic syndrome associated with inhaled allergens. *Lancet*, **1**, 542–543

57. Sandberg, D. H., McIntosh, R. M., Bernstein, C. W., Carr, R. and Strauss, J. (1977). Severe steroid-responsive nephrosis associated with hypersensitivity. *Lancet*, **1**, 388–391

58. Howanietz, H. and Lubec, G. (1985). Idiopathic nephrotic syndrome treated with steroids for five years, found to be allergic reaction to pork. *Lancet*, **2**, 450

59. Lagrue, G., Laurent, J., Belghiti, D. and Sainte-Laudy, J. (1985). Food sensitivity and idiopathic nephrotic syndrome. *Lancet*, **2**, 777

60. Stuhlinger, W. D., Verroust, P. J. and Morel-Maroger, L. (1976). Detention of circulating soluble immune complexes in patients with various renal diseases. *Immunology*, **30**, 43–47

61. Levinsky, R. J., Malleson, P. H., Barratt, T. M. and Soothill, J. F. (1978). Circulating immune complexes in steroid responsive nephrotics syndrome. *N. Engl. J. Med.*, **298**, 126–129

62. Cairns, S. A., London, R. A. and Mallick, N. P. (1980). Immune complexes in minimal change glomerulopathy. *N. Engl. J. Med.*, **302**, 1033

63. Pahmer, M. (1940). Pneumococcal peritonitis in nephritis and non-nephritic children: comparative clinical and pathologic study with brief review of literature. *J. Pediatr.*, **17**, 90–106

64. McVicar, M. I., Chandra, M., Mangouleff, D. and Zanzi, I. (1986). Splenic hypofunction in the nephrotic syndrome of childhood. *Am. J. Kidney Dis.*, **7**, 395–401

65. Schanper, H. W. and Aune, T. M. (1987). Steroid-sensitive mechanism of soluble immune response suppressor production in steroid responsive nephrotic syndrome. *J. Clin. Invest.*, **79**, 257–264

66. Schnaper, H. W. and Aune, T. M. (1985). Identification of the lymphokine soluble immune response suppressor in urine of nephrotic children. *J. Clin. Invest.*, **76**, 341–349

67. McClean, R. H., Forsgren, A., Bjorksten, B., Kim, Y., Quie, P. G. and Michael, A. F. (1977). Decreased serum factor B concentration associated with decreased opsonization of *Escherichia coli* in the idiopathic nephrotic syndrome. *Pediatr. Res.*, **11**, 910–916

68. Anderson, D. C., York, T. L., Rose, G. *et al.* (1979). Assessment of serum factor B, serum opsonins, granulocyte chemotaxis and infection in nephrotic syndrome of children. *J. Infect. Dis.*, **140**, 1–11

69. MacDonald, N. E., Wolfish, N., Mclaine, P., Phipps, P. and Rossier, E. (1986). Role of respiratory viruses in exacerbations of primary nephrotic syndrome. *J. Pediatr.*, **108**, 378–382

70. Naglo, O. (1928). Nefrospatient tillfrisknad efter morbilli. *Hygeia*, **90**, 980

71. Blumberg, R. W. and Cassady, H. A. (1974). Effect of measles on the nephrotic syndrome.

Am. J. Dis. Child, **73**, 151–166

72. Starr, S. and Berkovich, S. (1964). Effect of measles, gammaglobulin-modified measles and vaccine measles on the tuberculin test. *N. Engl. J. Med.*, **270**, 386–391
73. Pelton, B. K., Hylton, W. and Denman, A. M. (1982). Selective immunosuppressive effects of measles virus infection. *Clin. Exp. Immunol.*, **47**, 19–26
74. Lin, C-Y. and Hsu, H-C. (1986). Histological and immunological studies in spontaneous remission of nephrotic syndrome after intercurrent measles infections. *Nephron*, **42**, 110–115
75. Moorthy, A. V., Zimmerman, S. W. and Burkholder, P. M. (1976). Nephrotic syndrome in Hodgkins disease. *Am. J. Med.*, **61**, 471–477
76. Finkelstein, A., Fraley, D. S., Stachura, I., Feldman, H. A., Gandy, D. R. and Bourke, E. (1982). Fenoprofen nephropathy: Lipoid nephrosis and interstitial nephritis. *Am. J. Med.*, **72**, 81–87
77. Averbuch, S. D., Austin, H. A., Sherwin, S. A., Antonovych, T., Bunn, P. A. and Longo, D. L. (1984). Acute interstitial nephritis with the nephrotic syndrome following recombinant leukocyte A interferon therapy for mycosis fungoides. *N. Engl. J. Med.*, **310**, 32–35
78. Nair, R. B., Date, A., Kirubakaran, M. G. and Shastry, J. C. M. (1987). Minimal change nephrotic syndrome in adults treated with alternate-day steroid. *Nephron*, **47**, 209–210
79. Imbasciati, E., Gusmano, R., Edefonti, A., Zuchelli, P., Pozzi, C., Grassi, C., Della Volpe, M., Perfumo, F., Petrone, P., Picca, M., Claris Appiani, A., Pasquali, S. and Ponticelli, C. (1985). Controlled trial of methylprednisolone and low dose oral prednisolone for the minimal change nephrotic syndrome. *Br. Med. J.*, **291**, 1305–1308
80. Srivastava, R. N., Agarwal, R. K., Moudgil, A. and Bhuyan, U. N. (1986). Late resistance to corticosteroids in nephrotic syndrome. *J. Pediatr.*, **108**, 66–70
81. Walker, K. B., Potter, J. M. and House, A. K. (1987). Interleukin-2 synthesis in the presence of steroids: a model of steroid resistance. *Clin. Exp. Immunol.*, **68**, 162–167
82. Tejani, A., Phadke, K., Nicastri, A., Adamson, O., Chen, C. K., Trachtman, H. and Tejani, C. (1985). Efficacy of cyclophosphamide in steroid-sensitive nephrotic syndrome with different morphological lesions. *Nephron*, **41**, 170–173
83. Berns, J. S., Gaudio, K. M., Krassner, L. S., Anderson, F. P., Durante, D., McDonald, B. M. and Siegel, N. J. (1987). Steroid-responsive nephrotic syndrome of childhood: A long-term study of clinical course, histopathology, efficacy of cyclophosphamide and effects on growth. *Am. J. Kidney Dis.*, **IX**, 108–114
84. Cade, R., Mars, D., Privette, M., Thompson, R., Croker, B. and Peterson, J. (1986). Effect of long-term azathioprine administration in adults with minimal change glomerulonephritis and nephrotic syndrome resistant to corticosteroids. *Arch. Intern. Med.*, **146**, 737–741
85. Calne, R. Y. and White, D. J. G. (1982). The use of cyclosporin A in clinical organ grafting. *Ann. Surg.*, **196**, 330
86. Hoyer, P. F., Krull, F. and Brodehl, J. (1986). Cyclosporin in frequently relapsing minimal change nephrotic syndrome. *Lancet*, **1**, 335
87. Meyrier, A., Simon, P., Perret, G. and Condamin-Meyrier, M-C. (1986). Remission of idiopathic nephrotic syndrome after treatment with cyclosporin A. *Br. Med. J.*, **292**, 789–792
88. Tejani, A., Butt, K., Trachtman, H., Suthanthiran, M. and Madras, P. N. (1987). Cyclosporin-induced remission of relapsing nephrotic syndrome in children. *J. Pediatr.*, **111**, 1056–1061
89. Niaudet, P., Habib, R., Tete, M-J., Hinglais, N. and Broyer, M. (1987). Cyclosporin in the treatment of idiopathic nephrotic syndrome. *Pediatr. Nephrol.*, **1**, 566–573
90. Jordan, J. C., Querfeld, U., Toyoda, M. and Prehn, J. Serum interleukin-2 levels in a patient with focal segmental glomerulosclerosis: relationship to clinical course and cyclosporin A therapy. *Pediatr. Nephrol.* (In press)
91. Takahashi, N., Hayano, T. and Suzuki, M. (1989). Peptidyl-prolyl cis-trans isomerase is the cyclosporin A-binding protein cyclophilin. *Nature*, **337**, 473–475
92. Fischer, G., Wittmann-Liebold, B., Lang, K., Kiefhaber, T. and Schmid, F. X. (1989). Cyclophilin and peptidyl-prolyl cis-trans isomerase are probably identical proteins. *Nature*, **337**, 476–478
93. Tanphaichitr, P., Tanphaichitr, D., Sureeratanan, J. and Chatasingh, S. (1908). Treatment of nephrotic syndrome with levamisole. *J. Pediatr.*, **96**, 490–493
94. Mehta, K. P., Ali, U., Kutty, M. and Kolhatkar, U. (1986). Immunoregulatory treatment for minimal change nephrotic syndrome. *Arch. Dis. Child.*, **61**, 153–158

95. Hersey, P., Ho, K., Werkmeister, J. and Abele, U. (1981). Inhibition of suppressor T cells in pokeweed mitogen-stimulated cultures of T and B cells by levamisole in vitro and in vivo. *Clin. Exp. Immunol.*, **46**, 340–349

96. Aune, T. M. (1983). Inhibition of interferon or soluble immune response suppressor mediated suppression by levamisole. *Int. J. Immunopharmacol.*, **5**, 91–98

97. Niaudet, P., Drachman, R., Gagnadoux, M. F. and Broyer, M. (1984). Treatment of idiopathic nephrotic syndrome with levamisole. *Acta Paediatr. Scand.*, **73**, 637–641

98. McEnery, P. T. and Welch, T. M. (1989). Major histocompatibility complex antigens in steroid sensitive nephrotic syndrome. *Pediatr. Nephrol.*, **3**, 33–36

99. Kobayashi, Y., Chen, X-M., Hiki, Y., Fujii, K. and Kashiwagi, N. (1985). Association of HLA-DRw8 and DQw3 with minimal change nephrotic syndrome in Japanese adults. *Kidney Int.*, **28**, 193–197

100. Heslan, J. M., Branellec, A., Laurent, J. and Lagrue, G. (1986). The vascular permeability factor is a T lymphocyte product. *Nephron*, **42**, 187–188

101. Tomizawa, S., Mariiyama, K., Nagasawa, N., Suzuki, S. and Kuroumet (1985). Studies of vascular permeability factor derived from T lymphocytes and inhibitory effect of plasma on its production in minimal change nephrotic syndrome. *Nephron*, **41**, 157–160

102. Bakker, W. W., Beukoff, J. R., van Luyk, W. H. J. and van der Hem, G. K. (1982). Vascular permeability increasing factor in IgA nephropathy. *Clin. Nephrol.*, **18**, 165

103. Jones, J. M. B. and Simpson, S. (1980). Immunological studies of minimal change nephrotic syndrome. *Br. Med. J.*, **1**, 291–292

104. Lagrue, G., Xheneumont, S., Branellac, A. and Weil, B. (1975). Lymphocytes and nephrotic syndrome. *Lancet*, **1**, 271–272

105. Zimmerman, S. W. (1984). Increased urinary protein excretion in the rat produced by serum from a patient with recurrent focal glomerular sclerosis after renal transplantation. *Clin. Nephrol.*, **22**, 32–38

106. Wilkinson, A. H., Gillespie, C., Hartley, B. and Williams, D. G. (1988). Increase in proteinuria and reduction in number of anionic sites on the glomerular basement membrane in rabbits by infusion of human nephrotic plasma in vivo. *Clin. Sci.*, **77**, 43–48

107. Yoshizawa, N., Kusumi, Y., Matsumato, K., Oshima, S., Takeuchi, A., Kawamura, O., Kubota, T., Kondo, S. and Niwa, H. (1989). Studies of a glomerular permeability factor in patients with minimal change nephrotic syndrome. *Nephron*, **51**, 370–376

108. Jones, J. M. B., Tulloch, I., Dorte, B. and McLay, A. (1983). Changes in the glomerular capillary wall induced by lymphocyte products and serum of nephrotic patients. *Clin. Nephrol.*, **20**, 71–77.

109. Bakker, W. W., van Luijk, W. H. J., Hene, R. J., Desmit, E. M., van der Hem, G. K. and Vos, J. T. W. M. (1986). Loss of glomerular polyanion in vitro induced by mononuclear blood cells from patients with minimal change nephrotic syndrome. *Am. J. Nephrol.*, **6**, 107–111

9
IgA Nephropathies and Henoch–Schonlein Purpura

F. W. BALLARDIE

In the two decades since Berger's original description, insight into the immunopathogenesis of IgA-related nephropathies has provided our most direct evidence of induction of nephritis by infection, and has improved our understanding of the diverse interactions of the immune system with the environment and kidney. These nephropathies have become the most frequently detected renal diseases in developed countries[1]. Variations in policy towards renal biopsy are likely to account for the lower reported incidences in the UK and possibly in the USA[2-4]. Once considered benign, it is now recognized that inexorable progression of disease often occurs in the largest subgroup, those with low-grade urinary abnormalities[2,5], and that the IgA nephropathies are among the commonest causes of end-stage renal failure[6].

The cardinal symptom, in the early descriptions, of recurrent macroscopic haematuria of early onset in association with upper respiratory tract infections, is now recognized as a feature in only a minority of affected patients. The prerequisite for defining IgA nephropathy is accepted as immunoglobulin A deposited in glomerular mesangium, as the dominant or co-dominant immunoglobulin, in the absence of serological markers of SLE. This diagnostic criterion, and the designation IgA nephropathy, is now applicable to a diverse spectrum of renal disease[7,8], encompassing most clinical forms of glomerulonephritis (Table 1). The close temporal relationship between infection with environmental pathogens at mucosal surfaces and clinical evidence of nephritis, in some disease types, remains central in an explanation of the immunopathogenesis. Considerable recent advances in our understanding of the extent of perturbation in the immune system of patients have not yet precisely defined the immunopathogenetic factors responsible for this diversity of disease expression. The contributions of immune complexes, and recently described autoantibodies, to glomerular injury are the subject of considerable current research. Glomerular IgA itself

Table 1 Clinical presentations of IgA-related nephropathies

Primary		*Secondary*
Nephritic	*Nephrotic syndrome*	*Other*
Rapidly progressive nephritis	Steroid responsive	Nephropathy plus gastrointestinal disease:
	Steroid unresponsive	hepatic cirrhosis,
Haematuria with no		porta-caval shunt,
significant proteinuria:		Crohn's coeliac, disease.
recurrent macroscopic		*Complications*:
protracted microscopic		inflammatory arthropathies
Haematuria plus proteinuria		
Nephritis plus vasculitis:		
Henoch–Schonlein purpura		

does not appear a sufficient explanation[9], and experimental models of IgA nephropathy have to date not reproduced their intended counterpart in man, with macroscopic haematuria.

Conceptually, analysis of immune system dysfunction in IgA-related nephropathies has focused on two areas of regulatory disorder: the processes of local mucosal immunity and immune complex production as leading to nephritis; and the increasing evidence for involvement of systemic immune responses originating from bone marrow-derived cells in some forms of IgA-related nephropathy. Disease in man has features in common with experimental models of nephritis where polyclonal B cell activation occurs. Familial occurrence of the nephropathies, and the immune system abnormalities, also argues for an inherited mechanism of disease, although most genetic factors studied show weak associations and vary between populations. Patients exhibit hypersensitivity to environmental antigens with heterogenous characteristics; recently, evidence of autoreactivity of the immune system has been found, with autoantibodies of several isotypes recognizing self antigens on vascular endothelial cells, immunoglobulin constant regions, and mesangial cells of the glomerulus itself.

These emerging concepts in the pathogenesis of the IgA-related nephropathies have provided new avenues for clarification of their cause. Key developments in our understanding of the immunopathogenesis of the IgA nephropathies and the closely related Henoch–Schonlein purpura, and the implications for design of novel therapies for this important renal disease, will be examined in this chapter.

MUCOSAL IMMUNITY AND IgA NEPHROPATHY

IgA-related nephropathies as a mucosal serum sickness

A mucosal form of serum sickness, analogous to that initially described by Dixon as a consequence of BSA-derived immune complexes in rabbits more than 25 years ago[10], has become a widely held view of the pathogenesis of IgA-related nephropathies[11,12]. Pathogen-derived antigen from viral or bacterial infection[13] in upper respiratory and gastrointestinal tract is introduced by the mucosal route, eliciting a secretory IgA response from mucosal-associated lymphoid tissue (MALT), and leading to formation of immune complexes which deposit in the glomerular mesangium, thereby eliciting tissue injury. Increased intestinal permeability to low-molecular-weight tracers and carbohydrates has recently been shown in patients, where serum levels of IgA containing complexes are directly related to permeability defects[14,15]. Enhanced permeability is unlikely to be a primary event contributing to raised immune complex levels, since abnormalities are also found in unrelated bowel injuries[16]. Abnormal immune mechanisms at the mucosal surface as a primary defect will be considered in detail.

Abnormalities in mucosal surface immune mechanisms in IgA nephropathies

Quantitatively, IgA is the dominant immunoglobulin synthesized in man and distribution is largely restricted within mucosal surfaces and intravascular compartments[17]. Mucosal IgA is predominantly subclass 2, in contrast to that of serum, and is of dimeric (J-chain-linked) IgA, synthesized by B cells migrating through layers of the lamina propria[18]. A presumption is that specific antigen-directed immune responses of the IgA dimer are followed by established mechanisms of endocytosis of antibody–antigen complexes across the mucosal epithelial surface, initiated by, and linked to, secretory component (SC).

At the sites of mucosal antigen challenge, various isotype and subclass-specific disturbances of plasma cell numbers have been described. While there is no quantitative difference between patients and controls in the small intestine when examined for IgA-, M- or G-positive cells[19], and although IgA1 and IgA2 subclass plasma cells are reduced[20], tonsillar abnormalities have been found consistently. In patients with IgA nephropathy[21,22] and Henoch–Schonlein purpura[23], expansion occurs in the J-chain positive, dimeric IgA, secreting cell population compared with IgG positive cells, and similar findings have been reported in episclera[24]. Both subclasses, IgA 1 and 2, are found in pharyngeal secretions[25] of patients, and IgA containing lambda light chains dominates in tonsillar as well as glomerular deposits[26]. These findings in lymphoid tissue imply a local population expansion of IgA positive plasma cells. Clonal expansion seems unlikely since there is heterogeneity of pathogen-derived antigens in tonsillar tissue of patients when compared to controls[27]. Evidence for a mucosal surface origin of glomerular IgA deposits does not, however, receive support from immunochemical characteristics of the IgA subclass.

Glomerular deposits defined by monoclonal reagents are predominantly of IgA1 subclass, co-localizing with J-chain determinants, in the primary nephropathies, whereas SC is detectable in hepatic disease-related forms[28-33] (Table 2). The absence of SC in primary forms is indirect evidence that places doubt on the significance of mucosal surface-derived immune complexes

Table 2 Immunochemical characterization of mesangial IgA deposits in IgA-related nephropathies using monoclonal reagents

IgA-related nephropathy	IgA1	IgA2	J chain	SC	Light chains: κ:λ
Nephritic plus nephrotic	+ ≫	+/−	+	−	κ < λ
Hepatic cirrhosis	+	+	+	+	*

*Analysis not available
Adapted from refs. 28–33.

which might be transported via the systemic circulation in primary forms of IgA nephropathy. In IgA nephropathies secondary to hepatic and other forms of gastrointestinal disease, these links are more firmly established, but definitive studies using isotopically labelled, orally administered antigen have not been carried out in man.

INDUCTION OF IgA IMMUNE RESPONSE: HYPERSENSITIVITY TO ENVIRONMENTAL ANTIGENS

Phylogenetically, the selective induction of specific secretory IgA antibodies is desirable for prevention of infection due to pathogens encountered at mucosal surfaces. Antigen is potentially eliminated with minimal induction of local inflammation since IgA, unless in the form of aggregates, has little capability of complement fixation through the alternative pathway. Antigen-specific immune responses following oral immunization are detected in peripheral blood lymphocytes in normals, and responses of immunoglobulin isotypes G and M are detectable as well as IgA[34]. Classically, continued ingestion of foreign antigen results in systemic unresponsiveness[35], although local mucosal surface antigen-specific IgA responses persist[36]. Most antigens displayed by environmental pathogens require T–B cell cooperation for priming of B lymphocytes to synthesize dimeric IgA antibodies, but a minority—notably those with repetitive polysaccharide-containing epitopes— are capable of priming B lymphocytes in a T-independent manner. Populations of B lymphocytes migrate to blood via lymph and then to mucous or exocrine glands, where there is completion of maturation to IgA-dimer-secreting plasma cells[37]. The mechanisms of antigen transport and processing, sites of synthesis of specific antibodies, and mechanisms governing formation of polymeric as opposed to monomeric antibodies, are unknown in patients with IgA nephropathies.

Antibodies of isotypes G, A and M, with specificity for many microbial and food antigens, are found in normals[38,39], but in disease are predominantly of the IgA1 subclass, in both polymeric and monomeric forms. Immunization parenterally with tetanus toxoid results in both polymeric and monomeric IgA antibodies, the former persisting. After prolonged exposure to certain viral antigens, however, serum IgA antibodies shift from polymeric to monomeric[40,41], suggesting a change in site of production of antibodies, from mucosa where IgA subclass 2 B cells predominate, to bone marrow where there are mainly IgA1 positive B cells[42].

Patients with primary IgA nephropathies have altered kappa/lambda ratios of both IgA and IgG in serum[26], and enhanced IgA-lambda light-chain synthesis following mitogen stimulation of lymphocytes. Highly selective lambda light-chain deposition of immunoglobulins is found in glomerular mesangium[26,43]. These findings argue for a predilection of immunoregulatory disturbance, in patients with IgA nephropathies, for a selective population of IgA subclass 1 and IgG-secreting B cells. The implications of antigen specificity of immune responses for immunoglobulin deposition in the glomerulus will be considered further.

Hypersensitivity to environmental antigens

There are three mechanisms whereby serum antibodies to exogenous immunogens can result in glomerular injury. First, by formation of an immune complex capable of depositing in the glomerular mesangium; second, by cross-reactivity of antibody with endogenous determinants, within the glomerulus; and third by the so-called 'planted antigen' mechanism, where an extrinsic antigen is trapped within the glomerulus and binds circulating antibody in situ[44]. Each of these mechanisms receives support from work in experimental models of IgA nephropathy and disease in man.

In healthy adults, undegraded dietary antigens and associated IgG class antibodies are frequently detected in sera[45]. Increased responsiveness, mainly of IgA isotype antibodies, to environmental antigens in patients with primary IgA-related nephropathies is prima facie evidence for a fundamental regulatory defect in the immune system.

IgA antibodies in patients' sera have been detected with specificity for ubiquitous food and bacterial antigens: determinants present on ovalbumin[46], alpha-lactalbumin, gluten[47], bovine serum albumin[48], and pneumococcal polysaccharides[49], are capable of binding IgA; casein binds IgA1, IgG and IgM classes; and bovine gamma globulin binds IgG[38]. Although specific affinity of immunoglobulin through the antigen binding site has not been proved in most instances by appropriate F(ab')2 studies, and although not all papers confirm these findings[50], there is evidence implicating hypersensitivity of IgA class antibodies in patients. Enhanced immunity to gliadin has received most attention. Serum IgA binding to crude gliadin, and to a gliadin fraction, occurs with variable frequency[47,51]. IgA antibodies with activity to reticulin and endomyosin—markers of coeliac disease and dermatitis herpetiformis—are absent in IgA nephropathy[52], and IgA-containing complexes in sera are dependent on dietary gluten intake[53]. There is no association, however, between IgA nephropathy and coeliac disease[54], nor dependence of the activity of nephritis on these IgA-immune complexes. In contrast to these clinical observations, a gluten–mesangial cell complex is demonstrable in vitro[55], suggesting that glomerular deposition of IgA might be a consequence of in situ formation of a complex following systemic immunity to gluten.

The majority of analyses have not included examination of the specificity of immunoglobulins eluted from glomeruli of patients with IgA nephropathy. Preliminary evidence has shown polyspecific antibodies of isotypes A and G in glomerular deposits; antibody activity in eluants may be completely absorbed by one of wide range of food antigens (P. Druet, personal communication). Conceptually, it is difficult to formulate a mechanism by which chronic exposure to antigens, and the ensuing enhanced immunity, can result in the dramatic, infection-associated, recurrent macroscopic haematuria of subgroups of patients with IgA nephropathy, without invoking other factors exaggerating glomerular injury. The lack of longitudinal studies of patients' immunity to food antigens in relationship to the activity of nephritis reinforces this view. In patients with protracted low-grade urinary abnormalities, however, diet-induced renal injury cannot be ruled out.

AGGREGATES, COMPLEXES AND POLYMERS

Macromolecular aggregates in sera have been the subject of considerable research, but their nephritogenicity remains an unresolved issue. Attempts to detect IgA-containing aggregates in sera in the IgA nephropathies were initially unsuccessful, since complement-based assays often failed to capture these species from sera. At least ten distinct characteristics have been exploited for their detection (Table 3). Constituents have variously been described, including polymeric[56] and (by inference) monomeric IgA[46], fibronectin[57], IgM[61], IgG[61,62], and IgA antibodies with foreign antigen[58,60]. Early reservations about their significance, following detection of IgA-containing complexes in normals[63], were previously ameliorated by IgA subclass analysis. Macromolecular IgA1 is found exclusively in patients with primary IgA nephropathies, with increased total IgA1/IgA2 ratios in serum[64], providing further evidence for a selected B cell population proliferation.

The majority of circulating aggregates are of intermediate size on density gradient centrifugation (11 S to 21 S)[65], and instances of detection of foreign antigen suggest that at least some are immune complexes[66]. These properties of IgA-containing aggregates[67-71] (Table 3) give little insight into their potential to deposit and cause glomerular injury. Renal biopsy eluates have shown a more restricted range of features of deposited IgA aggregates, as characterized by size, IgA subclass and charge; it is clear that anionic IgA multimers deposit preferentially in glomeruli[73,74], and are predominantly of subclass IgA1. There is little information available on the idiotypic nature of the deposited IgA or other immunoglobulins, although one report suggests the absence of IgA-antiglobulin activity when assessed by a non-specific method[75]. Polymers of IgA are considered nephritogenic, since nephritis is associated with detection of IgA polymers in serum more commonly than with multimeric or monomeric IgA-containing complexes[76]. Polymeric IgA-producing lymphocytes are present in blood[77] and may be of intestinal origin[34,78]. These associations, however, are equally consistent with the possibility that other immune species, secreted at the time of IgA polymer synthesis, contribute to glomerular injury.

188

Table 3 Characteristics of immunoglobulin-containing aggregates in sera and glomeruli of patients with IgA-related nephropathies

Physicochemical characteristic	Circulating		Mesangial deposits	
	Assay	Size		
Solubility				
Cryoglobulin[59]		>21 S	17 to 21 S (<1%)	
Cryofibrinogen[57]				
Polyethylene glycol precipitate				
IgA				
Multimeric[61]	Raji cell, inhibitions;	7 S, 11 S	5–9 S (50%)	1000 kD to
Polymeric[46,56]	latex particle, anti-	to 21 S	10 S to 17 S	<160 Kd
Subclass 1[63]	IgA; conglutinin binding		(45%)	(ref. 75)
Antiglobulin activity[68]	Rheumatoid factor			
IgG, M				
Multimers[61,62,64,65,67,71,75]	C1q binding			
	Raji cell			
	Conglutinin binding			
	Fc receptor-related platelet agglutination			
	Inhibition of complement-dependent lymphocyte rosetting			
Complement binding				
Anti-C3: aggregate C3[68]	Anti-C3			
Anti-C3d: aggre-gate C3d[69]	Anti-C3d			
Complexed antigen				
Anti-BSA Antibodies[66]	Raji			
Fibronectin binding				
IgA-fibronectin/ collagen com-plex[70]	ELISA			
Erythrocyte complexed				
Aggregate affinity to erythrocyte CR1 receptor[72]	RBC–IgA binding			

Kinetics and clearances of aggregates

Clearance of the immune aggregates is poorly understood in man. In a murine model, there is renal deposition from sera of only a small fraction of dimeric IgA[79], the majority being cleared by the hepatic phagocytic activity of Kupffer cells. Size, charge and avidity are likely to alter considerably the tendency for mesangial deposition. There is a short half-life in the glomerulus of polymeric IgA complexes in a murine system, and although no analysis of glomerular turnover in man has been possible, clearance of IgA within weeks of deposition has occurred in a transplanted kidney with IgA deposits[80]. Delayed clearance of only polymeric IgA-containing complexes after food challenge in patients with IgA nephropathy, as compared to controls, suggests a defect in hepatic clearance of these species[46]; in normals and patients with coeliac disease, IgA polymeric antibodies to gluten have a shorter serum half-life than monomeric antibodies. Although clearances from blood of monomeric and polymer IgA-containing complexes have similar biphasic components, in a murine system, renal deposits contain only polymers[81,82]. This important abnormality of polymer, as opposed to monomer, deposition and clearance is poorly understood in man. The capability of primary deposits to accrete further monomeric immunoglobulin or other protein in the glomerulus, or to trap circulating proteins through non-specific means, has recently been demonstrated[83,84].

The erythrocyte CRI receptor has been shown to play an important role in transporting immune complexes which display the complement component C3b[72,85], and the disequilibrium between free and bound complexes has placed doubt on the significance of studies measuring free immune complexes in man[85]. IgA1-complex binding to erythrocytes via a complement and Fc-receptor-independent mechanism represents a small fraction only of the total[72]; thus, in patients with IgA nephropathies, IgA-erythrocyte binding does not assume major significance. The peripheral blood clearance of aggregates by polymorphonuclear cell and monocytes has not been quantified[86], although available data suggests that their efficacy at phagocytosis, as infiltrating cells within the glomerulus, is greater than that of the mesangial cell[87]. Stabilization of mesangial IgA deposits by patients' sera *in vitro* is less effective than that produced by normal human sera[88]. Complement may play a role, since C3b, a product of alternative pathway activation, enhances antigen–antibody aggregate solubility[89] by insertion into the lattice, thus limiting size and altering solubility characteristics. This phenomenon may contribute to impaired clearance of mesangial IgA aggregates, although the underlying mechanisms are not clear.

GLOMERULAR INJURY: EXPERIMENTAL IgA NEPHROPATHIES

The mechanisms by which immune reactants generate the great diversity of glomerular injury in the IgA nephropathies in man have remained controversial and poorly understood. Direct evidence for the roles of particular mediator systems is lacking, and current understanding is limited to inferences that the various immunoglobulin species present in sera and eluted from glomeruli are potentially capable of causing injury. Experimental models have focused principally on the means by which the characteristics, kinetics and clearances of the different forms of IgA can be altered to achieve glomerular deposition. It is clear that species containing IgA only are weakly phlogistic; the following discussion outlines our present knowledge of their role and of the ability of immunoglobulins G and M in circulation or complexed *in situ* with extrinsic or intrinsic antigen, complement, and effector cells to modify glomerular injury. In other experimental nephropathies, notably Masugi (or nephrotoxic) nephritis, glomerular injury is known to be mediated by distinct, but probably co-existing, mechanisms. These include, antibody binding alone to nephritogenic antigens of the glomerular basement membrane (GBM); the membrane attack complex of complement; and antibody- and complement-dependent polymorph- and macrophage-induced injury.

IgA complex-induced tissue injury in the alveolar epithelium of rats is complement dependent, occurs in the presence of activated macrophages and oxygen radicals, but is neutrophil independent[90]. Complexes containing other immunoglobulin isotypes, notably IgG, are capable of localizing neutrophils in a similar system[91], presumably because of more effective chemotaxis from complement cleavage products and more effective Fc-dependent mechanisms, although Fc-receptors for both IgA and IgG isotypes are present on neutrophils and mononuclear cells[39]. Glomerular inflammatory cell infiltrates in both IgA nephritis in man, and in experimental models, have frequently been described as nil or minimal[92,93]. During macroscopic haematuria in IgA nephritis in man, renal biopsy appearances show increased inflammatory cells, with extracapillary glomerular cell proliferation, fibrin deposition[13], and interstitial (but not glomerular), phagocyte infiltration. Interstitial changes are also present during quiescent phases of the disease[94,95]. These findings in man show some concordance with experimental IgA nephropathies, although in the latter the acute form of injury has not been reproduced.

Experimental IgA nephropathies

Generation of glomerular deposits: immune complex formation

In the first described model of IgA nephropathy, pre-formed complexes of specific IgA with DNP injected into Balb/c mice resulted in diffuse glomerular IgA deposits with mesangial expansion, but urinary abnormalities were minor and there was no apparent abnormality of glomerular filtration[96]. Multimeric fractions of the IgA complexes were essential for glomerular deposition, and variations in antigen:antibody ratio had no effect on nephritogenicity of the complexes. An active immunization model, that induced by intraperitoneal injection of dextran-derived polysaccharide antigens with anionic charge, resulted in an IgA-IgM mesangial proliferative nephropathy. More extensive glomerular morphological change was apparent, together with C3 deposition, with the use of a different dextran-derived antigen with a cationic charge[97]. Oral immunization of mice with bovine gamma globulin[98], bovine serum albumin, or ferritin[99] also induces serum IgA antibody responses and glomerular IgA deposition, but without detection of antigen or antibody in the glomerulus[100] and with only minor urinary abnormalities in the strains of mice studied.

Persistent virus infections are also capable of inducing glomerular IgA deposits. These include: lymphocytic choriomeningitis in mice (IgA and IgG)[101]; aleutian mink disease, a progressive multisystem parvovirus-induced disease (IgM, G and A)[93]; and oncorna virus-induced disease[102]. The ostensibly spontaneous deposition of immunoglobulins M, G and A in aging DDY mice[103] is now known to be associated with expression of a retroviral envelope glycoprotein (gp70) in lymphoid tissue, which accumulates with antibody in the glomerulus[104]. Systemic administration of lipopolysaccharide regulates the intensity and frequency of IgA deposits in affected mice, probably through a gut-associated lymphoreticular tissue (GALT)-related mechanism[105]. Immunoglobulins and antigen are present in glomeruli, and possible mechanisms include deposition of circulating complexes and complex formation *in situ* by circulating antibodies and a virus-infected glomerular cell. These models illustrate important conceptual advances in the pathogenesis of experimental IgA-related nephropathies. They will be discussed further in consideration of the role of retroviruses in IgA nephropathies in man, although glomerular injury in these models is minimal or absent.

Complement

Current evidence favours the role of complement activation by the alternative pathway in IgA nephropathy in man, which may be intraglomerular. Studies have been cross-sectional and it is not clear whether glomerular deposition of immune reactants other than IgA, at different phases of the disease, is also capable of inducing activation via the classical pathway. In passive murine models of IgA nephropathy, microscopic haematuria can be induced when IgA is complexed to anionic dextran which is independently capable of inducing localization of complement[97], or when complement-fixing IgG1–anti DNP containing complexes are administered[106]; complement depletion by cobra venom factor abrogates this minor glomerular injury. Multimeric IgA complexed with a variety of antigens, including pneumococcal polysaccharide, can induce glomerular complement deposition[107], although the potential nephritogenicity of the complexes is uncertain. In a murine system *in vitro*, dimeric IgA immune complexes activate guinea pig complement via the alternative pathway[108]. In man, the detection of glomerular properdin, and the infrequent detection of C1q and C4[109,110], suggests alternative pathway activation, and the presence of C9 neoantigen[111], C3c and C5[110] suggests terminal complement activation with participation of the membrane attack complex (MAC). Immunoelectron microscopy shows co-localization of IgA, IgG, C3, C5 and C9, but there was no relationship between glomerular protein leak and the intensity of MAC immunostaining[112]. Mesangial cells in culture can be stimulated to produce IL-I and prostaglandins by the MAC[113], but the significance of these findings *in vivo* is unknown. Intraglomerular IgA is detected frequently with components C3–9 and properdin, but early classical pathway components C1q and C4 are present only when IgG is also deposited; co-deposition of IgM does not further increase the classical pathway components[114].

Immune-mediated injury and urine sediment

There is a paucity of information relating immune reactants in sera and glomeruli, or morphological change, to urinary abnormalities in patients with IgA-related nephropathies. While an extensive literature exists on the mechanisms of selective passage of protein across the GBM—a consequence of structural changes and density of anionic sites on heparan sulphate proteoglycan—the mechanisms of haematuria are largely unknown. During episodic macroscopic haematuria, urinary red cell excretion usually exceeds 100 million per day, but urinary protein leak may be observed to be within normal limits (less than 0.3 g daily), implying a complete absence of selectivity for passage of whole blood constituents across the glomerulus to the urinary space. Such glomerular bleeding implies a mechanical disruption to the glomerular structure greater than that when proteinuria only is present. The sites of injury leading to glomerular bleeding in IgA nephropathies have not been identified, but in a modified Masugi nephritis model in rabbits, gaps in the GBM are proposed to be the source[115]. The propensity of subgroups of mesangial IgA nephropathy, in comparison with other acute nephritides, to exhibit this phenomenon suggests a mesangial or capillary loop site of injury.

Renal biopsies coincident with episodes of macroscopic haematuria in IgA nephropathy frequently show crescent formation[13], and patients with microscopic haematuria show increased urinary erythrocyte excretion following respiratory tract infection, in contrast to those with most other glomerular diseases[116]. Immunoglobulins A, G and M are present in glomeruli during active disease, whereas IgA is often the sole immunoglobulin during quiescence (F. P. Schena, personal communication), and IgG has been shown to be transiently present in some individuals[117,118]. These observations suggest a flux of immunoglobulins through the glomerulus. Urinary red cell morphology is variable and associated with histological changes of glomerular injury, increased mesangial and extracapillary proliferation leading to crenated and contracted erythrocytes[119], and urinary platelet excretion[120]. The degree of proteinuria is reflected in the severity of scarring and mesangial proliferative change, independent of renal function[121]. Urinary IgA and IgG characteristics do not reflect those in the serum of patients with IgA nephropathy and Henoch–Schonlein purpura—monomeric and not multimeric IgA is found[122]. The urinary low-molecular-weight protein content reflects tubulo interstitial injury[123].

These findings suggest that there are associated changes in immune-mediated injury, glomerular morphology, and urinary blood loss, with consequent erythrocyte deformity, but that protein loss is likely to be dependent on different constraints (also present in other glomerulopathies) which involve disruption changes to the GBM[124].

AUTOIMMUNITY

Autoimmunity, as recently described in the primary IgA nephropathies and Henoch–Schonlein purpura, has provided conceptual advances in our understanding of immune system perturbations, and allowed better comparisons of disease in man with experimental nephropathies. Glycoproteins and other structures within the glomerulus are a source of many potential antigens, although their characterization as autoantigens and demonstration of their nephritogenic role in man has proved technically difficult. Autoantibodies may be nephritogenic by interacting with discrete glomerular structures, thus initiating or compounding pre-existing injury by targeting mediators of inflammation such as complement or inflammatory cells.

Mechanisms

There are two plausible mechanisms by which autoreactive B cell clones are activated: first, by specific triggering in response to exogenous antigen challenge, with secretion of an antibody cross-reactive with endogenous determinants within the glomerulus; and second, by non-specific means, as in polyclonal B cell activation (PCBA) in response to exogenous mitogen—the B cell repertoire involves secreting autoreactive species of several immuno-globulin isotypes and subclasses. The evidence cited favours PCBA in the primary IgA nephropathies: hypersensitivity to environmental antigens, raised serum IgA, haematuria-associated B cell expansion within the IgA1 subclass in bone marrow[42], and IgG and IgA positive cells in peripheral blood[125,126].

The mechanisms of induction of B cell activation in the IgA nephropathies are unclear. Tolerance to self antigens is generally maintained at the T cell level, in some instances by T-suppressor cells and in others by clonal deletion. Transfer experiments, in the mercuric chloride-primed Brown Norway rat model, have shown that nephritogenic autoantibodies may be induced in naive recipients by autoreactive T cells[127]. In man, as in murine systems, PCBA can be triggered non-specifically by microbial products (lipopoly-saccharides, peptidoglycans and purified protein derivative), producing several autoantibodies from within the B cell repertoire, including rheumatoid factor and anti-DNA antibodies[128,129]. PCBA can also be triggered by various infectious agents, including Epstein–Barr virus, human immuno-deficiency virus, mycoplasma, and some parasites[130]. Within the spectrum of PCBA there is evidence for preferential immunoglobulin isotype production, lipopolysaccharide stimulation resulting in dominant IgM, IgG and E in some models (reviewed in ref. 130). These preferential B cell population expansions are likely to be substantially dependent on cytokines; interleukins 2 to 6 are known to promote specific B cell differentiation pathways (reviewed in ref. 131).

Autoantibodies

Autoimmunity was first suggested in IgA nephropathies when IgM class antinuclear factor was described, which was absent in patients with SLE and which was cold-reactive to nuclei in liver and renal tissue[132]. Subsequently, IgA eluted from renal biopsies was found to recombine with autologous tissue, but not with normal human tissue, in patients with IgA nephropathy and Henoch–Schonlein purpura[133,134]. Affinity of renal eluates for tonsillar cell nuclei, and of IgA in sera for nuclei of fibroblasts and Hel cells, has also been shown[135,136]. IgA from serum complexes with fibronectin and collagen, but not directly with collagen, to form aggregates; there is uncertainty whether this represents true antibody activity through the F(ab')2 site of IgA or non-specific binding to Fc pieces[70,137]. Affinity by ELISA of IgA and IgG for exogenous laminin and other potential antigens has also been reported[138]. IgA and IgG affinity has been found for D-galactose residues, present on human erythrocytes, as well as *E. coli* and mycoplasma pneumonia[139]; IgG antibodies are, however, also present in normals[140].

Autoimmunity directed at glomerular antigens—anti-mesangial cell autoantibodies of IgG isotype with specific F(ab')2 binding—was first described by our own group[141,142]. The autoantigen has components of 45–69 kD, and is apparently localized to the glomerular mesangium and capillary loops. We have recently shown that the target antigen is a human mesangial cell constituent[143], and initial studies suggest localization to the cell membrane. Anti-mesangial cell antibodies were detected in Henoch–Schonlein purpura and in primary IgA nephropathies[144], but not in patients with hepatic disease; there exists an isolated report of a patient with hepatic disease and an autoantibody binding to the mesangial region[145]. Anti-vascular endothelial cell antibodies, more commonly IgA than IgG class, have also been found, with binding in most instances to endothelial cell determinants other than HLA Class I antigens[146]; the antibody activity was not immune complex associated.

IgA autoantibodies with antiglobulin activity—IgA rheumatoid factors—have been detected in sera by several groups[147]. These autoantibodies have similar characteristics in both primary IgA nephropathies and Henoch–Schonlein purpura[148]; they are polymeric, of IgA1 subclass[68], appear to recognize determinants on the constant regions of human IgG, and are a component of polyethylene glycol-precipitable aggregates containing IgG and IgA rheumatoid factor[148]. The IgG subclass specificity of these polyclonal rheumatoid factors has not been determined.

The characteristics of IgA rheumatoid factors provide valuable insights into perturbations of the immune system in IgA nephropathies. Monoclonal rheumatoid factors derived from patients with B cell neoplasms display cross-reactive idiotypes (the Wa group)[149], recently shown to be derived from germ-line L-chain gene segments[150,151]. Studies of hypervariable VH gene elements suggest that autoantibody is expressed early, in a limited way, in B cell differentiation[151]. Rheumatoid factors may be part of a primitive immune system; the relationship between monoclonal rheumatoid factors and the polyclonal rheumatoid factors of the IgA nephropathies is unclear, but they may represent secretion products of polyclonally stimulated and partially differentiated B cell populations.

Nephrotoxicity of autoantibodies: experimental and clinical associations

The human glomerulus contains a multiplicity of potentially antigenic structures, but those which may function as autoantigens are limited. This is dependent on the genetic constitution of the individual, synthesis of autoantibody, and accessibility and display of the relevant epitopes. Hyper-reactivity of the immune system and sensitivity to environmental antigens in IgA nephropathies introduce difficulties in interpreting the growing array of apparent autoantigenic substances. A number of immunoassays have used substrates derived from other mammalian species, although those using substrates extracted from the human glomerulus are more likely to measure antibodies implicated in autoimmune processes. Further analysis of cross-reactivity and polyspecificity of serum and eluted antibody in man and in experimental models is needed. Current work has not yet proved the direct nephrotoxicity of autoantibodies cross-reactive with environmental antigens.

IgG anti-mesangial cell antibodies, in IgA nephropathies and Henoch–Schonlein purpura, were intermittently detected in sera from patients who had IgG present in most renal biopsies, and were found with a high frequency during macroscopic haematuria[143]. In one study, IgA anti-vascular endothelial cell antibody levels correlated with the degree of proteinuria[146]. Longitudinal data on clinical-pathological correlations between immune reactants in sera and disease in man have provided circumstantial evidence for the role of autoantibodies in glomerular injury. In experimental models, Wistar rats receiving murine, complement-fixing IgG1 class monoclonal antibody specific for the Thy-1 antigen present on mesangial cells and other body tissues developed a crescentic nephritis with mesangial cell lysis, followed by mesangial proliferation and heavy proteinuria[152]. Similar effects have been observed with anti-thymocyte serum in Lewis rats[153]. Nephritogenicity is critically dependent on antibody characteristics, including ability to fix complement; other monoclonals recognizing Thy-1 were unable to induce glomerular injury[152].

Autoantibodies and immune reactants: potential synergism in glomerular injury

The contributions and interdepenence of the immune reactants in glomerular injury in IgA nephropathy remains uncertain. Patients may rarely enter complete clinical remission with no urinary abnormality, yet have significant, but reduced, IgA deposits present on renal biopsy[9]. During episodes of acute glomerular inflammation, immunoglobulins G and M are commonly, but not always, present[13,118]. The immunochemistry of eluates from serial biopsies has not yet been examined. Studies of several experimental nephropathies have revealed that the kinetics, dose, and clearance of immune reactants, as well as their intrinsic phlogistic potential, determine glomerular injury. In IgA nephropathies, contributions from each species are likely.

Our patients who were positive for IgG anti-mesangial cell antibodies during a minimum of a 2-year screening period were more likely to have impaired renal function (Table 4). Another study has shown no correlation between nephritis and detection of IgA rheumatoid factor[154]. We have also examined the interdependence of IgG anti-mesangial cell antibody and IgA rheumatoid factor; patients may secrete IgG anti-mesangial cell antibodies together with, or distinct from, IgA rheumatoid factor[155] (Figure 1). Patients with episodic macroscopic haematuria more frequently secrete these two autoantibodies concurrently, whereas there is dissociation in those with microscopic haematuria. These results provide evidence for a contribution

Table 4 Renal function and autoimmunity

	Renal function	
IgG antimesangial cell antibody	Impaired or declining	Normal
+	19	7
−	5	35

$$\chi^2 = 34.5; p < 0.001$$

Primary IgA nephropathies in 66 patients, autoantibody screening > 2 years; no patients had accelerated hypertension
Manchester Royal Infirmary, Department of Medicine

to glomerular injury from IgG autoantibodies in both acute and chronic phases of disease activity, and suggest that these IgG and IgA autoantibodies may produce distinct and additive glomerular injury, potentially via an *in situ* complex formation. Detailed assessment of immunoglobulins present in renal biopsies is required to substantiate these possible mechanisms of injury.

Longitudinal studies of autoantibody secretion have also provided insight into the extent of diversity of polyclonal B cell activation and differentiation. We found that IgG anti-mesangial cell antibodies were more frequently secreted than IgA rheumatoid factor[156] (Table 5). There may also be a role for components of the idiotypic network. Polyclonal B cell activation may be expected to produce perturbation in the idiotypic network, as first suggested by Jerne[157]. For example, in the T15 idiotype system in Balb/c mice, anti-idiotype-containing complexes are deposited in glomeruli but represent only a fraction of the total immune deposits[158]. Disturbance of a component of a putative idiotypic network involving epitopes present on bovine serum albumin has recently been described in IgA nephropathies[159].

Table 5 Differential secretion of autoantibody immunoglobulin isotypes in IgA nephropathy

			Autoantibodies	
Patients	Haematuria	Detection episodes	IgG–anti-mesangial cell Associated	IgA rheumatoid factor Dissociated
9	Macro	21	11	10
7	Micro	11	1*	10

*χ^2; $p < 0.05$
Longitudinal study of 16 patients over 3.6 ± 2.1 years[151]. Patients with episodic macroscopic haematuria secreted both autoantibodies simultaneously more often than those with microscopic haematuria. IgG antimesangial antibodies were also detected as the sole autoantibody more frequently than IgA rheumatoid factor (18 vs 2 of 32 episodes; $p < 0.01$)

Viruses and autoantigens

Intercurrent and persistent virus infection is capable of inducing or modifying nephritis through distinct mechanisms. Each is exemplified in experimental

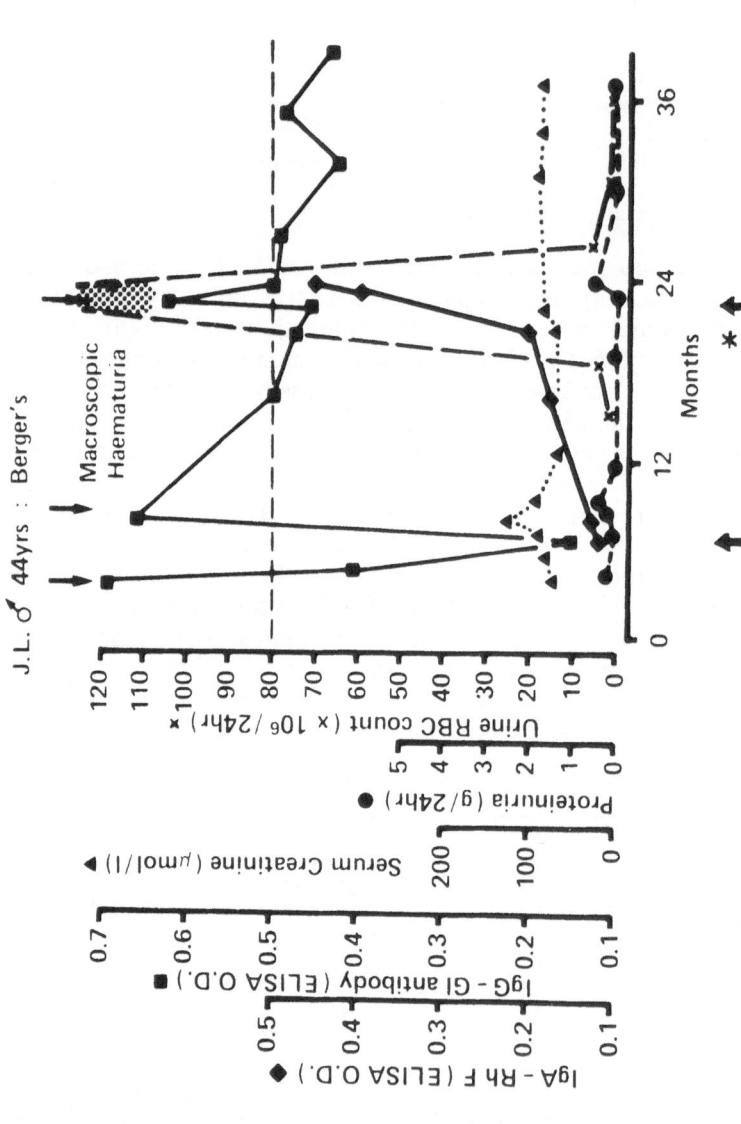

Figure 1 Products of B cell activation and differentiation in IgA nephropathy: dissociated and associated (*) secretion of IgG–anti-mesangial cell antibodies and IgA-rheumatoid factor[151]. Macroscopic haematuria was present only when both autoantibodies were secreted together

human nephritis, and include: polyclonal B cell activation; perturbation of T cell-mediated immunity, including T cell-dependent regulatory circuits; immune complex formation from viral antigen, either formed in the circulation or *in situ*; *in situ* complex formation with virus-encoded glomerular neoantigens; or up-regulated intrinsic glomerular antigens.

In IgA nephropathy, there are several abnormalities associated with viral infection. Haematuria with intercurrent virus infection is well described. Patients have preferential virus-specific IgA1 antibody synthesis in response to vaccination with influenza virus[160]. In an endemic area, persistent hepatitis B antigenaemia is more common in patients with IgA nephropathy than in the general population; virus antigen and DNA are present in glomeruli[161,162]. Cytomegalovirus has been the focus of recent attention. In one series, 31 patients with IgA nephropathy were found to have cytomegalovirus antigen in glomeruli, as detected by antisera[163]. These findings have not been reproduced in identical conditions[164], but non-specific mesangial staining is probably present[165], and CMV-specific monoclonal antibodies in most cases fail to detect viral antigens in glomeruli[166]. Rheumatoid factor autoantibodies might be cross-reactive with CMV antigens since there is considerable amino acid homology between monoclonal (IgM) rheumatoid factor and monoclonal CMV antibody. In addition, cytomegalovirus DNA, if inserted into the host genome, could mimic polymorphisms present in the DQB region; homology or coding for at least six amino acids is described[167], with potential consequences for immunoregulation. Glomerular cytomegalovirus antigen and DNA can be present, however, without glomerulopathy, or with only minor IgG deposits during active infection[168]. This important facet of the pathogenesis of IgA nephropathy merits further scrutiny.

IMMUNOREGULATION: GENETIC FACTORS

Analysis of immunoregulatory defects in primary IgA nephropathies, including Henoch–Schonlein purpura, should be viewed within the constraints imposed by the absence of a specific disease marker or precise description of the role of immune reactants to gomerular injury. There is a need for a better understanding of the immunobiology of stimulatory factors resulting in the selective responses of IgA1, IgA2 and IgG to antigen challenge. The role of cytokines with respect to differential immunoglobulin secretions needs to be defined. The remarkable absence of constant HLA associations in these diseases, although definable as clinically homogeneous subgroups, necessitates extended examination of non-HLA genetic systems.

General

Our current understanding of regulatory networks, essential background for developments in IgA nephropathies, is summarized here. In the normal Balb/c mouse, immunoglobulin production in gut-associated lymphoid tissue (GALT) is governed by regulatory T cell populations with immunoglobulin class-specific helper and suppressor activity. Gut-derived T cell subpopulations are capable of inducing class switching of B cell isotype expression, from IgM to IgA, before maturation to IgA-producing plasma cells[169]. Initial B cell activation requires help from MHC-restricted, antigen-specific Th cells, before division and maturation under the influence of T cell-derived B cell growth and differentiation factors. Subsets of Th cells can support either idiotype, allotype or isotype-specific B cell responses to T-dependent antigens, and T cells from GALT are isotype specific for IgA + B cells[170]. In contrast, spleen-derived cell populations contain so-called T 'contrasuppressor' cells, which support IgM and IgG production, but not IgA responses[171].

In peripheral blood, regulatory Tα cells with Fc receptors for immunoglobulin A (FcαR) have specific helper activity for pokeweed mitogen-induced, differentiated IgA-producing B cells[172]. In man, expression of Fcα receptors on T and B cells is upregulated by infecting pathogens or their products (e.g. *Staphylococcus aureus* and lipopolysaccharide), interleukins, and exposure to dimeric or polymeric IgA[173]. The dependence of these processes on cytokines is the subject of intense research; factors responsible for activation, growth and differentiation have been characterized[174]. Differentiation of certain B cells to IgA + is interleukin-4-induced, and secretion of IgA is IL-5-dependent[175]; specific gene segments of the immunoglobulin heavy-chain switch region, Cu and Ch, are transcribed during these processes[176]. IgA responses from murine GALT B cells are enhanced by combined IL-4 and IL-5[177]. Interleukin-5 induces high rates of IgA synthesis in IgA positive GALT B cells stimulated with lipopolysaccharide[178], but this effect is absent in cells that have not undergone isotype switch[179]. B cell differentiation is also enhanced by the complement breakdown product C3dg, independent of T cells[180]. Interleukin-6, in part responsible for acute-phase responses and enhanced thymocyte proliferation, is also implicated in selective B cell population expansion in certain autoimmune diseases[181,182].

IgA nephropathies

The role of these complex regulatory circuits is exemplified by autoantibody production in experimental nephropathies. T cell contrasuppression is known to facilitate polyclonal B cell activation and synthesis of nephritogenic autoantibodies in a murine model of interstitial nephritis[183] and autoimmunity can be induced by primed T cells only[127]. In IgA nephropathies, activation of the IgA-secreting system occurs during haematuria[126], but studies of cell function and phenotype at the population level have provided conflicting results and it has not been possible to define a central mechanism of regulatory dysfunction. Analysis of circulating IgA and IgG-bearing lymphocytes, T cells with helper and suppressor function, T and B alpha cells (with receptors for Fc of IgA), and spontaneous and mitogen-stimulated immunoglobulin synthesis *in vitro*, has been the subject of a recent review. Receptor up-regulation for Fcα on T and B cells, and IL-2 on T cells, is found in patients[184,185]. Fcα expression is inducible *in vitro* by co-culture with IgA, and reduced expression in patients with selective IgA deficiency is correctable by cell-free conditioned medium[186]. In contrast, patients with IgA nephropathy show maximal expression of Fcα density. These findings suggest that changes in receptor expression are secondary to defects in cytokine production.

The inconsistent reporting of enhanced T-helper cell function, reduced T-suppressor cell function, and increased IgA production (with or without concanavalin A or pokeweed mitogen) has not been resolved by correlations of these analyses with phasic activity of nephritis[126,186,187]. In the mouse, some autoreactive T cell clones are known to support B cell differentiation and proliferation into distinct IgA and IgG isotype-positive secretory cells through soluble factors in murine systems[188]. The variable associations of T cell populations with IgA nephropathy may be explicable by future clonal analyses. Patterns of IgG production parallel those of IgA[189,190], particularly in patients with marked glomerular injury[191]. Pokeweed mitogen-stimulated polymeric IgA synthesis is increased[192], and found more frequently in patients with macroscopic haematuria[193].

Genetic factors potentially influencing expression of these disturbances in the immune system in IgA nephropathies have recently been reviewed[194]. The apparently weak association with Class I and II HLA antigens (BW35 and DR4) may be a consequence of the variable composition of patient groups analysed (see Chapter 1). The marked influence of the tendency to perform renal biopsies for diagnostic purposes[3] is likely to bias groups towards those with particular clinical characteristics. Familial occurrences of disease without association with HLA antigens supports non-HLA linkages. Polymorphisms within the immunoglobulin heavy-chain switch region are associated with primary IgA nephropathy with recurrent macroscopic haematuria[195]; a significant decrease in cu-related phenotype and increase in Cα1 are present. Transcription from polymorphisms in these loci, which are of importance in immunoglobulin isotype switching, is likely to influence expression of gene products in IgA nephropathies.

HEPATIC DYSFUNCTION AND IgA NEPHROPATHIES

Hepatic dysfunction in cirrhosis in man induces elevated total serum IgA and low-grade proliferative and glomerulosclerotic lesions, with IgA deposition in 33–90% of cases and IgG or IgM in 4–10%[196−200]. Clinical evidence of nephropathy—significant proteinuria or microscopic haematuria—is present in only a minority, typically 5–10% of those with immune deposits[201]. Loss of renal function is generally a consequence of renal haemodynamic factors and not glomerulopathy. The distinction from the primary IgA nephropathies is further supported by immunochemical differences in glomerular deposits (Table 2), and absence of evidence for overactivity of the systemic immune system[142]. Much information on the clearance kinetics of IgA and aggregates has originated from studies of experimental and human hepatic dysfunction. The liver is the major site of catabolism for both polymeric and monomeric IgA in the mouse[202,203].

Parenchymal liver disease in man, but not biliary obstruction, results in a preferential rise in serum polymeric IgA, accompanied by a reduction in fractional catabolic rate[204]. In a murine system, cholestasis also promotes deposition of circulating IgA complexes, with specific antigen detectable in glomeruli[205]. In cirrhotic rats, there is a rise in IgA- and IgM-containing aggregates, with glomerular deposition[206] which may include IgG[207]. Foreign antigen complexed with oligomeric IgA is cleared via hepatocyte receptors which have affinity for both Fc and secretory component (whereas Kupffer cells express Fcγ only)[208-210]. Polymeric IgA and polymeric IgA antigen complexes are transported by the same mechanism[211].

Glomerular morphological abnormalities at the light-microscopic level, and proteinuria, do not occur in these experimental systems unless there is additional non-specific blockage of the hepatic reticuloendothelial system; this results in greater intensity of staining of immunoglobulin deposits[212,213]. Findings in these animal models appear to resemble the minor glomerular disease found in the secondary IgA nephropathies in man.

HENOCH–SCHONLEIN NEPHRITIS

Henoch–Schonlein purpura (HSP) is a systemic disease with leukocytoclastic vasculitis proven on cutaneous biopsy or suggested by bowel and joint symptoms. The diagnosis generally requires detection of immunoglobulin A in an organ of injury[214]; when found in glomeruli, with urinary abnormality, the term Henoch–Schonlein nephritis is properly applied. The concept of HSP as a vasculitis superimposed on the nephritis of primary IgA nephropathy has important implications in our understanding of the pathogenesis and interdependence of autoimmune vascular and glomerular injury. In adults, HSP is rare in contrast to its frequency in paediatric practice, but is now recognized to carry a higher long-term risk of renal dysfunction[215] than was previously considered[214,216,217]. Mortality may be significant[215], although bowel vasculitis has been reported to be steroid responsive or self-limiting in some cases[217].

Serological abnormalities found in patients with HSP closely reflect those of primary IgA nephropathies: total serum IgA is increased; spontaneous IgA, IgG and IgM synthesis *in vitro* by peripheral blood mononuclear cells is increased, and can be suppressed by pokeweed mitogen and allogeneic but not autologous T cells[218]; aggregates, polymers and immune complexes containing IgA as well as IgG are present (Table 3); and polyclonal IgA rheumatoid factor is found[219]. In addition, glomerular and cutaneous IgA1 and J-chain deposition is similar to that in primary IgA nephropathy (reviewed in ref. 220). Circulating IgG autoantibodies recognizing glomerular antigenic components of the same molecular weight as IgA nephropathies are detectable in HSP[144], and we recently localized the autoantigen to the mesangial cell as in IgA nephropathy[143a,143b].

These comparisons of immune perturbations do not explain the disparity in organ injury between HSP and IgA nephropathy. HSP with microscopic haematuria is described in a patient with a history of recurrent macroscopic haematuria due to IgA nephropathy (ref. 141 and unpublished observations of Ballardie). Each disease is described in twins, precipitated by the same antecedent infection[221], and there exist *formes frustes* of HSP with IgA nephritis and related uveitis[222]. Recent findings suggest a pathogenetic mechanism for the differences between the two diseases. We found that IgG anti-mesangial cell antibodies were present in sera during active Henoch–Schonlein nephritis, but were absent when only other (non-renal) organs were affected[223]. The vasculitis of HSP may be accompanied by IgA and IgG autoantibodies recognizing anti-neutrophil cytoplasmic antigens[224,225]. The relationship between these two autoantibody systems may hold the key to expression of organ injury.

TREATMENT OF IgA NEPHROPATHIES

Therapeutic intervention in the various forms of IgA nephropathy has been designed to arrest inexorable or rapid decline in renal function, to induce remission in nephrotic syndrome, or to suppress the more severe forms of vasculitis in adults with Henoch–Schonlein nephritis. Treatments include: reduction in load of foreign antigen, by eradication of chronic infection or dietary manipulation; removal of immunocompetent tissue; immunosuppression with drugs and plasma exchange in rapidly progressive nephritis; and modification of glomerular inflammation with corticosteroids or other therapies.

Tonsillectomy reduced episodic macroscopic haematuria and proteinuria compared with controls[226], and also reduced serum total IgA, polymeric IgA and PEG-precipitable immune complexes[227]. Cyclophosphamide reduces GALT IgA responses to cholera toxin in murine systems, but only when administered at high dose prior to antigen challenge[228]. It has been used at conventional dosage with anti-platelet agents and warfarin in IgA nephropathies. Decline in renal function over periods of up to 3 years was less than in controls; there was a reduction in proteinuria[229]; and repeated renal biopsies showed reduction in progressive scarring[230]. Corticosteroids administered for up to 19 months and followed by non-steroidal anti-inflammatory or anti-platelet drugs reduced persistent proteinuria and decline in renal function in patients with creatinine clearances greater than 70 ml/min[231]. Haemodynamic effects of treatment in these uncontrolled studies cannot, however, be discounted. Remission can be induced in patients with severe nephrotic syndrome with steroids, but without long term benefit on renal function[232,233]. Anti-platelet agents[234], non-steroidal anti-inflammatory drugs[235], eicosapentanoic acid[236], danazol[237], dapsone[238], and phenytoin[239,240], are of unproven or no benefit.

Five children with rapidly progressive nephritis due to IgA nephropathy proved resistant to pulse corticosteroids[6]. There are anecdotal reports of recovery of renal function using plasma exchange, cyclophosphamide and prednisolone[241]. Our experience in this rare form of IgA nephropathy is less encouraging; two adults with 80% and 95% crecentic change failed to improve after similar therapy (Ballardie, unpublished data). Plasma exchange without immunosuppressive drugs had no effect on patients with slowly progressive IgA nephropathy, but led to improvement in two with rapidly progressive Henoch–Schonlein nephritis, one of whom also received prednisolone[242]. Severe Henoch–Schonlein nephritis is reported to be steroid responsive[243,244]. Vasculitis affecting the bowel in HSP can be dramatically improved with corticosteroids alone[217]. Anti-mesangial cell autoantibodies in individual patients with persistently active Henoch–Schonlein purpura were rapidly suppressed during treatment with corticosteroids only, in association with remission of nephritis and vasculitis. Relapse and recurrence of antibodies followed withdrawal of therapy[141], but longer-term benefit in these patients remains in doubt[223].

The design and application of future treatment regimens are likely to be radically influenced by our rapidly expanding knowledge of immune system perturbations and processes of immune injury in the IgA nephropathies and Henoch–Schonlein purpura.

References

1. D'Amico, G. (1987). The commonest glomerulonephritis in the world: IgA nephropathy. *Q. J. Med.*, **64**(245), 709–727
2. Ballardie, F. W., O'Donoghue, D. J. and Feehally, J. (1987). Increasing frequency of adult IgA nephropathy in the UK? *Lancet*, **2**, 1205
3. Feehally, J., O'Donoghue, D. J. and Ballardie, F. W. (1989). Current nephrological practice in the investigation of haematuria: relationship to incidence of IgA nephropathy. *J. R. Coll. Physicians.*, **23**, 228–231
4. Julian, B. A., Waldo, F. B. and Rifai, A. (1988). IgA nephropathy, the most common glomerulonephritis worldwide. A neglected disease in the United States? *Am. J. Med.*, **84**, 129–132
5. Emancipator, S. N., Gallo, G. R. and Lamm, M. E. (1985). IgA nephropathy: perspectives on pathogenesis and classification. *Clin. Nephrol.*, **24**(4), 161–179
6. Simon, P., Bramee, M. S. and Ang, K. S. (1988). Idiopathic IgA mesangial nephropathy is the main cause of end stage renal failure in a French area. *Kidney Int.*, **34**(4), 566 (Abstract)
7. Welch, T. R., McAdams, A. J. and Berry, A. (1988). Rapidly progressive IgA nephropathy. *Am. J. Dis. Child.*, **142**, 789–793
8. Brouhard, B. H. (1988). The spectrum of IgA nephropathy. *Am. J. Dis. Child.*, **142**, 709–710
9. Costa, R. S., Droz, D. and Noel, L. H. (1987). Long-standing spontaneous clinical remission and glomerular improvement in primary IgA nephropathy (Berger's disease). *Am. J. Nephrol.*, **7**, 440–444
10. Dixon, F. J., Feldeman, J. D. and Vazquez, J. J. (1961). Experimental glomerulonephritis: pathogenesis of a laboratory model resembling the spectrum of human glomerulonephritis. *J. Exp. Med.*, **113**, 899–920
11. Lamm, M. E. (1987). The mucosal immune system and IgA nephropathy. *Semin. Nephrol.*, **VII**(4), 280–282
12. Bene, M. C. and Faure, G. C. (1987). Mucosal immunity and IgA nephropathies. *Semin. Nephrol.*, **VII**(4), 297–300
13. Nicholls, K. M., Fairley, K. F. and Dowling, J. P. (1984). The clinical course of mesangial IgA associated nephropathy in adults. *Q. J. Med.*, **210**, 227–250
14. Davin, J. C., Forget, P. and Mahieu, P. R. (1988). Increased intenstinal permeability to (51 Cr) EDTA is correlated with IgA immune complex-plasma levels in children with IgA-associated nephropathies. *Acta Paediatr. Scand.*, **77**, 118–124
15. Jenkins, D. A. S., Bell, G. M. and Ferguson, A. (1988). Intestinal permeability in IgA nephropathy. *Nephron*, **50**, 390
16. Forget, P., Sodoyez-Goffauz, F. and Zappitelli, A. (1984). Permeability of the small intestine to (51 Cr) EDTA in children with acute gastroenteritis or eczema. *J. Pediatr. Gastroenterol. Nutr.*, **4**, 393–396
17. Conley, M. E. and Delacroix, D. L. (1987). Intravascular and mucosal immunoglobulin A: two separate but related systems of immune defense? *Ann. Intern. Med.*, **106**, 892–899
18. Lawton, A. R., III and Mage, R. G. (1969). Synthesis of secretory IgA in the rabbit, I. Evidence for synthesis as an 11S dimer. *J. Immunol.*, **102**, 693–697
19. Westberg, N. G., Baklien, K. and Schmekel, B. (1983). Quantitation of immunoglobulin-producing cells in small intestinal mucosa of patients with IgA nephropathy. *Clin. Immunol. Immunopathol.*, **26**, 442–445

20. Hene, R. J., Schuurman, H. and Kater, L. (1988). Immunoglobulin A subclass-containing plasma cells in the jejunum in primary IgA nephropathy and in Henoch–Schonlein purpura. *Nephron*, **48**, 4–7

21. Bene, M. C., Faure, G. and Hurault de Ligney, B. (1983). Quantitative immunohistomorphometry of the tonsillar plasma cells evidences an inversion of the immunoglobulin A versus immunoglobulin G secreting cell balance. *J. Clin. Invest.*, **71**, 1342–1347

22. Egido, J., Blasco, R. and Lozano, L. (1984). Immunological abnormalities in the tonsils of patients with IgA nephropathy: inversion in the ratio of IgA: IgG bearing lymphocytes and increased polymeric IgA synthesis. *Clin. Exp. Immunol.*, **57**, 101–106

23. Bene, M. C., Hurault de Ligny, B. and Faure, G. (1986). Histoimmunological discrepancies in primary IgA nephropathy and anaphylactoid purpura sustain relationships between mucosa and kidney. *Nephron*, **43**, 214–216

24. Bene, M. C., Hurault de Ligny, B. and Sirbat, D. (1984). IgA nephrology: dimeric IgA-secreting cells are present in episcleral infiltrate. *Am. J. Clin. Pathol.*, **82**, 608–611

25. Tomino, Y., Endoh, M. and Kaneshige, H. (1983). Increase of IgA in pharyngeal washings from patients with IgA nephropathy. *Am. J. Med. Sci.*, **286**(2), 15–21

26. Lai, K.-N., Chui, S.-H. and Lai, F. M.-M. (1988). Predominant synthesis of IgA with lambda light chain in IgA nephropathy. *Kidney Int.*, **33**, 584–589

27. Tomino, Y., Sakai, H. and Hashimoto, K. (1987). Antigenic heterogeneity in patients with IgA nephropathy. *Semin. Nephrol.*, **VII**(4), 294–296

28. Andre, C., Berthoux, F. C. and Andre, F. (1980). Prevalence of IgA2 deposits in IgA nephropathies. *N. Engl. J. Med.*, **303**(23), 1343–1346

29. Lomax-Smith, J. D., Zabrowarny, L. A. and Howarth, G. S. (1983). The immunochemical characterization of mesangial IgA deposits. *Am. J. Pathol.*, **113**(3), 359–370

30. Conley, M. E., Cooper, M. D. and Michael, A. F. (1980). Selective deposition of immunoglobulin A1 in immunoglobulin A nephropathy, anaphylactoid pupura nephritis, and systemic lupus erythematosus. *J. Clin. Invest.*, **66**, 1432–1436

31. Tomino, Y., Endoh, M. and Nomoto, Y. (1981). Immunoglobulin A1 in IgA nephropathy. *N. Engl. J. Med.*, **305**, 1159–1160

32. Donini, U., Casanova, S. and Zini, N. (1982). The presence of J chain in mesangial immune deposits of IgA nephropathy. *Proc. EDTA*, **19**, 655–661

33. Coppo, R., Basolo, B. and Mazzucco, G. (1983). IgA1 and IgA2 in circulating immune complexes and in renal deposits of Berger's and Schonlein–Henoch glomerulonephritis. *Proc. EDTA*, **19**, 648–654

34. Forrest, B. D. (1988). Identification of an intestinal immune response using peripheral blood lymphocytes. *Lancet*, **1**, 81–83

35. Wells, G. H. (1911). Studies on the chemistry of anaphylaxis IV. Experiments with isolated proteins, especially those of hens eggs. *J. Infect. Dis.*, **9**, 147–154

36. Challacombe, S. J. and Tomasi, T. B. (1980). Systemic intolerance and secretory immunity after oral immunisation. *J. Exp. Med.*, **153**, 1459–1472

37. Solari, R.l and Kraehenbuhl J.-P. (1985). The biosynthesis of secretory component and its role in the transepithelial transport of IgA dimer. *Immunol. Today*, **6**(1), 17–20

38. Russell, M. W., Mestecky, J. and Julian, B. A. (1986). IgA-associated renal diseases: antibodies to environmental antigens in sera and deposition of immunoglobulins and antigens in glomeruli. *J. Clin. Immunol.*, **6**(1), 74–86

39. Mestecky, J. and McGhee, J. R. (1987). Immunoglobulin A (IgA): molecular and cellular interactions involved in IgA biosynthesis and immune response. *Adv. Immunol.*, **40**, 153–245

40. Mestecky, J., Czerkinsky, C. and Russell, M. W. (1987). Induction and molecular properties of secretory and serum IgA antibodies specific for environmental antigens. *Ann. Allergy*, **59**, 54–59

41. Negro-Ponzi, A., Merlino, C. and Angeretti, A. (1985). Virus-specific polymeric immunoglobulin A antibodies in serum from patients with rubella, measles, varicella and herpes zoster virus infections. *J. Clin. Microbiol.*, **22**, 505–509

42. van den Wall Bake, A. W. L., Daha, M. R. and Radl, J. (1988). The bone marrow as production site of the IgA deposited in the kidneys of patients with IgA nephropathy. *Clin. Exp. Immunol.*, **72**, 321–325

43. Lai, K.N., Chan, K. W. and Lai, F. M.-M. (1985). The immunochemical characterization of the light chains in the mesangial IgA deposits in IgA nephropathy. *Am. J. Clin. Pathol.*,

85(5), 548–551
44. Mauer, S. M., Sutherland, D. E. R. and Howard, R. J. (1973). The glomerular mesangium. Acute immune mesangial injury: a new model of glomerular nephritis. *J. Exp. Med.*, **137**, 8553–8570
45. Husby, S., Jensenius, J. C. and Svehag, S.-E. (1986). Passage of undergraded dietary antigen into the blood of healthy adults. Further characterization of the kinetics of uptake and the size distribution of the antigen. *Scand. J. Immunol.*, **24**, 447–455
46. Sancho, J., Egido, J. and Rivera, F. (1983). Immune complexes in IgA nephropathy: presence of antibodies against diet antigens and delayed clearance of specific polymeric IgA immune complexes. *Clin. Exp. Immunol.*, **54**, 194–202
47. Nagy, J., Scott, H. and Brandtzaeg, P. (1988). Antibodies to dietary antigens in IgA nephropathy. *Clin. Nephrol.*, **29**(5), 274–279
48. Egido, J., Sancho, J. and Hernando, P. (1984). Presence of specific IgA immune complexes in IgA nephropathy. *Contrib. Nephrol.*, **40**, 80–86
49. Drew, P. A., Nieuwhof, W. N. and Clarkson, A. R. (1987). Increased concentration of serum IgA antibody to pneumococcal polysaccharides in patients with IgA nephropathy. *Clin. Exp. Immunol.*, **67**, 124–129
50. Fornasieri, A., Sinico, R. A. and Maldifassi, P. (1988). Food antigens, IgA-immune complexes and IgA mesangial nephropathy. *Nephrol. Dial. Transplant.*, **3**, 738–743
51. Fornasieri, A., Sinico, R. A. and Maldifassi, P. (1987). IgA-antigliadin antibodies in IgA mesangial nephropathy (Berger's disease). *Br. Med. J.*, **295**, 78–80
52. Rostoker, G., Laurent, J. and Andre, C. (1988). High levels of IgA antigliadin antibodies in patients who have IgA mesangial glomerulonephritis but not coeliac disease. *Lancet*, **1**, 356–357
53. Coppo, R., Basolo, B. and Rollino, C. (1986). Mediterranean diet and primary IgA nephropathy. *Clin. Nephrol.*, **26**(2), 72–82
54. Kumar, V., Sieniawska, M. and Beutner, E. H. (1988). Are immunological markers of gluten-sensitive enteropathy detectable in IgA nephropathy? *Lancet*, **2**, 1307
55. Amore, A., Emancipator, S. and Coppo, R. (1988). Specific binding of gliadin to rat mesangial cells in culture. *Proc. EDTA-ERA, XXV Congress*, p. 47 (Abstract)
56. Sanchio, J., Gido, J. and Gonzalis, E. (1983). Simplified method for determining polymeric IgA-containing immune complexes. *J. Immunol. Method.*, **60**, 305–317
57. Nagy, J., Ambrus, M. and Paal, M. (1987). Crylroglobulinaemia and cryofibrinogenaemia in IgA nephropathy: a follow-up study. *Nephron*, **46**, 337–342
58. Mascart-Lemone, F., Van den Broeck, S. C. and Dive, C. (1988). IgA immune response patterns to gliadin in serum. *Int. Arch. Allergy Appl. Immunol.*, **86**, 412–419
59. Garcia-Fuentes, M., Chantler, C.l and Williams, D. G. (1977). Cryoglobulinaemia in Henoch–Schonlein purpura. *Br. Med. J.*, **2**, 163–165
60. Egido, J., Sancho, J. and Blasco, R. (1983). Immunopathogenetic aspects of IgA nephropathy. *Adv. Nephrol.*, **12**, 103–137
61. Woodruffe, A. J., Gormly, A. A. and McKenzie, P. E. (1980). Immunologic studies in IgA nephropathy. *Kidney Int.*, **18**, 366–374
62. Egido, J., Sancho, J. and Rivera, F. (1984). The role of IgA and IgG immune complexes in IgA nephropathy. *Nephron*, **36**, 52–59
63. Cairns, S. A., London, R. A. and Mallick, N. P. (1981). Circulating immune complexes following food: delayed clearance in idiopathic glomerulonephritis. *J. Clin. Lab. Immunol.*, **6**, 121–126
64. Valentijn, R. M., Radl, J. and Haaijman, J. J. (1984). Circulating and mesangial secretory component-binding IgA-1 in primary IgA nephropathy. *Kidney Int.*, **26**, 760–766
65. Valentijn, R. M., Kauffmann, R. H. and de la Riviere, G. B. (1983). Presence of circulating macromolecular IgA in patients with hematuria due to primary IgA nephropathy. *Am. J. Med.*, **74**, 375–381
66. Yap, H. K., Sakai, R. S. and Woo, K. T. (1987). Detection of bovine serum albumin in the circulating IgA immune complexes of patients with IgA nephropathy. *Clin. Immunol. Immunopathol.*, **43**, 395–402
67. Coppo, R., Basolo, B. and Martina, G. (1982). Circulating immune complexes containing IgA, IgG and IgM in patients with primary IgA nephropathy and with Henoch–Schonlein nephritis. Correlation with clinical and histologic signs of activity. *Clin. Nephrol.*, **18**(5), 230–239

68. Czerkinsky, C., Koopman, W. J. and Jackson, S. (1986). Circulating immune complexes and immunoglobulin A rheumatoid factor in patients with mesangial immunoglobulin A nephropathies. *J. Clin. Invest.*, **77**, 1931–1938

69. Doi, T., Kanatsu, K. and Seceta, K. (1984). Detection of IgA class circulating immune complexes bound to anti-C3d antibody in patients with IgA nephrology. *J. Immunol. Meth.*, **69**, 95–104

70. Cederholm, B., Wieslander, J. and Byren, P. (1986). Patients with IgA nephropathy have circulating anti-basement membrane antibodies reacting with structures common to collagen I, II, and IV. *Proc. Natl Acad. Sci. USA*, **83**, 6151–6155

71. Levinsky, R. J. and Barratt, T. M. (1979). IgA immune complexes in Henoch–Schonlein purpura. *Lancet*, **2**, 1100–1103

72. Matsuda, S., Waldo, F. B. and Czerkinsky, C. (1988). Binding of IgA to erythrocytes from patients with IgA nephropathy. *Clin. Immunol. Immunopathol.*, **48**, 1–9

73. Monteiro, R. C., Halbwachs-Mecarelli, L. and Roque-Barreira, M. C. (1985). Charge and size of mesangial IgA in IgA nephropathy. *Kidney Int.*, **28**, 666–671

74. Sinico, R. A., Fornasieri, A. and Paterna, L. (1987). Studies on IgA antiglobulins in IgA nephropathy. *Semin. Nephrol.*, **VII**(4), 325–328

75. Egido, J., Sancho, J. and Blasco, R. (1983). Immunopathogenetic aspects of IgA nephropathy. *Adv. Nephrol.*, **12**, 103–137

76. Hernando, P., Egido, J. and de Nicolas, R. (1986). Clinical significance of polymeric and monomeric IgA complexes in patients with IgA nephropathy. *Am. J. Kidney Dis.*, **VIII**(6), 410–416

77. Lozano, L., Garcia-Hoyo, R. and Egido, J. (1987). IgA nephropathy: association of a history of macroscopic haematuria episodes with increased production of polymeric IgA. *Nephron*, **45**, 98–103

78. Kutteh, W. H., Prince, S. J. and Mestecky, J. (1982). Tissue origins of human polymeric and monomeric IgA. *J. Immunol.*, **128**(2), 990–995

80. Silva, F. G., Chander, P. and Pirani, C. (1982). Disappearance of glomerular mesangial IgA deposits after renal allograft transplantation. *Transplantation*, **33**(2), 214–216

81. Rifai, A. and Mannik, M. (1983). Clearance kinetics and fate of mouse IgA immune complexes prepared with monomeric or dimeric IgA. *J. Immunol.*, **130**(4), 1826–1832

82. Rifai, A. and Millard, K. (1985). Glomerular deposition of immune complexes prepared with monomeric or polymeric IgA. *Clin. Exp. Immunol.*, **60**, 363–368

83. Chen, A., Wong, S. S. and Rifai, A. (1988). Glomerular immune deposits in experimental IgA nephropathy. A continuum of circulating and in situ formed immune complexes. *Am. J. Pathol.*, **130**(1), 216–222

84. Bellon, B., Belair, M. F. and Kuhn, J. (1982). Trapping of circulating proteins in immune deposits of Heymann nephritis. *Lab. Invest.*, **46**(3), 306–312

85. Herbert, L. A. and Cosio, F. G. (1987). The erythrocyte-immune complex-glomerulonephritis connection in man. *Kidney Int.*, **31**, 877–885

86. Tomino, Y., Miura, M. and Suga, T. (1984). Detection of IgA1 dominant immune complexes in peripheral blood polymorphonuclear cells by double immunofluorescence in patients with IgA nephropathy. *Nephron*, **37**, 137–139

87. Sinniah, R. (1988). Mesangial handling of immune deposits in IgA nephropathy. *Nephrology, Proc. Xth International Congress on Nephrology*, Vol. 1, pp. 558–573

88. Tomino, Y., Sakai, H. and Woodroffe, A. J. (1987). Studies on glomerular immune solubilization by complement in patients with IgA nephropathy. *Acta Pathol. Jpn*, **37**(2), 1763–1767

89. Miller, G. W. and Nussenzweig, V. (1975). A new complement function: solubilisation of antigen-antibody aggregate. *Proc. Natl Acad. Sci. USA*, **72**, 418–422

90. Johnson, K. J., Ward, P. A. and Kumkel, R. G. (1986). Mediation of IgA induced lung injury in the rat: role of macrophages and reactive oxygen products. *Lab. Invest.*, **154**, 499–504

91. Johnson, K. J., Wilson, B., S. and Till, G. O. (1984). Acute lung injury in the rat caused by immunoglobulin A immune complexes. *J. Clin. Invest.*, **74**, 358–363

92. Emancipator, S. N. and Lamm, M. E. (1986). Pathways of tissue injury initiated by humoral immune mechanisms. *Lab. Invest.*, **54**(5), 475–478

93. Rifai, A. (1987). Experimental models for IgA-associated nephritis. *Kidney Int.*, **31**, 1–7

94. Lupo, A., Rugiu, C. and Cagnoli, L. (1987). Acute changes in renal function in IgA

nephropathy. *Semin. Nephrol.*, **VII**(4), 359–362
95. Alexopoulos, E., Seron, D. and Cameron, J. S. (1988). Role of interstitial infiltrates in IgA nephropathy: a study with monoclonal antibodies. *Nephrol. Dial. Transplant.*, **3**(4), 521–522 (Abstract)
96. Rifai, A., Small, P. A. and Teague, P. O. (1979). Experimental IgA nephropathy. *J. Exp. Med.*, **150**, 1161–1173
97. Isaacs, K. L. and Miller, F. (1982). Role of antigen size and charge in immune complex glomerulonephritis. I. Active induction of disease with dextran and its derivatives. *Lab. Invest.*, **47**(2), 198–205
98. Emancipator, S. N., Gallo, G. R. and Lamm, M. E. (1983). Experimental IgA nephropathy induced by oral immunization. *J. Exp. Med.*, **157**, 572–582
99. Genin, C., Laurent, B. and Sabatier, J. C. (1986). IgA mesangial deposits in C3H/HeJ mice after oral immunization with ferritin or bovine serum albumin. *Clin. Exp. Immunol.*, **63**, 385–394
100. Sato, M., Ideura, T. and Koshikawa, S. (1986). Experimental IgA nephropathy in mice. *Lab. Invest.*, **54**(4), 377–384
101. Oldstone, M. B. A. and Dixon, F. G. (1972). Disease accompanying in utero viral infection. The role of maternal antibody in tissue injury after transplacental infection with lymphocytic choriomeningitis virus. *J. Exp. Med.*, **135**, 827–838
102. Markham, R. V., Sutherland, J. C. and Mardiney, M. R. (1973). The ubiquitous occurrence of immune complex localisation in the glomeruli of normal mice. *Lab. Invest.*, **129**, 111–120
103. Imai, H., Nakamoto, Y. and Asukara, K. (1985). Spontaneous glomerular IgA deposition in ddY mice: an animal model of IgA nephritis. *Kidney Int.*, **27**, 756–761
104. Takeuchi, F., Doi, T. and Shimada, E. (1989). Retroviral gp70 antigen in ddY mice, a spontaneous murine model of IgA nephropathy. *Kidney Int.* (In press)
105. Kamaguchi, S., Tanaka, H. and Hoshine, K. (1988). Suppression of glomerular IgA deposits through periodic injections of lipopolysaccharides. *Clin. Immunol. Immunopathol.*, **48**, 362–370
106. Emancipator, S. N., Ovary, Z. and Lamm, M. E. (1987). The role of mesangial complement in the hematuria of experimental IgA nephropathy. *Lab. Invest.*, **57**(3), 269–276
107. Rifai, A., Chen, A. and Imai, H. (1987). Complement activation in experimental IgA nephropathy: an antigen-mediated process. *Kidney Int.*, **32**, 838–844
108. Pfaffenbach, G., Lamm, M. E. and Gigli, I. (1982). Activation of the guinea pig alternative complement pathway by mouse IgA immune complexes. *J. Exp. Med.*, **155**, 231–247
109. Sissons, J. G. P., Woodrow, D. F. and Curtis, J. R. (1975). Isolated glomerulonephritis with mesangial IgA deposits. *Br. Med. J.*, **3**, 611–614
110. Chen, A., Ho, Y.-S. and Tu, Y.-C. (1988). C5 component: immunopathological index for the activity of IgA nephropathy. *Nephron*, **49**, 255
111. Rauterberg, E. W., Lieberknecht, H. M. and Wingen, A. M. (1987). Complement membrane-attack complex (MAC) in idiopathic IgA-glomerulonephritis. *Kidney Int.*, **31**, 820–829
112. Miyamoto, H., Yoshioka, K. and Takemura, T. (1988). Immunohistochemical study of the membrane attack complex in IgA nephropathy. *Virchows Archiv. A. Pathol. Anat.*, **413**, 77–86
113. Lovett, D. H., Haensch, G. M. and Goppelt, M. (1987). Activation of glomerular mesangial cells by the terminal membrane attack complex of complement. *J. Immunol.*, **138**, 2473–2480
114. Tomino, Y. (1980). Complement system in IgA nephropathy. *Tokai J. Exp. Clin. Med.*, **5**(1), 15–22
115. Makino, H., Nishimura, S. and Takaoka, M. (1988). Mechanism of hematuria. *Nephron*, **50**, 143–150
116. Miura, M., Tomino, Y. and Suga, T. (1984). Increase in proteinuria and/or microhematuria following upper respiratory tract infections in patients with IgA nephropathy. *Tokai J. Exp. Clin. Med.*, **9**(1), 139–145
117. Feltis, J. T., Churg, J. and Holley, K. M. (1984). Active and chronic phases of Berger's disease (IgA nephropathy). *Am. J. Kidney Dis.*, **III**, 349–355
118. Nakamoto, Y., Asano, Y. and Kazuhiro, D. (1978). Primary IgA glomerulonephritis and Schonlein–Henoch purpura nephritis: clinicopathological and immunohistological characteristics. *Q. J. Med.*, **188**, 495–516
119. Kaneko, Y., Tomino, Y. and Ikeda, T. (1987). Comparative studies among morphological changes of urinary sediments and histopathological injuries in patients with IgA nephropathy. *Tokai J. Exp. Clin. Med.*, **12**(2), 103–108
120. Tomino, Y., Ma, Y. and Sakai, H. (1988). Detection of platelets in urinary sediments

from patients with 'advanced' stages of immunoglobulin A nephropathy. *J. Clin. Lab. Anal.*, **2**, 241–244

121. Neelakantappa, K., Gallo, G. R. and Baldwin, D. S. (1988). Proteinuria in IgA nephropathy. *Kidney Int.*, **33**, 716–721

122. Galla, J. H., Spotswood, M. F. and Harrison, L. A. (1985). Urinary IgA in IgA nephropathy and Henoch-Schoenlein purpura. *J. Clin. Immunol.*, **5**(5), 298–306

123. Nagy, J., Miltenyi, M. and Dobos, M. (1987). Tubular proteinuria in IgA glomerulonephritis. *Clin. Nephrol.*, **27**(2), 76–78

124. Morita, M. and Sakaguchi, H. (1988). A quantitative study of glomerular basement membrane changes in IgA nephropathy. *J. Pathol.*, **154**, 7–18

125. Schena, F. P., Mastrolitti, G. and Fracasso, A. R. (1986). Increased immunoglobulin secreting cells in the blood patients with active idiopathic IgA nephropathy. *Clin. Nephrol.*, **26**, 163–168

126. Feehally, J., Beattie, J. T. and Brenchley, P. E. C. (1986). Sequential studies of the IgA system in relapsing IgA nephropathy. *Kidney Int.*, **30**, 924–931

127. Pelletier, L., Pasquier, R. and Rossert, J. (1988). Autoreactive T cells in mercury-induced autoimmunity. Ability to induce the autoimmune disease. *J. Immunol.*, **140**(3), 750–754

128. Gronowicz, E., Coutinho, A. and Miller, G. (1974). Differentiation of B cells: sequential appearance of responsiveness to polyclonal activators. *Scand. J. Immunol.*, **3**, 413–420

129. Dziarski, R. (1982). Preferential induction of autoantibody secretion in polyclonal activation by peptidoglycan and lipopolysaccharides II in vivo studies. *J. Immunol.*, **128**, 1026–1030

130. Goldman, M., Baran, D. and Druet, P. (1988). Polyclonal activation and experimental nephropathies. *Kidney Int.*, **34**, 141–150

131. Cooper, M. D. (1987). B. lymphocytes. Normal development and function. *N. Engl. J. Med.*, **317**(23), 1452–1456

132. Nomoto, Y. and Sakai, H. (1979). Cold-reacting antinuclear factor in sera from patients with IgA nephropathy. *J. Lab. Clin. Med.*, **94**, 76–87

133. Tomino, Y., Endoh, M. and Nomot, Y. (1982). Specificity of eluted antibody from renal tissues of patients with IgA nephropathy. *Am. J. Kidney Dis.*, **1**(5), 276–280

134. Tomino, Y., Sakai, H., Endoh, M. (1983). Cross-reactivity of eluted antibodies from renal tissues of patients with Henoch–Schonlein purpura nephritis and IgA nephropathy. *Am. J. Nephrol.*, **3**, 315–318

135. Tomino, Y., Sakai, H. and Endoh, M. (1983). Cross-reactivity of IgA antibodies between renal mesangial areas and nuclei of tonsillar cells in patients with IgA nephropathy. *Clin. Exp. Immunol.*, **51**, 605–610

136. Tomino, Y., Sakai, H. and Miura, M. (1985). Specific binding of circulating IgA antibodies in patients with IgA nephropathy. *Am. J. Kidney Dis.*, **VI**(3), 149–153

137. Cederholm, B., Wieslander, J. and Bygren, P. (1988). Circulating complexes containing IgA and fibronectin in patients with primary IgA nephropathy. *Proc. Natl Acad. Sci. USA*, **85**, 4865–4868

138. Frampton, G., Harada, T. and Cameron, J. S. (1988). IgA autoantibodies in Berger's disease. *Nephrol. Dial. Transplant.* (Abstract)

139. Davin, J.-C., Malaise, M. and Foidart, J. (1987). Anti-alpha-galactosyl antibodies and immune complexes in children with Henoch–Schonlein purpura or IgA nephropathy. *Kidney Int.*, **31**, 1132–1139

140. Galili, U., Rachmilewitz, E. A. and Peleg, A. (1984). A unique natural human IgG antibody with anti-alpha-galactosyl specificity. *J. Exp. Med.*, **160**, 1519–1531

141. Ballardie, F. W., Williams, S. and Brenchley, P. E. C. (1987). IgG antibodies to glomerular antigens in IgA nephropathy: detection and clinical significance. *Nephrol. Dial. Transplant.*, **2**, 422 (Abstract)

142. Ballardie, F. W., Brenchley, P. E. C. and Williams, S. (1988). Autoimmunity in IgA nephropathy. *Lancet*, **2**, 598–592

143a. O'Donoghue, D. J., Darvill, A. and Brenchley, P. E. C. (1989). Mesangial cell autoantigens in IgA nephropathy and Henoch–Schonlein purpura. *Kidney Int.*, **35**(1), 372 (Abstract)

143b. O'Donoghue, D. J., Darvill, A. and Ballardie, F. W. (1991). Mesangial cell autoantigens in IgA nephropathy and Henoch–Schonlein purpura. *J. Clin. Invest.* (in press)

144. O'Donoghue, D. J., Brenchley, P. E. C. and Ballardie, F. W. (1988). Autoimmunity to glomerular antigens in adult Henoch–Schonlein nephritis and IgA nephropathy. *Clin. Sci.*,

75, 52 (Abstract)

145. Batsford, S. R., Rohrbach, R. and Takamiya, H. (1979). Autoantibody specific for the glomerular mesangium and Bowman's capsule in man. *Clin. Nephrol.*, **12** (4), 163–167

146. Yap, H. K., Sakai, R. S. and Bahn, L. (1988). Anti-vascular endothelial cell antibodies in patients with IgA nephropathy: frequency and clinical significance. *Clin. Immunol. Immunopathol.*, **49**, 450–462

147. Sinico, R. A., Fornasieri, A. and Oreni, N. (1986). Polymeric IgA rheumatoid factor in idiopathic IgA mesangial nephropathy (Berger's disease). *J. Immunol.*, **137**(2), 536–541

148. Saulsbury, F. T. (1987). The role of IgA rheumatoid factor in the formation of IgA-containing immune complexes in Henoch–Schonlein purpura. *J. Clin. Lab. Immunol.*, **23**, 123–127

149. Kunkel, H. G., Winchester, R. J. and Joslin, F. G. (1974). Similarities in the light chains of anti-gamma globulins showing cross-idiotypic specificity. *J. Exp. Med.*, **139**, 128–135

150. Crowley, J. J., Goldfien, R. D. and Schrohenlocker, R. E. (1988). Incidence of free cross-reactive idiotypes on human rheumatoid factor paraproteins. *J. Immunol.*, **140**, 3411–3416

151. Sanz, I. and Capra, J. D. (1988). The genetic origin of human autoantibodies. *J. Immunol.*, **140**, 328–335

152. Bagchus, W. M., Hoedemaeker, Ph. J. and Rozing, J. (1986). Glomerulonephritis induced by monoclonal anti-Thy 1.1 antibodies. A sequential histological and ultrastructural study in the rat. *Lab. Invest.*, **55**(6), 680–687

153. Wilson, C. B., Yamamoto, T. and Moullier, P. (1988). Selective glomerular mesangial cell immune injury—antimesangial cell antibodies. In Davidson, A. M. (ed.) *Nephrology*, Vol. 1, pp. 509–522 (London: Baillière Tindall)

154. Sinico, R. A., Fornasieri, A. and Maldifassi, P. (1988). The clinical significance of IgA rheumatoid factor in idiopathic IgA mesangial nephropathy (Berger's disease). *Clin. Nephrol.*, **30**(4), 182–186

155. Ballardie, F. W., Brenchley, P. E. C. and O'Donoghue, D. J. (1988). Autoantibodies in IgA nephropathy: differential secretion of immunoglobulin isotypes during haematuria. *Nephrol. Dial. Transplant.*, **3**(4), 524–525 (Abstract)

156. Izui, S., Lambert, P. H. and Fourni, G. J. (1977). Features of SLE in mice injected with bacterial lipopolyusaccharides. Identification of circulating DNA and renal localisation of DNA–anti DNA complexes. *J. Exp. Med.*, **145**, 1115–1130

157. Jerne, K. (1974). Towards a network theory of the immune system. *Ann. Immunol. (Paris)*, **1125**, 373–379

158. Goldman, M., Rose, L. M. and Hochmann, A. (1982). Deposition of idiotypes—anti-idiotype immune complexes in renal glomeruli after polyclonal B cell activation. *J. Exp. Med.*, **155**, 1385–1399

159. Gonzalez-Cabrero, J., Egido, J. and Sancho, J. (1987). Presence of shared idiotypes in serum and immune complexes in patients with IgA nephropathy. *Clin. Exp. Immunol.*, **68**, 694–702

160. Van den Wall Bake, A. W. L., Beyer, W. E. and Jeanette, H. (1989). Immune response to influenza virus in primary IgA nephropathy. *7th International Congress on Immunology* (Abstract)

161. Lai, K. N., Lai, F. M. and Tam, J. S. (1988). Strong association between IgA nephropathy and hepatitis B surface antigenaemia in endemic areas. *Clin. Nephrol.*, **29**(5), 229–235

162. Magil, A., Webber, D. and Chan, V. (1986). Glomerulonephritis associated with hepatitis B surface antigenaemia. *Nephron*, **42**, 335–339

163. Gregory, M. C., Hammond, M. E. and Brewer, E. D. (1988). Renal deposition of cytomegalovirus antigen in immunoglobulin A nephropathy. *Lancet*, **1**, 11–14

164. Sato, M., Kojima, H. and Shinkai, Y. (1988). Cytomegalovirus and IgA nephropathy. *Lancet*, **2**, 1251

165. Waldo, F. B., Britt, W. J. and Tomana, M. (1989). Nonspecific mesangial staining with antibodies against cytomegalovirus in immunoglobulin A nephropathy. *Lancet*, **1**, 129–131

166. Jassani, D. and Griffiths, D. F. R. (1988). Cytomegalovirus and IgA nephropathy. *Lancet*, **2**, 1251

167. Newkirk, M. M., Ostberg, L. and Wasserman, R. W. (1987). Human rheumatoid factors of the Wa idiotypic family appear to use highly homologous variable region genes as a human anti-cytomegalovirus antibody. *Fed. Proc.*, **46**, 916

168. Battergay, E. J., Mihatsch, M. and Mazzacchelli, H. U. (1988). Cytomegalovirus and kidney. *Clin. Nephrol.*, **30**(5), 239–247

169. Kawanishi, H., Saltzman, L. E. and Strober, W. (1983). Mechanisms regulating IgA

class-specific immunoglobulin production in murine gut-associated lymphoid tissues. 1. T cells derived from Peyer's patches that switch sIgM B cells to sIgA B cells in vitro. *J. Exp. Med.*, **157**, 433–450

170. Kiyono, H., Cooper, M. D. and Kearney, J. F. (1984). Isotype specificity of helper T cell clones. Peyer's patch Th cells preferentially collaborate with mature IgA B cells for IgA responses. *J. Exp. Med.*, **159**, 798–811

171. Kitamura, K., Kiyono, H. and Fujihashi, K. (1988). Isotype-specific immunoregulation. Systemic antigen induces splenic T contrasuppressor cells which support IgM and IgG subclass but not IgA responses. *J. Immunol.*, **140**(5), 1385–1392

172. Endoh, M., Sakai, H. and Nomoto, Y. (1981). IgA-specific Helper activity of Tα cells in human peripheral blood. *J. Immunol.*, **127**(6), 2612–2613

173. Millet, I., Briere, F. and de Vries, J. (1988). Up-regulation of receptors for IgA on activated human B lymphocytes. *Immunol. Lett.*, **19**, 153–158

174. Gordon, J. and Guy, G. R. (1987). The molecules controlling B lymphocytes. *Immunol. Today*, **8**(11), 339-344

175. Beagley, K. W., Eldridge, J. H. and Kiyonon, H. (1988). Recombinant murine IL-5 induces high rate IgA synthesis in cycling IgA-positive Peyer's patch B cells. *J. Immunol.*, **141**(6), 2035–2042

176. Stavnezer, J., Sirlin, S. and Abbott, J. (1985). Induction of immunoglobulin isotype switching in culture lymphoma cells. *J. Exp. Med.*, **161**(3), 577–601

177. Lebman, D. A. and Coffman, R. L. (1988). The effects of IL-4 and IL-5 on the IgA response by murine Peyer's patch B cell subpopulations. *J. Immunol.*, **141**(6), 2050–2056

178. Kunimoto, D. Y., Harriman, G. R. and Strober, W. (1988). Regulation of IgA differentiation in CH12LX B cells by lymphokines. IL-4 induces membrane IgM-positive CH12LX cells to express membrane IgA and IL-5 induces membrane IgA-positive CH12LX cells to secrete IgA. *J. Immunol.*, **141**(3), 713–720

179. Harriman, G. R., Kunimoto, D. Y. and Elliott, J. F. (1988). The role of IL-5 in IgA B cell differentiation. *J. Immunol.*, **140**(9), 3033–3039

180. Bohnsack, J. F. and Cooper, N. R. (1988). CR2 ligands modulate human B cell activation. *J. Immunol.*, **141**(8), 2569–2576

181. O'Garra, A. (1989). Interleukins and the immune system. *Lancet*, **1**, 943–946

182. Hodgkin, P. D., Bond, M. W. and O'Garra, A. (1988). Identification of IL-6 as a T cell-derived factor that enhances the proliferative response of thymocytes to IL-4 and phorbol myristate acetate. *J. Immunol.*, **141**(1), 151–157

183. Kelly, C. J. and Neilson, E. G. (1987). Contrasuppression in autoimmunity. Abnormal contrasuppression facilitates expression of nephritogenic effector T cells and interstitial nephritis in kdkd mice. *J. Exp. Med.*, **165**, 107–116

184. Endoh, M. (1984). Increases in lymphocytes with Fc receptors for IgA and rates of spontaneous IgA synthesis in patients with IgA nephropathy. *Jpn J. Nephrol.*, **26**(9), 1179–1185

185. Lai, K. N., Leung, J. C. K. and Mac-Moune Lai, F. (1988). In vitro study of expression of interleukin-2 receptors in T-lymphocytes from patients with IgA nephropathy. *Clin. Nephrol.*, **30**(6), 330–334

186. Adachi, M., Yodoi, J. and Masuda, T. (1983). Altered expression of lymphocyte Fcα receptor in selective IgA deficiency and IgA nephropathy. *J. Immunol.*, **131**(3), 1246–1251

187. Wyatt, R. J., Valenski, W. R. and Stapleton, F. B. (1988). Immunoregulatory studies in patients with IgA nephropathy. *J. Clin. Lab. Immunol.*, **25**, 109–114

188. Maghazachi, A. A. and Phillips-Quagliata, J. M. (1988). Con A-propagated, auto-reactive T cell clones that secrete factors promoting high IgA responses. *Int. Arch. Allergy Appl. Immunol.*, **86**, 147–156

189. Casanueva, B., Rodriguez-Valverde, V. and Arias, M. (1986). Immunoglobulin-producing cells in IgA nephropathy. *Nephron*, **43**, 33–37

190. Hale, G. M., McIntosh, S. L. and Hiki, Y. (1986). Evidence for IgA-specific B cell hyperactivity in patients with IgA nephropathy. *Kidney Int.*, **29**, 718–724

191. Cosio, F. G., Lam, S. and Folami, A. O. (1982). Immune regulation of immunoglobulin production in IgA-nephropathy. *Clin. Immunol. Immunopathol.*, **23**, 430–436

192. Egido, J., Blasco, R. and Sancho, J. (1982). Increased rates of polymeric IgA synthesis by circulating lymphoid cells in IgA mesangial glomerulonephritis. *Clin. Exp. Immunol.*, **47**, 309–316

193. Lozano, L., Garcia-Hoyo, R. and Egido, J. (1987). IgA nephropathy: association of a history

of macroscopic hematuria episodes with increased production of polymeric IgA. *Nephron*, **45**, 98–103

194. Egido, J., Julian, B. A. and Wyatt, R. J. (1987). Genetic factors in primary IgA nephropathy. *Nephrol. Dial. Transplant.*, **2**, 134–142

195. Demaine, A. G., Rambausek, M. and Knight, J. F. (1988). Relation of mesangial IgA glomerulonephritis to polymorphism of immunoglobulin heavy chain switch region. *J. Clin. Invest.*, **81**, 611–614

196. Callard, P., Feldman, G. and Prandi, P. (1975). Immune complex type glomerulonephritis in cirrhosis of the liver. *Am. J. Pathol.*, **80**, 329–340

197. Nochy, D., Callard, P. and Bellon, B. (1976). Association of overt glomerulonephritis and liver disease. A study of 34 patients. *Clin. Nephrol.*, **6**, 422–427

198. Berger, J., Yaneva, H. and Navarra, B. (1977). Glomerular changes in patients with cirrhosis of the liver. *Adv. Nephrol.*, **7**, 3–14

199. Nakamoto, Y., Idia, H. and Kobayashi, K. (1981). Hepatic glomerulonephritis. Characteristics of hepatic IgA glomerulonephritis as the major part. *Virchows Arch. (Pathol. Anat.)*, **392**, 45–54

200. Sinniah, R. (1984). Heterogeneous IgA glomerulonephropathy in liver cirrhosis. *Histopathology*, **8**, 947–962

201. Bene, M. C., de Korwin, J. D. and de Ligny, B. H. (1988). IgA nephropathy and alcoholic liver cirrhosis. A prospective necropsy study. *Am. J. Clin. Pathol.*, **89**, 769–773

202. Sancho, J., Gonzalez, E. and Rivera, F. (1984). Hepatic and kidney uptake of soluble monomeric and polymeric IgA aggreagates. *Immunology*, **52**, 161–167

203. Moldoveanu, Z., Epps, J. M. and Thorpe, S. R. (1988). The sites of catabolism of murine monomeric IgA. *J. Immunol.*, **141**(1), 208–213

204. Edlacroix, D. L., Elkon, K. B. and Geubel, A. P. (1982). Changes in size, subclass, and metabolic properties of serum immunoglobulin A in liver diseases and in other diseases with high serum immunoglobulin A. *J. Clin. Invest.*, **71**, 358–367

205. Emancipator, S. N., Gallo, G. R. and Razaboni, R. (1983). Experimental cholestasis promotes the deposition of glomerular IgA immune complexes. *Am. J. Pathol.*, **113**, 19–26

206. Gormly, A. A., Smith, P. S. and Seymour, A. E. (1981). IgA glomerular deposits in experimental cirrhosis. *Am. J. Pathol.*, **104**(1), 50-54

207. Iida, H., Izumino, K. and Matsumoto, M. (1985). Glomerular deposition of IgA in experimental hepatic cirrhosis. *Acta Pathol. Jpn*, **35**(3), 561–567

208. Russell, M. W., Brown, T. A. and Mestecky, J. (1982). Role of serum IgA. Hepatobiliary transport of circulating antigen. *J. Exp. Med.*, **153**, 968-976

209. Sancho, J., Gonzalez, E. and Egido, J. (1986). The importance of the Fc receptors for IgA in the recognition of IgA by mouse liver cells: its comparison with carbohydrate and secretory component receptors. *Immunology*, **57**, 37–42

210. Rifai, A. and Mannik, M. (1984). Clearance of circulating IgA immune complexes is mediated by a specific receptor on Kupffer cells in mice. *J. Exp. Med.*, **160**, 125–137

211. Phillips, J. O., Komiyama, K. and Epps, J. M. (1988). Role of hepatocytes in the uptake of IgA and IgA-containing immune complexes in mice. *Mol. Immunol.*, **25**(9), 873–879

212. Ogata, I., Fujiwara, K. and Nishi, T. (1988). Contribution of hepatic reticuloendothelial system to glomerular IgA deposition in rat liver injury. *Am. J. Pathol.*, **131**(3), 411–417

213. Sato, M., Ideura, T. and Koshikawa, S. (1986). Experimental IgA nephropathy in mice. *Lab. Invest.*, **54**(4), 377–384

214. Knight, J. F. and Cameron, J. S. (1987). Henoch–Schonlein nephritis in adults: a report from the UK MRC glomerulonephritis registry. *Nephrol. Dial. Transplant.*, **2**, 415 (Abstract)

215. Fogazzi, G. B., Pasqualim, S. and Moriggi, M. (1988). Long-term outcome of Schonlein–Henoch nephritis in the adult. *Clin. Nephrol.*, **198**, 60–66

216. Lee, H. S., Koh, H. I. and Kim, M. J. (1986). Henoch–Schonlein nephritis in adults: a clinical and morphological study. *Clin. Nephrol.*, **26**, 215–222

217. Roth, D. A., Wilz, D. R. and Theil, G. B. (1985). Schonlein–Henoch syndrome in adults. *Q. J. Med. New Ser.*, **55**(217), 145–152

218. Beale, M. G., Nash, G. S. and Bertovich, M. J. (1983). Evidence of enhanced immunoglobulin synthesis and defective immune regulation in Henoch–Schonlein purpura. *Contrib. Nephrol.*, **35**, 46–60

219. Saulsbury, F. T. (1986). IgA rheumatoid factor in Henoch–Schonlein pupura. *J. Paediatr.*, **108**(1), 71–76

220. Feehally, J. (1988). Immune mechanisms in glomerular IgA deposition. *Nephrol. Dial. Transplant.*, 3(4), 361–378

221. Meadow, S. R. and Scott, D. G.(1985). Berger disease: Henoch–Schonlein syndrome without the rash. *J. Pediatr.*, **106**, 27–32

222. Yamabe, H., Ozawa, K. and Fukushi, K. (1988). IgA nephropathy and Henoch–Schonlein purpura nephritis with anterior uveitis. *Nephron*, **50**, 368–370

223. O'Donoghue, D. J., Brenchley, P. E. C. and Ballardie, F. W. (1988). Autoimmunity to glomerular antigens in adult Henoch–Schonlein nephritis. *Nephrol. Dial. Transplant.*, 3(4), 512 (Abstract)

224. van den Waal Bake, A. W. L., Lobatta, S. and Jonges, L. (1988). IgA antibodies directed against cytoplasmic antigens of polymorphonuclear leucocytes in patients with Henoch–Schonlein purpura. *Adv. Exp. Biol.*, 1593–1598

225. Penning, C. A., Jones, S. and Lockwood, C. M. (1988). Antibody binding profiles of sera from systemic vasculitis patients. *Nephrol. Dial. Transplant.*, 3(4), 527 (Abstract)

226. Lozano, L., Garcia-Hoyo, R. and Egido, J. (1985). Tonsillectomy decreases the synthesis of polymeric IgA by blood lymphocytes and clinical activity in patients with IgA nephropathy. *Proc. EDTA-ERA*, **22**, 800–804

227. Masuda, Y., Terazawa, K. and Kawakami, S. (1988). Clinical and immunological study of IgA nephropathy before and after tonsillectomy. *Acta Otolaryngol. (Stockholm)*, **454**, 248–255

228. Karacic, J. J. and Cowdery, J. S. (1988). The effect of single dose, intravenous cyclophosphamide on the mouse intestinal IgA response to cholera toxin. *Immunopharmacology*, **16**, 53–60

229. Woo, K. T., Edmondson, R. P. S. and Yap, H. K. (1987). Effects of triple therapy on the progression of mesangial proliferative glomerulonephritis. *Clin. Nephrol.*, **27**, 56–64

230. Woo, K. T., Chaing, G. S. C. and Yap, H. K. (1988). Controlled therapeutic trial of IgA nephritis with follow-up renal biopsies. *Am. Acad. Med.*, **17**(2), 226–231

231. Kobayashi, Y., Fujii, K. and Hiki, Y. (1986). Steroid therapy in IgA nephropathy: a prospective pilot study in moderate proteinuric cases. *Q. J. Med. New Ser.*, **61**(234), 935–943

232. Kobayashi, Y., Fujii, K. and Hiki, Y. (1988). Steroid therapy in IgA nephropathy: a retrospective study in heavy proteinuric cases. *Nephron*, **48**, 12–17

233. Lai, K. N., Lai, E. M. and Ho, C. P. (1986). Corticosteroid therapy in IgA nephropathy with nephrotic syndrome: a long-term controlled trial. *Clin. Nephrol.*, **26**(4), 174–180

234. Chan, M. K., Kwan, S. Y. L. and Chan, K. W. (1987). Controlled trial of antiplatelet agents in mesangial IgA glomerulonephritis. *Am. J. Kidney Dis.*, **9**(5), 417–421

235. Lagrue, G., Sadreux, T. and Laurent, J. (1981). Is there a treatment of mesangial IgA glomerulonephritis? *Clin. Nephrol.*, **16**, 161–166

236. Bennett, W. M., Walker, R. G. and Kincaid-Smith, P. (1989). Treatment of IgA nephropathy with eicosapentanoic acid (EPA): a two-year prospective trial. *Clin. Nephrol.*, **3**, 128–131

237. Tomino, Y., Sakai, HY. and Miura, M. (1984). Effect of danazol on solubilization of immune deposits in patients with IgA nephropathy. *Am. J. Kidney Dis.*, **9**(2), 135–140

238. Deteix, P., Colon, S. and Leitienne, Ph. (1984). Prospective controlled therapeutic trial with diaminodiphenylsulfone-dapsone (DDS) in primitive IgA nephropathy (IgAN). *Kidney Int.*, **26**, 493 (Abstract)

239. Clarkson, A. R., Seymore, A. E. and Woodroffe, A. J. (1980). Controlled trial of phenytoin therapy in IgA nephropathy. *Clin. Nephrol.*, **13**, 215–218

240. Egiod, J., Rivera, F. and Sancho, J. (1984). Phenytoin in IgA nephropathy: a long-term controlled trial. *Nephron*, **38**, 30–39

241. Coppo, R., Basolo, B. and Giachino, O. (1985). Plasmapheresis in a patient with rapidly progressive idiopathic IgA nephropathy: removal of IgA-containing circulating immune complexes and clinical recovery. *Nephron*, **40**, 488–490

242. Hene, R. J. and Kater, L. (1983). Plasmapheresis in nephritis associated with Henoch–Schonlein purpura and in primary IgA nephropathy. *Plasma Ther. Transfus. Technol.*, **4**, 165–173

243. Rose, G. M., Cole, B. R. and Robson, A. M. (1981). The treatment of severe glomerulopathies in children using high dose intravenous methylprednisolone pulses. *Am. J. Kidney Dis.*, **1**(3), 148–156

244. Austin, H. A. and Barlow, J. E. (1983). Henoch–Schonlein nephritis: prognostic features and the challenge of therapy. *Am. J. Kidney Dis.*, **2**, 512–620

10
C3 Nephritic Factor and Membranoproliferative Glomerulonephritis

Y. C. NG

C3 nephritic factor (NeF) is an IgG autoantibody that is directed against neoantigenic determinants on the alternative pathway C3 convertase, C3bBb. It stabilizes the enzyme, thereby causing complement activation, and is characteristically associated with profound hypocomplementaemia. Clinically, NeF has striking associations with partial lipodystrophy and membrano-proliferative glomerulonephritis (MPGN), particularly type II MPGN or dense deposit disease.

HISTORICAL BACKGROUND

A subgroup of patients with chronic nephritis and decreased serum complement was described by Fischel[1] in 1952. Lange and colleagues[2] subsequently observed that persistently decreased serum complement was associated with a poor renal prognosis. However, it was not until 1965 that membrano-proliferative glomerulonephritis, with its characteristic histological appearance and clinical features, was recognized when Gotoff[3] and West[4] independently described a group of patients with chronic glomerulonephritis, persistent hypocomplementaemia and a 'lobulated, proliferative' glomerulonephritis. Further study of serum from such a patient with hypocomplementaemic glomerulonephritis led Spitzer and colleagues in 1969 to describe the presence of a factor, which they called C3 nephritic factor, that caused the breakdown of C3 in normal human serum[5]. The reaction required Mg^{2+} but not Ca^{2+}, and they recognized that it also required the presence of 'cofactors' in normal human serum. They concluded that the 'cofactors' required were not part of the complement system as they knew it (at that time only the classical pathway

215

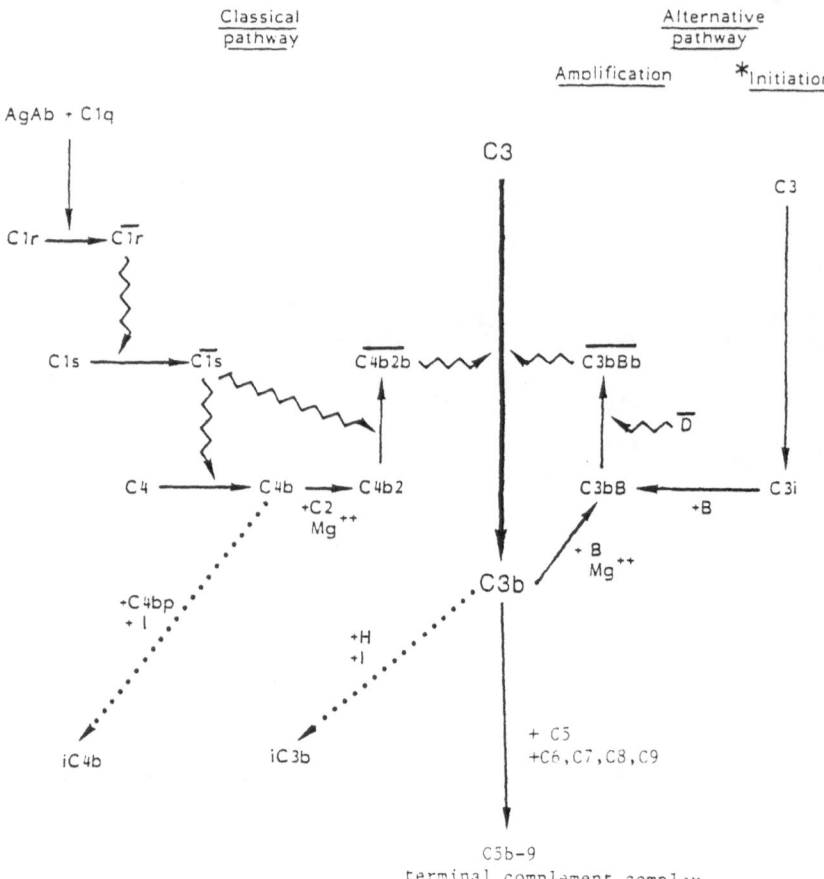

Figure 1 Complememt activation. C1q, C1r and C1s associate in a calcium-dependent non-covalent interaction. *: Initiation of alternative pathway activation occurs by spontaneous generation of C3i either by hydrolysis of C3 or by direct condensation of C3 with substrate acceptor groups. X̄ denotes activated enzyme ＭＭ denotes enzymatic cleavage. → denotes activation reaction. ⋯→ denotes inactivation reaction. C3 nephritic factor stabilizes C3bBb.

of complement activation had been identified). The C3 nephritic factor was found in the pseudoglobulin fraction of patient serum and was extremely stable, retaining its C3 converting activity for 7 days at 37°C.

Clear demonstration of the existence of a second pathway of complement activation, accordingly named the alternative pathway, came in the early 1970s. The proteins involved in this pathway were rapidly identified (Figure 1) and in 1977 NeF was shown to bind to the C3 convertase of the alternative pathway, C3bBb[6].

In 1978, NeF was shown by two independent groups to be an IgG molecule[7,8]. Its activity in stabilization of the alternative pathway C3 convertase was retained in the (Fab)'2 and Fab fragments[8,9] and specificity was to neoantigenic determinants on the alternative pathway C3 convertase, C3bBb. NeF has a higher apparent molecular weight than normal IgG and is heavily glycosylated. The attached carbohydrate groups are functionally important, since their chemical removal was associated with loss of activity[10].

MECHANISM OF ACTION OF NeF

This is best described following an account of the alternative pathway of complement activation, since NeF acts to perturb the normal control of this pathway (Figure 1).

The central event in complement activation is cleavage of C3 to C3b. This is achieved by enzymes, C3 convertases, which are generated by activation of either the classical pathway or the alternative pathway. Both pathways require the presence of Mg^{2+}; the classical pathway, in addition, requires the presence of Ca^{2+}. Unlike the classical pathway, activation of the alternative pathway does not require an immunologically specific mechanism. Instead, the pathway turns over continuously, forming a positive feedback cycle that is normally held firmly in check by three control mechanisms: (1) the extreme lability of the convertase; (2) factor H, which binds to the convertase and accelerates its decay-dissociation; and (3) factor I, which degrades C3b to iC3b. Activators of the alternative pathway, such as zymosan and bacterial endotoxin, interfere with these control mechanisms by increasing the affinity of surface-bound C3b for factor B relative to factor H[11,12]. This allows the positive feedback loop of complement activation to proceed unchecked. NeF binds to the C3 convertase and stabilizes the enzyme, i.e. decreases the spontaneous rate of decay of the enzyme[13]. It also protects the C3 convertase from factor H-enhanced decay-dissociation[14]. These effects result in activation of the alternate pathway.

METHODS FOR DETECTION OF NeF

The presence of NeF is suspected in the presence of markedly decreased serum concentrations of C3 with normal concentrations of C4. The serum concentrations of C5 are usually normal[15,16], although there is a subgroup of patients with an unusual NeF in whom the serum C5 is significantly lowered[17,18]. Other properties of these unusual nephritic factors will be described later.

Screening methods

Screening methods are relatively simple to perform and the older, well-established methods all measure in various ways the cleavage of C3 following incubation of NeF-containing serum with normal human serum at 37°C. Normal human serum provides the complement components required for generation of the alternative pathway C3 convertase, C3bBb. The necessary controls are:

(1) Demonstration that the reaction is abolished in the presence of 10 mM EDTA (ethylenediaminetetra-acetic acid) but persists in the presence of 5 mM Mg^{2+}/10 mM EGTA (ethylene glycol-bis(aminoethylether)-

N,N'-tetra-acetic acid). EDTA chelates both Ca^{2+} and Mg^{2+}, thereby preventing complement activation. EGTA, on the other hand, chelates Ca^{2+} preferentially to Mg^{2+} and so allows alternative pathway complement activation while abolishing classical pathway function.

(2) Demonstration that the factor responsible is stable to heat at 56°C, which is consistent with its being an IgG molecule.

Two dimension crossed immunoelectrophoresis[19]

Native C3 is separated from converted C3 in agarose by electrophoresis, the converted C3 being more anodic. The amounts of native and converted C3 are then quantitated by immunoelectrophoresis run in the perpendicular direction. Following reaction of test serum with normal human serum at 37°C for 30 minutes, an NeF-containing serum usually gives a clearly positive result, i.e. 80–100% C3 conversion compared with 5–10% C3 conversion of control normal serum.

Loss of B antigen[20]

B antigen is lost when native C3 is cleaved; it may be quantitated using radial immunodiffusion.

Production of complexes containing factor B and C3[21]

Since NeF stabilizes the C3 convertase, C3bBb, its reaction with normal human serum is accompanied by generation of increased quantities of the enzyme. D3bBb molecules may be measured semiquantitatively using antibodies to factor B and C3 as the first and second antibodies respectively in an enzyme-linked immunoabsorbent assay.

By-stander deposition of C3bBb on indicator erythrocytes[22]

Increased generation of C3b in the fluid phase in the presence of NeF is accompanied by by-stander fixation of C3b to neighbouring surfaces, such as unsensitized sheep erythrocytes. Alternative pathway C3 convertase molecules form by reaction of fixed C3b with factor B and factor D, resulting in lysis of C3bBb-bearing erythrocytes when a source of C5b-9 is added.

While all these screening assays are relatively simple to perform, there is some loss of specificity. False positive results occur in the presence of non-NeF alternative pathway activators such as endotoxin, molecules that appear to be complexed to factor H[23,24], and heat-labile factors[25,26]. False negative results using C3 conversion occur with a variant of NeF which is unusual in that stabilization of cell-bound alternative pathway C3 convertase is accompanied by only weak fluid-phase C3 conversion[17] (see later).

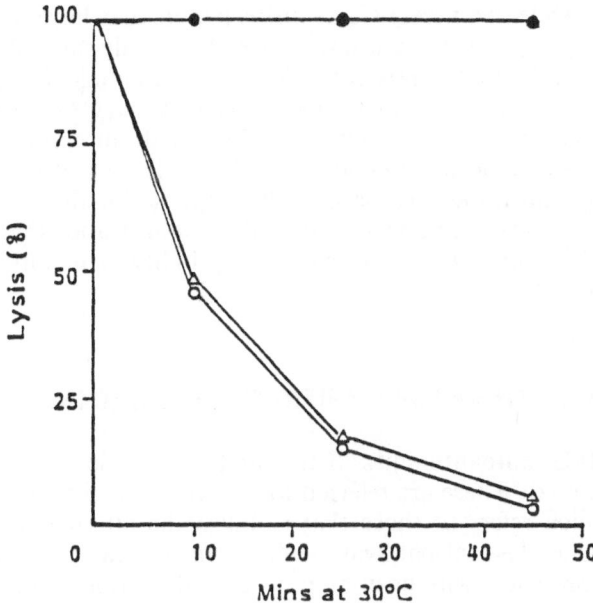

Figure 2 Stabilization assay. Lysis of sheep erythrocytes bearing alternate pathway C3 convertase, C3bBb, incubated in the presence of NeF IgG (●), normal IgG (△) or buffer (○).

Stabilization assay

The definitive detection of NeF requires the demonstration of stabilization activity of cell-bound C3bBb[13] (Figure 2). In brief, cell-bound alternative pathway C3 convertase is generated on sensitized sheep erythrocytes (EA) bearing classical pathway C3 convertase which is formed from purified guinea pig C1, C4 and C2. Purified human C3 is cleaved by this to form EAC43b (C2 and C1 having decayed). Addition of purified human factor B and factor D generates EAC3bBb, the intermediate for the assay.

Decay in activity of the C3bBb is measured in the presence or absence of NeF–IgG, surviving EAC3bBb sites being developed at various time intervals with a source of C5b-9 (commonly guinea pig complement in 10 mM EDTA). The lysis measured is proportional to the number of active C3bBb sites (Figure 2). Purified patient IgG is required in this assay since patient serum, even when inactivated at 56°C, would provide a source of C5b-9.

ATYPICAL C3 NEPHRITIC FACTORS

These nephritic factors are atypical in that they cause only weak, slow fluid-phase C3 conversion[17,27], in spite of demonstrable stabilization activity of cell-bound C3bBb[17]. They are associated with markedly decreased serum concentrations of C5, increased circulating terminal complement complex consistent with increased activation of the terminal complement pathway *in vivo*[28], and increased C5 activation *in vitro*[27]. The molecular basis for these differences is unclear; different C3 nephritic factors may have different modes of interaction with the C3 convertase, which allows only some of the stabilized enzymes to cleave C5 efficiently in the fluid phase. Binding of C5 to additional C3b molecules is a prerequisite for its cleavage by the C3 convertase[29,30]. It is possible that these atypical NeFs combine with an epitope revealed on C3b when it is complexed to either C5 or factor B, so that they are capable of stabilizing C3b-Bb as well as C5-C3b. Support for the heterogeneity of NeF interactions with C3bBb comes from the demonstration that stabilization activities of different NeFs vary in their susceptibility to inhibition by purified C3b receptor (CR1)[31].

CLASSICAL PATHWAY NEPHRITIC FACTORS (C4NeF)

These are IgG autoantibodies that stabilize the classical pathway C3 convertase, C4b2b. These are referred to as C4NeF, as distinct from C3NeF (or NeF), which refers to those that stabilize the alternative pathway C3 convertase. The classical pathway nephritic factor was first described in a patient who presented with post-streptococcal glomerulonephritis[32], but has since been demonstrated in some patients with systemic lupus erythematosus (SLE)[33]. The mechanism of action of classical pathway nephritic factor is analogous to that of the alternative pathway nephritic factor. Thus, classical pathway nephritic factor stabilizes the C4b2b enzyme, inhibits the action of C4-binding protein (the classical pathway analogue of factor H) on the decay of the enzyme, and inhibits the cleavage of C4b by factor I[34]. Like the alternative pathway nephritic factor, the stabilization activity is retained in the (Fab)'2 and Fab fragments[32] and the autoantibody has an increased apparent molecular weight as estimated by SDS-PAGE[32,35].

CLINICAL ASSOCIATIONS OF NeF

NeF is an acquired autoantibody, the best evidence for this being its discordant occurrence in identical twins[36]. No strong genetic susceptibility factor has, as yet, been identified, although it has been detected in family members[75] and an increased incidence of HLA-DR7 has been described in patients with NeF[37].

NeF is detected in approximately 30% of patients with MPGN type I and 60–70% of patients with MPGN type II[38,39]. It is also found in a significant proportion of patients with partial lipodystrophy; some of these patients also have glomerulonephritis, which, interestingly, tends to be dense-deposit disease[40]. There are also case reports of NeF being associated with conditions such as herpes gestiationis[41] and idiopathic RPGN[42]. Patients with NeF may also suffer from recurrent bacterial infection, presumably secondary to the associated hypocomplementaemia[43–46]. However, NeF has also been described in apparently healthy individuals with no evidence of glomerulonephritis or partial lipodystrophy[47,48].

MPGN TYPE I (SUBENDOTHELIAL DEPOSITS)

This is most probably an immune complex disease, with glomerular deposits consistently shown to contain immunoglobulin, often, but not always, with C3. While some cases are idiopathic, others are associated with conditions such as SLE, essential mixed cryoglobulinaemia, subacute bacterial endocarditis and shunt nephritis, all of which are examples of immune complex diseases. The association of NeF with this variant of MPGN is weaker than that with dense-deposit disease, and it is unclear whether NeF contributes in an independent way to the pathogenesis of nephritis in these circumstances. NeF may interfere with the normal clearance of immune complexes, which will be discussed in greater detail in the following section.

MPGN TYPE II (DENSE-DEPOSIT DISEASE)

In contrast to MPGN type I, the pathological basis underlying this disease is completely unclear. There is no firm evidence that this is an immunologically mediated disease, since immunoglobulin is rarely seen in the deposits, although C3 is usually demonstrated in the vicinity. However, studies of experimental immune-complex nephritis show that C3 may persist where antigen and antibody are removed[49]. The nature and composition of dense deposits is unclear.

There is a notable association of NeF with dense-deposit disease. However, it appears that NeF is neither necessary nor sufficient as a pathogenetic mechanism, since it may occur without clinical or pathological evidence of nephritis[47,48,50], and not all patients with dense-deposit disease have NeF.

PATHOGENETIC MECHANISMS

There are several difficulties in trying to elucidate the role of NeF in MPGN. First, any associations that may occur between serum concentrations of either NeF or C3 and disease characteristics may be blurred by a number of confounding factors which will be discussed later. Second, primary pathological events that initiate tissue injury should be distinguished from secondary events that perpetuate this process, some of which may be non-immune, e.g. hypertension. Third, MPGN is a histological diagnosis that represents a common pathway of renal injury induced by a variety of stimuli.

It is, nevertheless, of interest to consider the various pathological mechanisms that have been proposed for NeF and the evidence for and against each of these hypotheses. The main pathogenetic mechanisms proposed are:

(1) The systemic hypocomplementaemia that is associated with NeF predisposes to nephritis.
(2) NeF acts as a complement activator locally to cause tissue injury.
(3) Normal clearance mechanisms for immune complexes by erythrocyte CR1 (complement receptor of type I) are disrupted by a combination of hypocomplementaemia and the molecular interactions of NeF with CR1.

Systemic hypocomplementaemia

The systemic hypocomplementaemia that is characteristically seen with NeF is striking and is due to hypercatabolism combined with hyposynthesis[51]. Evidence to suggest the possible significance of decreased serum C3 concentrations comes from the association of MPGN with systemic hypocomplementaemia occurring independently of NeF. Thus, MPGN has been described in members of a family with hypocomplementaemia due to increased catabolism of C3; this was accompanied by an inherited variant of C3 with decreased affinity for factor H and increased affinity for factor B[52,53]. MPGN has also been described in association with a functional hypocomplementaemia occurring with an inherited hypomorphic variant of C3[54].

The mechanisms by which hypocomplementaemia might predispose to nephritis are unknown. It has been suggested that the increased susceptibility to infection results in increased frequency of antigen exposure, leading to increased formation of immune complexes in these subjects[55]. Alternatively, the erythrocyte transport mechanism for immune complexes may be disrupted (see later).

Other evidence, however, suggests that systemic hypocomplementaemia is not sufficient in itself to cause MPGN; attempts to produce renal damage in experimental animals rendered hypocomplementaemic by non-immune mechanisms have been uniformly unsuccessful[56,57]. Furthermore, it is now apparent that NeF in the context of nephritis may coexist with normo-complementaemia[58], which suggests that hypocomplementaemia is not necessary, at least for the perpetuation of nephritis. It does not, however, exclude a role for systemic hypocomplementaemia in initiation of the disease process.

NeF as a cause of local complement activation

Renal deposits of alternate pathway activators may be associated with histological evidence of renal injury similar to that seen in MPGN; for example, renal tissue from a patient with systemic candidiasis, hypo-complementaemia and MPGN was shown to contain deposits of *Candida albicans* antigen associated with C3. *Candida* is an alternative pathway activator, and treatment with antifungal agents was followed by clinical resolution of the nephritis[59]. Some rabbits injected repeatedly with zymosan (another activator of the alternative pathway) developed deposits of zymosan associated with C3 in glomerular and peritubular capillary walls, which were accompanied by endocapillary and mesangial proliferation[56]. Further, heat-killed kidney cells have been shown (albeit only under certain conditions *in vitro*) to be capable of activating complement and binding C3 convertase, which, in certain circumstances, may be stabilized by NeF[60].

However, evidence from clinical studies in support of such a role for NeF is, at best, circumstantial and comes from the demonstration that treatment of some patients with plasma exchange was followed by decrease in circulating levels of NeF accompanied by improvement of renal function[61].

Unfortunately, the elucidation of a directly pathogenic role for NeF has been hampered by the absence of a suitable animal model. The recent description of monoclonal antibodies against factor B and C4, which have demonstrable stabilizing activity of the alternative and classical pathway C3 convertases respectively[62,63], may allow the development of suitable experimental systems for investigation of this hypothesis, as may the generation of NeF *in vitro* from Epstein–Barr virus-transformed human B cells[64].

Defects in transport of immune complexes

Recent experiments on the clearance of injected immune complexes in baboons[65] have focused attention on the possible role of erythrocyte CR1 in the normal processing and clearance of circulating immune complexes[66] — see Chapter 4 for further details. Briefly, the postulated pathway involves first the fixation of C3b to immune complexes (opsonization), through which they then bind to CR1 on circulating erythrocytes. The immune complexes are prevented from being deposited in vessel walls and are transported to the fixed macrophage system where they are stripped off the erythrocytes. In addition, CR1 enhances the catabolism of C3b bound to the immune complexes by acting as a cofactor for factor I in the successive cleavages of C3b to iC3b and then C3dg. Complexes processed in this way appear to lose their ability to activate complement further[67].

NeF may interfere with this process by inhibiting the function of CR1 in the degradation of bound C3b[68]. Interestingly, CR1 is also found on glomerular podocytes[69], although its function is unknown. In addition, the hypocomplementaemia occurring in association with NeF may reduce the efficiency of opsonization. The potential consequences of these effects are an increased availability of circulating complexes for deposition in small vessels. These complexes, having escaped processing by factor I, would retain their phlogistic potential. The effects of hypocomplementaemia on the erythrocyte–immune complex transport mechanism have been demonstrated in baboons rendered hypocomplementaemic by injection of cobra venom factor[70]. However, the relevance of these findings to patients with NeF is not clear.

To date, only a limited number of studies have been performed to evaluate this potential pathogenetic role for NeF in patients and, so far, no supporting evidence has been obtained. Hypocomplementaemic serum from patients with NeF had no demonstrable defect in opsonization and binding of radiolabelled immune complexes to normal human erythrocytes *in vitro* (Y. C. Ng, unpublished). Similarly, clearance of radiolabelled immune complexes injected intravenously into two patients with NeF and hypocomplementaemia followed normal kinetics, and there was no detectable defect in binding of these immune complexes to erythrocytes *in vivo*[71]. However, the immune complexes used in these studies (respectively, bovine serum albumin (BSA)–rabbit anti-BSA and tetanus toxoid–human anti-tetanus toxoid) may be of limited pathological relevance, and there is ample evidence that the biological properties of an immune complex vary with its nature and composition.

CLINICAL STUDIES

Clinical studies have yielded conflicting results on the associations between serum C3 concentrations and levels of NeF[20,39,72], the presence of NeF and the rate of progression of nephritis[20,39], and the relationship between the reappearance of NeF and recurrence of MPGN in renal allografts[73,74]. Possible reasons for this confusion include: (1) the spontaneous waxing and waning of autoantibodies; (2) the occurrence of atypical nephritic factors that give false negative results in methods of detection used in screening of patients in clinical studies[17]; (3) the fact that plasma concentrations are a combination of both synthetic and catabolic rates and are affected by changes in extravascular distribution; and (4) the imprecise nature of such 'macroscopic' systemic measurements when used as indicators of local events occurring at sites of tissue injury.

SUMMARY

C3 nephritic factor is an IgG autoantibody that stabilizes the alternative pathway C3 convertase, thereby causing complement activation. Its pathogenetic significance in membranoproliferative glomerulonephritis has been discussed.

References

1. Fischel, E. E. and Gajdusek, D. C. (1952). Serum complement in acute glomerulonephritis and other renal diseases. *Am. J. Med.*, **12**, 190–196
2. Lange, K., Wasserman, E. and Slobody, L. B. (1960). The significance of serum complement levels for the diagnosis and prognosis of acute and subacute glomerulonephritis and lupus erythematosus disseminatus. *Ann. Intern. Med.*, **53**, 636–646
3. Gotoff, S. P., Fellers, F. X., Vawter, G. F., Janeway, C. A. and Rosen, F. S. (1965). The Beta-1c globulin in childhood nephrotic syndrome. *N. Engl J. Med.*, **273**, 524–529
4. West, C. D., McAdams, A. J., McConville, J. M., Davis, N. C. and Holland, N. H. (1965). Hypocomplementemic and normocomplementemic persistent (chronic) glomerulonephritis; clinical and pathologic characteristics. *J. Pediatr.*, **67**, 1089–1112
5. Spitzer, R. E., Vallota, E. H., Forristal, J., Sudora, E., Stitzel, A., Davis, N. S. and West, C. D. (1969). Serum C3 lytic system in patients with glomerulonephritis. *Science*, **164**, 436–437
6. Daha. M. R., Austen, K. F. and Fearon, D. T. (1977). The incorporation of NeF into a stabilised C3 convertase, C3bBb (C3NeF) and its release after decay of convertase function. *J. Immunol.*, **119**, 812–817
7. Davis, A. E., Ziegler, J. B., Gelfand, E. W., Rosen, F. S. and Alper, C. A. (1977). Heterogeneity of nephritic factor and its identification as an immunoglobulin. *Proc. Natl Acad. Sci. USA*, **74**, 3980–3983
8. Scott, D. M., Amos, N., Sissons, J. G. P., Lachmann, P. J. and Peters, D. K. (1978). The immunoglobulin nature of nephritis factor (NeF). *Clin. Exp. Immunol.*, **32**, 12–24
9. Daha, M. R. and van Es, L. A. (1979). Further evidence for the antibody nature of C3 nephritic factor. *J. Immunol.*, **123**, 755–758
10. Scott, D. M., Amos, N. and Bartolotti, S. R. (1981). The role of carbohydrate in the structure and function of nephritic factor. *Clin. Exp. Immunol.*, **46** 120–129
11. Kazatchkine, M. D., Fearon, D. T. and Austen, K. F. (1979). Human alternate complement pathway: membrane associated sialic acid regulates the competition between B and β1H for cellbound C3b. *J. Immunol.*, **122**, 75–80
12. Pangburn, M. K. and Muller-Eberhard, H. J. (1978). Complement C3 convertase: cell surface restriction of β1H control and generation of restriction on neuraminidase treated cells. *Proc. Natl Acad. Sci. USA*, **75**, 2416–2420

13. Daha, M. R., Fearon, D. T. and Austen, K. F. (1976). C3 nephritic factor (C3NeF): stabilisation of fluid phase and cell bound alternative pathway convertase. *J. Immunol.*, 116, 1–7
14. Weiler, J. M., Daha, M. R., Austen, K. F. and Fearon, D. T. (1976). Control of the amplification convertase of complement by the plasma protein β1H. *Proc. Natl Acad. Sci. USA*, 73, 3268–3272
15. Williams, D. G., Peters, D. K., Fallows, J., Petrie, A., Kourilsky, O., Morel-Maronger, L. and Cameron, J. S. (1974). Studies of serum complement in the hypocomplementaemic nephritides. *Clin. Exp. Immunol.*, 18, 391–405
16. Sissons, J. G. P., Leibowitch, J., Amos, N. and Peters, D. K. (1977). Metabolism of C5 and its relation to C3 in patients with complement activation. *J. Clin. Invest.*, 59, 704–715
17. Ng, Y. C. and Peters, D. K. (1986). C3 nephritic factor (C3NeF): dissociation of cell-bound and fluid phase stabilization of alternative pathway C3 convertase. *Clin. Exp. Immunol.*, 65, 450–457
18. Ohi, H., Watanabe, S., Seki, M., Fujita, T., Ohmori, F. and Hatano, M. (1987). C5 measurement in membranoproliferative glomerulonephritis patients with C3 nephritic factor. *Nephron*, 46, 217–218
19. Peters, D. K., Martin, A., Weinstein, A., Cameron, J. S., Barratt, T. M., Ogg, C. S. and Lachmann, P. J. (1972). Complement studies in membranoproliferative or other glomerulonephritis. *Clin. Exp. Immunol.*, 11, 311–320
20. Vallota, E. H., Forristal, J., Davis, N. C. and West, C. D. (1972). The C3 nephritic factor and MPGN: correlation of serum levels of nephritic factor with C3 levels, with treatment and with progression of disease. *J. Pediatr.*, 80, 947–959
21. Seino, J., Fukuda, K., Kinoshita, Y., Sudo, K., Horigome, I., Sato, H., Saito, T. and Furuyama, T. (1987). Quantitation of C3 nephritic factor of alternative complement pathway by an enzyme-linked immunosorbent assay. *J. Immunol. Methods*, 105, 119–125
22. Rother, U. (1982). A new screening test for C3 nephritic factor based on a stable cell bound convertase on sheep erythrocytes. *J. Immunol. Meth.*, 51, 101–107
23. Roberts, J. L., Levy, M., Chioros, P. G., Bartlow, B. G., Forristal, J., West, C. D., Habib, R. and Lewis, E. J. (1981). A serum C3-activating factor: its characterisation and its presence in glomerular deposits. *J. Immunol.*, 127, 1131–1137
24. Bartlow, B. G., Roberts, J. L. and Lewis, E. J. (1979). Non-immunoglobulin C3 activating factor in MPGN. *Kidney Int.*, 15, 294–302
25. Craddock, C. F., Richards, N. P., Powell, R. J. and Morgan, A. G. (1987). Novel C3 nephritic factor activity in the glomerulonephritis of staphylococcal endocarditis. *Q. J. Med.*, 65, 895–898
26. Meri, S. (1985). Complement activation in circulating serum factors in human glomerulonephritis. *Clin. Exp. Immunol.*, 59, 276–284
27. Clardy, C. W., Forristal, J., Strife, C. F. and West, C. D. (1989). A properdin dependent nephritic factor slowly activating C3, C5 and C9 in membranoproliferative glomerulonephritis types I and III. *Clin. Immunol. Immunopathol.*, 50, 333–347
28. Mollnes, T. E., Ng, Y. C., Peters, D. K., Lea, T., Tschopp, J. and Harboe, M. (1986). Effect of nephritic factor on C3 and on the terminal pathway of complement in vivo and in vitro. *Clin. Exp. Immunol.*, 65, 73–79
29. Vogt, W., Schmidt, G., von Buttlar, B. and Diemingler, L. (1978). A new function of the activated third component of complement: binding to C5, an essential step for C5 activation. *Immunology*, 34, 29–40
30. Isenman, D. E., Podack, E. R. and Cooper, N. R. (1980). The interaction of C5 with C3b in free solution: a sufficient condition for cleavage of a fluid phase C3/C5 convertase. *J. Immunol.*, 124, 326–331
31. Daha, M. R., Kok, D. J. and van Es, L. A. (1982). Regulation of C3 nephritic factor stabilised C3/C5 convertase of complement by purified human C3b receptor. *Clin. Exp. Immunol.*, 50, 209–217
32. Halbwachs, L., Leveille, M., Lesavre, P., Wattels, S. and Leibowitch, J. (1980). Nephritic factor of the classical pathway of complement. Immunoglobulin autoantibody directed against the classical pathway C3 convertase enzyme. *J. Clin. Invest.*, 65, 1249–1256
33. Daha, M. R., Hazevoet, H. M., Es, L. A. van and Katz, A. (1980). Stabilisation of the classical pathway convertase C42 by a factor (F-42) isolated from sera of patients with SLE. *Immunology*, 40, 417–424
34. Gigli, I., Sorvillo, J., Mecarelli-Halbwachs, L. and Leibowitch, J. (1981). Deregulation of

the classical pathway C3 convertase. *J. Exp. Med.*, **154**, 1–12

35. Daha, M. R., Hazevoet, H. M. and Es, L. A. van (1984). Heterogeneity, polypeptide chain composition and antigenic reactivity of autoantibodies (F-42) that are directed against the clasical pathway C3 convertase of complement and isolated from sera of patients with systemic lupus erythematosus. *Clin. Exp. Immunol.*, **56**, 614–620

36. Reichel, W., Kobberling, J., Fischbach, H. and Scheler, F. (1976). Membranoproliferative glomerulonephritis with partial lipodystrophy: discordant occurrence in identical twins. *Klin. Wochenschr.*, **54**, 75–81

37. Rees, A. J. (1984). The HLA complex and susceptibility to glomerulonephritis. *Plasma Ther. Trans. Technol.*, **5**, 455

38. Cameron, J. S., Turner, D. R., Heaton, J., Williams, D. G., Ogg, C. S., Chantler, C., Haycock, G. B. and Hicks, J. (1983). Idiopathic mesangiocapillary glomerulonephritis. Comparison of types I and II in children and adults and long-term prognosis. *Am. J. Med.*, **74**, 175–192

39. Schena, F. P., Pertosa, G., Stanziale, P., Vox, E., Pecoraro, C. and Andreucci, V. E. (1982). Biological significance of the C3 nephritic factor in membranoproliferative glomerulonephritis. *Clin. Nephrol.*, **18**, 240–246

40. Sissons, J. G. P., West, R. J., Fallows, J., Williams, G. D., Boucher, B. J., Amos, N. and Peters, D. K. (1976). The complement abnormalities of lipodystrophy. *N. Engl J. Med.*, **294**, 461–465

41. Grimwood, R. (1980). Herpes gestationis associated with C3 nephritic factor. *Arch. Dermatol.*, **116**, 1045–1047

42. Davis, C. A., McAdams, A. J., Wyatt, R. J., Forristal, J. and West, C. D. (1979). Idiopathic rapidly progressive glomerulonephritis with C3 nephritic factor and hypocomplementaemia. *J. Pediatr.*, **94**, 559–563

43. Thompson, R. A., Yap, P. L., Brettle, R. B., Dunmow, R. E. and Chapel, H. (1983). Meningococcal meningitis associated with persistent hypocomplementaemia due to circulating C3 nephritic factor. *Clin. Exp. Immunol.*, **52**, 153–156

44. Edwards, K. M., Alford, R., Gewurz, H. and Mold, C. (1983). Recurrent bacterial infections associated with C3 nephritic factor and hypocomplementemia. *N. Engl J. Med.*, **308**, 1138–1141

45. Teisner, B., Elling, P., Svehag, S. E., Poulsen, L., Lamm, L. U. and Sjoholm, A. (1984). C3 nephritic factor in a patient with recurrent *Neisseria meningitidis* infections. *Acta Pathol. Microbiol. Immunol. Scand [C]*, **92**, 341–349

46. Wahn, V., Muller, W., Rieger, C. and Rother, U. (1987). Persistently circulating C3 nephritic factor (C3 NeF)-stabilized alternative pathway C3 convertase (C3 CoF) in serum of an 11-year-old girl with meningococcal septicemia—simultaneous occurrence with free C3 NeF. *Pediatr. Res.*, **22**, 123–129

47. Gewurz, A. T., Imherr, S. M., Strauss, S., Gewurz, H. and Mold, C. (1983). C3 nephritic factor and hypocomplementaemia in a clinically healthy individual. *Clin. Exp. Immunol.*, **54**, 253–258

48. Tedesco, F., Tovo, P. A., Tamaro, G., Basaglia, M., Perticarari, S. and Villa, M. A. (1985). Selective C3 deficiency due to C3 nephritic factor in an apparently healthy girl. *Ric. Clin. Lab.*, **15**, 323–329

49. Wilson, C. B. and Dixon, F. J. (1971). Quantitation of acute and chronic serum sickness in rabbits. *J. Exp. Med.*, **134**, 7s–18s

50. Bennett, W. M., Bardana, E. J., Wuepper, K., Houghton, G., Border, W. A., Gotze, O. and Schreiber, R. (1977). Partial lipodystrophy, C3 nephritic factor and clinically inapparent mesangiocapillary glomerulonephritis. *Am. J. Med.*, **62**, 757–760

51. Charlesworth, J. A., Williams, D. G., Sherington, E., Lachmann, P. J. and Peters, D. K. (1974). Metabolic studies of the third component of complement and the glycine-rich β glycoprotein in patients with hypocomplementaemia. *J. Clin. Invest.*, **53**, 1578–1587

52. Marder, H. K., Coleman, T. H., Forristal, J., Beischel, L. and West, C. D. (1983). An inherited defect in the C3 convertase C3bBb associated with glomerulonephritis. *Kidney Int.*, **23**, 749–758

53. Linshaw, M. A., Stapleton, F. B., Cuppage, F. E., Forristal, J., West, C. D., Schreiber, R. D. and Wilson, C. B. (1987). Hypocomplementemic glomerulonephritis in an infant and mother. Evidence for an abnormal form of C3. *Am. J. Nephrol.*, **7**, 470–477

54. McLean, R. H. and Hoefnagel, D. (1980). Partial lipodystrophy and familial C3 deficiency. *Hum. Hered.*, **30**, 149–154

55. Peters, D. K. and Williams, D. G. (1974). Complement and mesangiocapillary glomeruloneph-

ritis: role of complement deficiency in the pathogenesis of nephritis. *Nephron*, **13**, 189–197

56. Verroust, P. J., Wilson, C. B. and Dixon, F. J. (1974). Lack of nephritogenicity of systemic activation of the alternative complement pathway. *Kidney Int.*, **6**, 157–169

57. Simpson, I. J., Moran, J., Evans, D. J. and Peters, D. K. (1978). Prolonged complement activation in mice. *Kidney Int.*, **13**, 467–471

58. Venning, M. C., Ng, Y. C., Amos, N. and Peters, D. K. (1989). Normocomplementaemia associated with glomerulonephritis, partial lipodystrophy and C3 nephritic factor. Submitted for publication.

59. Chesney, R. W., Oregan, S., Guyda, H. J. and Drummond, K. N. (1976). Candida endocrinopathy syndrome with membranoproliferative glomerulonephritis: demonstration of glomerular candida antigen. *Clin. Nephrol.*, **5**, 232–238

60. Baker, P. J., Adler, S., Yang, Y. and Couser, W. G. (1984). Complement activation by heat-killed human kidney cells: formation, activity, and stabilization of cell-bound C3 convertases. *J. Immunol.*, **133**, 877–881

61. Chalopin, J. M., Tanter, Y., Wenning, M. and Rifle, G. (1984). Immunosuppression and plasma exchange in dense deposit disease. *Ann. Int. Med.*, **135**, S31

62. Daha, M. R., Deelder, A. M. and Es, Z. A. van (1984). Stabilisation of the amplification convertase of Ce by monoclonal antibodies against human factor B. *J. Immunol.*, **132**, 2538–2542

63. Ichihara, C., Nakamura, T., Nagasama, S. and Koyama, J. (1986). Monoclonal anti-human C4b antibodies: stabilisation and inhibition of the classical pathway C3 convertase. *Mol. Immunol.*, **23**, 151–158

64. Hiramatsu, M., Balow, J. E. and Tsokos, G. C. (1986). Production of nephritic factor of the alternate complement pathway by Epstein–Barr virus-transformed B cell lines derived from a patient with MPGN. *J. Immunol.*, **136**, 4451–4455

65. Cornacoff, J. B., Hebert, L. A., Smead, W. L., Vanaman, M. E., Birmingham, D. J. and Waxman, F. J. (1983). Primate erythrocyte-immune complex-clearing mechanism. *J. Clin. Invest.*, **71**, 236–247

66. Schifferli, J. A., Ng, Y. C. and Peters, D. K. (1986). The role of complement and its receptor in the elimination of immune complexes. *N. Engl J. Med.*, **315**, 488–495

67. Medof, M. E., Prince, G. M. and Oger, J. J-F. (1982). Kinetics of interactions of immune complexes with complement receptors on human blood cells: modification of complexes during interaction with red cells. *Clin. Exp. Immunol.*, **48**, 715–725

68. Mold, C. and Medof, M. E. (1985). C3 nephritic factor protects bound C3bBb from cleavage by factor I and human erythrocytes. *Mol. Immunol.*, **22**, 507–512

69. Fearon, D. T. (1980). Identification of the membrane glycoprotein that is the C3b receptor of the human erythrocyte, polymorphonuclear leucocyte, B lymphocyte and monocyte. *J. Exp. Med.*, **152**, 20–30

70. Waxman, F. J., Hebert, L. A., Cornacoff, J. B., Vanaman, M. E., Smead, W. L., Kraut, E. H., Birmingham, D. J. and Taguiam, J. M. (1984). Complement depletion accelerates the clearance of immune complexes from the circulation of primates. *J. Clin. Invest.*, **74**, 1329–1340

71. Schifferli, J. A., Ng, Y. C., Paccaud, J. P. and Walport, M. J. (1989). The role of hypocomplementaemia and low erythrocyte complement receptor type 1 numbers in determining abnormal immune complex clearance in human. *Clin. Exp. Immunol.*, **75**, 329–335

72. Berthoux, F. C., Carpenter, C. B., Freyria, A. M., Traeger, J. and Merrill, J. P. (1976). Human glomerulonephritis and C3 nephritic factor (C3NeF). *Clin. Nephrol.*, **5**, 93–100

73. Curtis, J. J., Wyatt, R. J., Bhathena, D., Lucas, B. A., Holland, N. H. and Luke, R. G. (1979). Renal transplantation for patients with type I and type II MPGN: serial complement and nephritic factor measurements and the problem of recurrence of disease. *Am. J. Med.*, **66**, 216–225

74. Liebowitch, J., Halbwachs, L., Wattel, S., Failland, M. H. and Droz, D. (1979). Recurrence of dense deposits in transplanted kidney II. Serum complement and nephritic factor profiles. *Kidney Int.*, **15**, 396–403

75. Power, D. A., Ng, Y. C. and Simpson, J. G. (1990). Familial incidence of C3 nephritic factor, partial lipodystrophy and membranoproliferative glomerulonephritis. *Q. J. Med.*, **75**, 387–398

11
Anti-glomerular Basement Membrane Disease

N. TURNER and C. D. PUSEY

Human anti-glomerular basement membrane (anti-GBM) disease is a rare disorder characterized by rapidly progressive glomerulonephritis (RPGN) and lung haemorrhage. However, it is the cause of only about one third of the cases of this clinical syndrome, and lung haemorrhage does not occur in all patients. The autoantibodies which define the disorder are directed towards a component of the glomerular basement membrane that is also found in a restricted range of other basement membranes, although renal and pulmonary disease are the only clinically important consequences of their presence.

Some confusion has been generated by the use of Ernest Goodpasture's name in association with this disorder. He described an 18-year-old man who had lung haemorrhage and crescentic nephritis at autopsy during the influenza epidemic of 1918[1]. Stanton and Tange later used the term 'Goodpasture's syndrome' to describe a group of patients with the same combination of renal disease and lung haemorrhage[2]. Only later did the immunological disturbance underlying a proportion of these cases become clear, when linear deposition of immunoglobulin on the GBM was demonstrated in the kidneys of patients with the syndrome[3]. It is now clear that systemic vasculitis of several types accounts for most of the remaining cases of Goodpasture's syndrome, although in these disorders there is commonly evidence of pre-existing or simultaneous disease in other organ systems.

Some authors have restricted the term 'Goodpasture's syndrome' to those cases with anti-GBM antibodies, and the molecular target of these autoantibodies has become known as the Goodpasture antigen. The term 'anti-GBM disease' has been widely used to avoid this possible confusion, but it has become apparent that antibodies to a variety of GBM components apart from the Goodpasture antigen may be formed in other types of glomerulonephritis[4-6]. In none of these other disorders is there evidence that the antibodies are important in the pathogenesis of the disease, but there is an expanding literature on the phenomenon and an increasing interest in the possible role of such antibodies. We will try to follow the least confusing course by calling the disease associated with autoantibodies to the Goodpasture antigen *Goodpasture's disease*, to avoid confusion with the clinical syndrome of lung haemorrhage and RPGN, or with other disorders in which 'non-Goodpasture anti-GBM antibodies'[6] are formed.

The immunopathology of Goodpasture's disease is the best-characterized of all the human nephritides. Despite its rarity, this has led to a great deal of clinical and research interest since its course and immunological features were first described. A number of remarkable features are worth emphasizing here before some of them are described in greater detail.

(1) The autoantibodies seem to be particularly closely involved in tissue injury, and there is an unusually close correlation between presence of circulating antibody and clinical disease when compared with other autoimmune disorders. The demonstration that the antibodies cause renal injury when injected into another primate species provides additional evidence for their importance in mediating, as well as characterizing the disease.

(2) The combination of immunosuppression and plasma exchange to remove circulating antibodies has proved very effective in arresting the disease—and Goodpasture's disease was among the first types of nephritis to show a convincing response to any therapy.

(3) There is a strong genetic influence on susceptibility to the disease, suggesting the necessity of T lymphocyte recognition of an autoantigenic target for the disease to occur (discussed in Chapter 1).

(4) The GBM of patients with hereditary nephritis of the Alport type usually have deficiency or absence of the target 'Goodpasture antigen' on immunohistochemical studies. Furthermore, when such patients are transplanted with a normal kidney, they may develop antibodies to the Goodpasture antigen and occasionally RPGN.

These features make Goodpasture's disease a good subject for the application of modern immunological, biochemical and molecular biological techniques in order to discover more about the mechanisms underlying the disease. It seems likely that the precise structure of the autoantigen will emerge in the near future, and it is hoped that this will pave the way for greater understanding of the autoimmune perturbation, as well as opening new avenues for more specific therapy.

CLINICAL ASPECTS

Incidence

Goodpasture's disease has an incidence of about 0.5 cases per million in Great Britain, but it is probably much rarer in many populations. Successive series over the years since the disease was first described have shown a progressively greater incidence in females, a greater distribution of age, and a lower incidence of lung haemorrhage. These changes have generally been attributed to increased recognition of the disease with greater use of immunoassays in patients with crescentic nephritis. Although originally described as a disease of young men, it is now clear that it can affect all age groups and that there is only a slight male predominance[7,8]. Our data show a bimodal distribution of incidence by age, the major peaks being in the 20–30 years and 50–60 years age groups. Both peaks contain about the same number of patients and have a similar sex ratio. Men are more likely to have lung haemorrhage, perhaps because of differences in smoking habits and occupational exposures (see below).

Genetic factors and susceptibility

There are several reports of Goodpasture's disease occurring in siblings[2,9] and in identical twins [10,11], although there are also cases of identical twins who did not contract the disease (ref. 12 and two pairs in our series). In the last decade the importance of the major histocompatibility antigens, particularly the Class II molecules, in susceptibility to autoimmune diseases has been increasingly appreciated. Rees and colleagues[13] observed a strong association with HLA DR2 by serotyping, and these observations have been extended by more reliable and extensive RFLP typing at DR and DQ loci by Burns et al. (Chapter 1). There is no difference in the HLA associations between older and younger patients, as has been noted for myasthenia gravis. An association between HLA-B7 and more severe disease was described by Rees et al.[14], and an association with specific Gm allotypes of the IgG heavy-chain constant region has also been reported[15].

Environmental and other influences

Since Goodpasture's observations on one patient during an influenza epidemic, there have been attempts to link Goodpasture's disease with a variety of infections and environmental factors. As well as the usual difficulties in deciding whether an association is causal or coincidental, there is the additional complicating possibility in this setting that some of the reported exposures or infections could have revealed the presence of the disease, rather than causing it. This applies particularly to patients presenting with pulmonary haemorrhage, the occurrence and even timing of which has been strongly associated with cigarette smoking[16,17] and exposure to other pulmonary irritants. Other factors, particularly infections, may non-specifically exacerbate tissue injury in subacute disease, bringing to light disease which has been worsened but not caused by the apparent precipitant. Possible mechanisms underlying this phenomenon are discussed in the section on immunopathogenesis.

Several observations of clusters of cases[18–20] suggest that an infective or other environmental agent might be important; we recently learnt of two unrelated patients who presented with acute Goodpasture's disease on the same day to a district hospital on the British south coast. In none of these reports has there been a strong case for any particular precipitant. Following Goodpasture's original report, several workers have looked for associations of the disease with viral infections. No relationship with any specific virus or other infection has been demonstrated[8,21]. In case reports and epidemiological surveys, exposure to hydrocarbon or solvent fumes has frequently been implicated in the aetiology of glomerulonephritis, and of Goodpasture's disease in particular. The number of reports is persuasive, but awareness of the possible association may have made reporting more likely, and some of the series are not well controlled. Several reports concern renal disease alone[22-24], while others lend more support to the 'pulmonary irritant' hypothesis[25]. How hydrocarbons could affect the incidence of nephritis is unknown.

Several lines of evidence suggest that pulmonary haemorrhage only occurs when there is an additional insult to the lung. In practice this is commonly cigarette smoking, which has been strongly associated with the occurrence of lung haemorrhage in Britain[17]. Fluid overload[18,26-28] or chest infections[18,26,27], and sometimes remote infections[29,30], may achieve the same effect. Antibodies (and presumably other effectors of the immune response) do not normally have access to the alveolar basement membrane, and these factors may act by disrupting the endothelial barrier and exposing the alveolar basement membrane to the circulation. It is interesting to note that the relationship between smoking and lung haemorrhage does not hold in Goodpasture's syndrome caused by systemic vasculitis[31]. This presumably reflects differences in the pathogenetic mechanisms.

Disease associations

Goodpasture's disease has been described in association with a number of other conditions (Table 1). The list is notable for the rarity of associations with other autoimmune diseases, although there are isolated observations of occurrence with several such disorders. The associations with cases of microscopic polyarteritis and Wegener's granulomatosis, which can both themselves cause RPGN and lung haemorrhage, are particularly interesting. Recent work has suggested that, immunologically at least, there is some overlap between the groups of patients with systemic vasculitis and Goodpasture's disease. In our laboratory about 8% of patients with specific antibodies to the Goodpasture antigen also have antibodies to neutrophil cytoplasm (ANCA), and about 5% of patients with ANCA have anti-Goodpasture antibodies. The Cambridge group found a much higher incidence of overlap[54] (see also Chapter 12), but this may reflect different referral patterns. The ANCA associated with the anti-GBM antibodies may be cytoplasmic or perinuclear (with anti-myeloperoxidase antibodies) in pattern (unpublished observations). The clinical and pathological significance of these laboratory observations is not yet clear. The majority of these patients have clinical and/or pathological evidence of systemic vasculitis, and the course of their disease and outcome seems to be more consistent with a primary diagnosis of systemic vasculitis. However, there are at least two examples of patients with distinct disorders separated in time—and this association has been noted before, as well as after, the availability of assays for ANCA[33,55]. In the more common patients with a single episode of disease, anti-GBM antibodies may be present only fleetingly. It is possible that anti-Goodpasture antibodies are raised as a secondary phenomenon following

Table 1 Disease associations of Goodpasture's disease

Disease	Reference
Autoimmune disorders	
Microscopic polyarteritis	[32]
Wegener's granulomatosis	[33]
Hashimoto's thyroiditis	[34]
Myasthenia gravis	Lightstone, unpublished
Coeliac disease	[7]
Partial lipodystrophy	[35]
Penicillamine therapy	Lechler, unpublished
Other renal diseases	
Membranous nephropathy	[36–40]
Cortical necrosis	[41]
Post-lithotripsy	[42]
Obstructive uropathy	[43]
Malignant disease	
Hodgkin's disease/lymphoma	[23, 44, 45]
Thymoma	Turner, unpublished
Inherited disorders	
Nail-patella syndrome	[46]
Alport's syndrome	[47–53] (after renal transplantation)

damage to basement membranes caused by systemic vasculitis: such a hypothesis has been raised previously to explain the uncommon but striking occurrence of crescentic nephritis in patients with membranous nephritis. However, only about half of the reported cases of crescentic deterioration in membranous nephritis have had anti-GBM antibodies; whether the remainder have ANCA is not yet known. Similar mechanisms could underly the recently reported temporal associations of the disease with lithotripsy and urinary obstruction. A genetic susceptibility is likely to be critical, and it is interesting that both these patients carried HLA-DR2[42,43].

Penicillamine, a known polyclonal activator that has associations with several other autoimmune disorders, has repeatedly been associated with RPGN and lung haemorrhage[56–58]. Most reports antedate the ANCA era, but a single case seen by us recently had antibodies to myeloperoxidase with a perinuclear ANCA (Gaskin et al., unpublished observation). We know of one case of Goodpasture's disease in association with the drug; unfortunately, an ANCA assay was not available.

Of the six patients with Hodgkin's disease or other lymphoma who are reported to have developed Goodpasture's disease, scanty information is published on two. Both developed the disease after successful treatment of their lymphoma, and neither had evidence of residual malignancy. One had been treated by upper-mantle radiotherapy alone. It is possible that any influence of the lymphoma or the treatment on the occurrence of Goodpasture's disease may be through disordered regulation of immunity, rather than through effects on the glomerular or other basement membranes.

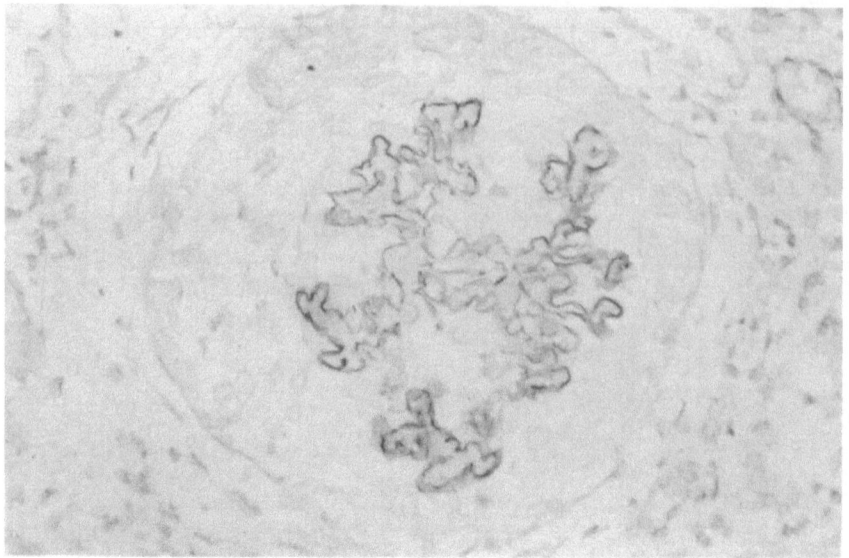

Figure 1 Photomicrograph of a glomerulus with a near-circumferential crescent, and immunoperoxidase staining showing IgG bound in a linear fashion to the basement membrane. (Courtesy of Dr E. M. Thompson.)

Clinical and laboratory features

The clinical features have been described in a number of series and reviews[8,45,59-61]. Patients usually present acutely, although occasional cases present with intermittent episodes of haemoptysis, or with chronic iron-deficiency anaemia caused by lung haemorrhage. About two-thirds of patients have pulmonary haemorrhage at the time of diagnosis, and this has often been the presenting problem. Those who present with renal disease alone often have more advanced glomerular damage, as there are frequently only non-specific symptoms until those of renal failure develop. The renal lesion can progress extremely rapidly once significant glomerular damage has occurred, so that a patient with a normal creatinine may lose all renal function within a few days or even hours. A deterioration of pulmonary haemorrhage often occurs at the same time, so that the patient may develop simultaneous acute renal and respiratory failure. This is the classical case of 'Goodpasture's syndrome', although as mentioned above, the clinical features of the same syndrome caused by systemic vasculitis are indistinguishable. A few patients present subacutely with lung haemorrhage and no overt renal disease, although they usually have haematuria, and renal biopsy shows linear fixation of IgG despite the lack or triviality of morphological changes[62].

The diagnosis is usually suspected clinically because of the finding of a nephritic urine sediment in a patient with acute renal failure and/or pulmonary haemorrhage. The finding of linear binding of IgG to the GBM (Figure 1) by direct immunofluorescence or immunoperoxidase is almost pathognomic in the setting of RPGN, but has been described in other circumstances, including diabetes mellitus, systemic lupus erythematosus, and some renal transplant biopsies and autopsy kidneys[49,63]. Additional granular deposits have been noted in some biopsies, and in occasional patients a progression from a linear to a granular pattern has been noted[64]. It is now clear that the pattern of immunoglobulin binding in renal biopsies does not necessarily reflect the natural distribution of the target antigen[65], and it remains to be seen whether these granular deposits are a result of antibodies to a different target or whether they are a phase of accumulation or clearance of antibodies to the usual target.

The measurement of circulating anti-GBM antibodies has become an invaluable aid to rapid diagnosis and the tailoring of treatment. Most of the available assays have used a collagenase-solubilized preparation of human GBM as the ligand for a radioimmunoassay or ELISA[45,66-68]. The expertise required to prepare good enough antigen, and to perform inhibition assays and Western blots where appropriate, has restricted these assays to a few centres. Recently the antigenic component has been further purified from the GBM of cows[69] or sheep[70] for use in ELISA, with apparently equal or greater sensitivity and reliability, and with more specific results. These assays are robust and probably could be used more widely, although the rarity of the disease makes it likely that their availability will remain restricted.

Anti-Goodpasture autoantibodies are largely made up of IgG1 and IgG4 subclasses[71-73]. Other classes of antibody may coexist; IgA and IgM may bind to the GBM in some patients, and circulating IgA antibodies have been demonstrated in several, usually in low titre. One patient is described who apparently had no detectable circulating IgG antibodies but had circulating and bound IgA antibodies in association with severe disease of lungs and kidney[74]. Linear C3 is seen on the GBM in 40–70% of cases. Similar binding can often be demonstrated in the lungs of patients with pulmonary haemorrhage, but may be patchy. Bound IgG can occasionally be demonstrated in other locations where the Goodpasture antigen is known to be present (Table 2), notably in the choroid plexus and the eye, but it has only rarely been associated with disease manifestations at these sites[75-78]. There are no abnormalities of serum complement or total immunoglobulin levels, and rheumatoid factors or other autoantibodies are not generally found.

Table 2 Distribution of the Goodpasture antigen by indirect immunofluorescence and immunoperoxidase studies[77,89,90]

Kidney	GBM, distal tubular basement membrane, Bowman's capsule
Lung	Alveolar basement membrane
Eye	Choroid, ciliary body, Bruch's membrane, basement membranes of retinal capillaries, lens capsule and cornea
Ear	Cochlear basement membrane
Brain	Basement membrane of choroidal epithelium
Liver	Hepatic arteries in portal tract
Other	Adrenal, breast (ducts), pituitary, thyroid gland (follicular basement membrane)

Treatment

Since the mid-1970s, when treatment by powerful immunosuppression with cyclophosphamide and prednisolone in conjunction with plasma exchange was introduced[30,79], there have been only minor alterations to the recommended therapy. This treatment was found to be effective in arresting pulmonary haemorrhage and preventing the progression of renal damage, while previous thereapy with corticosteroids and sometimes immunosuppressive agents in varying doses had inconsistent effects on pulmonary haemorrhage and had little effect on renal disease[45,59,80]. Which components are essential and what doses of the combination therapy are optimal has not been thoroughly examined, as such trials are difficult in a rare disease with many confounding variables. Plasma exchange seems rational for accelerating the removal of antibodies, but it is not effective as sole treatment[81]. It is the only component that has been subjected to a controlled trial[82], but the results, while favourable, illustrated the difficulties of mounting and interpreting such a trial rather better than they demonstrated a beneficial effect[8]. Immunoadsorption with staphylococcal protein A has been successfully used as a more efficient way of removing large amounts of immunoglobulin without depleting clotting factors and complement, or the need for large volumes of colloid replacement solutions[83].

It is a depressing observation that while mortality has been substantially reduced since the development of methods for rapid diagnosis and effective treatment, a large proportion of patients (50% or more) still develop end-stage renal failure. This appears to be because of the rapidity of progression and the severity of the renal damage. The renal lesion appears to be relatively non-reversible when compared with histologically similar lesions in patients with RPGN caused by systemic vasculitis. Dialysis-dependent renal failure associated with a large percentage of crescents on renal biopsy is frequently recoverable when caused by systemic vasculitis, but almost never when caused by Goodpasture's disease[8,84]. There is great interest therefore in the mechanism underlying these differences, and in ways of developing still more effective treatments.

Resolution

Even in untreated patients, autoantibody levels tend to decline and to reach background levels over 1–2 years[45,84]. Renal transplantation seems to carry little risk of recurrent disease if the autoantibody levels have been at background levels for 6 months or more. Treatment with cyclophosphamide, corticosteroids and plasma exchange accelerates the decline in antibody levels to around 8 weeks to disappearance, and levels only rarely rise significantly after the completion of 3 months' treatment[7,82]. This modulation of the autoimmune response seems to be unusual in other diseases in which there is autoantibody production, but the phenomenon makes a short period of intensive treatment justifiable and effective. However, this therapeutic or spontaneous regulation of antibody production has only been observed after a distinct severe episode of disease. A non-progressive course may be seen in early disease; individuals are described with a long history (up to 12 years[85]) of recurrent episodes of haemoptysis in the presence of anti-GBM antibodies before they presented with fulminant lung and renal disease.

Goodpasture's disease after renal transplantation

There are two possible explanations for this phenomenon. First, the patient had Goodpasture's disease as their original diagnosis. This is likely to occur if circulating antibodies are still present at the time of transplantation, and unlikely to occur if they have been proved to be absent for a period[18,59] (as long as immunosuppression is used after transplantation[12]). Second, the allograft has introduced the Goodpasture antigen to a patient who lacked it in their native basement membranes—the only known example of this occurs in patients with Alport's syndrome[47,52,53]. This is quite a rare phenomenon, and many patients with Alport's syndrome have had successful allografts. Where it recurs in a first transplant the graft has always been lost, but successful retransplantation can be achieved. The appearance of anti-GBM antibodies without overt disease in this situation may be quite common.

THE GOODPASTURE ANTIGEN

Knowledge of the target of autoimmune attack makes Goodpasture's disease unique among nephritides and better understood than most other autoimmune diseases. The major antibody response is probably restricted towards a part of one molecule, an antigen which has become known as the Goodpasture antigen. Although patients' sera may contain low titres of antibodies to other GBM components[6,86-88], immunohistochemical and Western blotting studies always show reactivity with this specific minority constituent of GBM. The immunohistochemical and immunoblotting patterns can be replicated by single monoclonal antibodies[77,89,90] (Figures 2 and 3).

Distribution and localization

Indirect immunohistochemical studies show that the antigen is normally present in a number of basement membranes, but that it cannot be detected elsewhere in tissue sections. The major locations are in the glomeruli and in the alveolar basement membrane, as predicted from the manifestations of the disease, but it is interesting that the other basement membranes in which it is found (Table 2) are also usually of specialized function and formed by fusion of basement membranes from epithelial cell and endothelial cell layers[91,92]. Recent studies with monoclonal antibodies that appear to recognize the antigenic molecule confirm the earlier finding[93] that it is found in the lamina densa, on the epithelial side of the staining for the ubiquitous $\alpha 1$ and $\alpha 2$ chains[94,95].

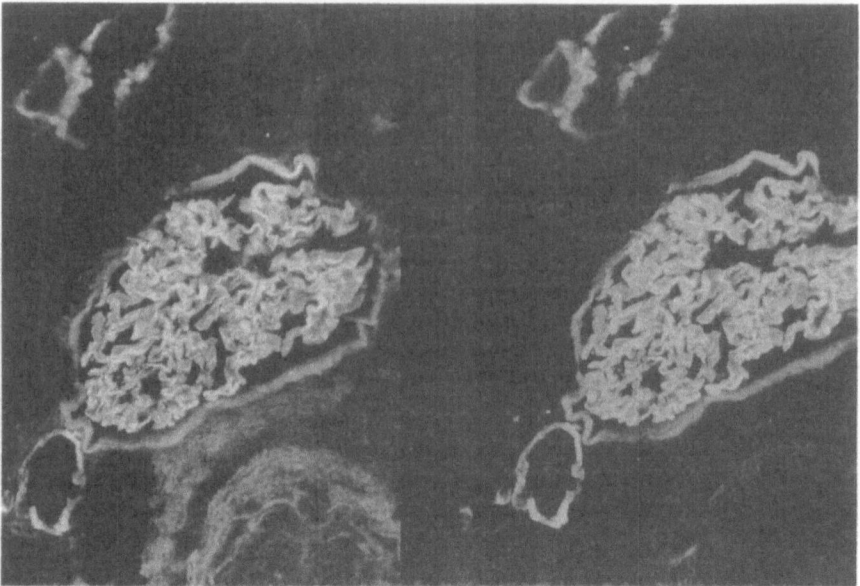

Figure 2 Double-stained indirect immunofluorescence of a single section of a normal human glomerulus. Left panel shows the pattern obtained with autoantibodies eluted from a patient's kidney, with fluorescein-conjugated secondary antibody. Right panel shows the pattern obtained with the monoclonal antibody P1, with rhodamine-conjugated secondary antibody. (Courtesy of S. J. Cashman.)

The nature of the antigen

Basement membranes have been intensively studied in order to define their composition, structure and properties[96,97]. The glomerular basement membrane is composed of largely the same constituents as other basement membranes, but is particularly modified to fulfil its specialized role[91]. Morphologically, it is a fused basement membrane separating the endothelial cells of the glomerular capillaries from the visceral epithelial cells of Bowman's space. The endothelial surface is pitted with *fenestrae* so that the capillary contents do not have to traverse the endothelial cells, or their intercellular junctions, in order to reach the basement membrane. Circulating or injected antibodies to basement membrane components appear to have direct access to the glomerular basement membrane, whereas this is not the case in the unfenestrated capillaries of, for instance, the lung[75,98,99] or elsewhere in the kidney[98] (notably the distal tubules), where the antigen can be demonstrated by indirect immunofluorescence. These barriers may be important in limiting the manifestations of the disease—their role in pulmonary haemorrhage has been discussed above.

Glomerular basement membranes can be prepared by sieving glomeruli from fresh or frozen kidney and sonicating and lysing to remove attached cells. The antigen can then be released from lyophilized membranes by digestion with collagenase. Extraction with salt solutions fails to release the antigenic component, while other methods of digestion destroy it. Reduction

238

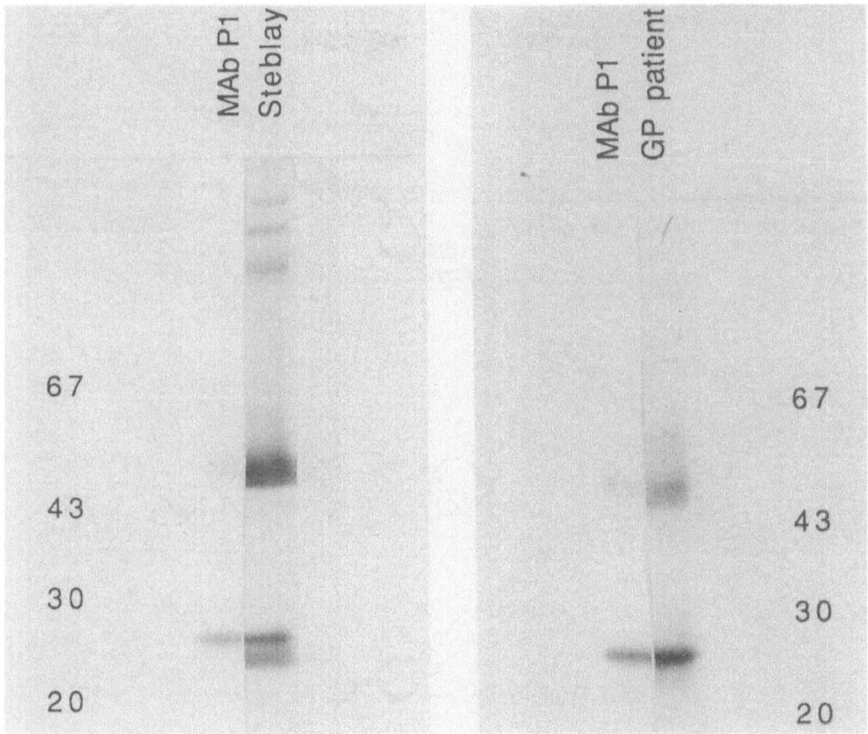

Figure 3 Western blots of collagenase-solubilized human GBM separated by SDS-PAGE in non-reducing conditions. Positions of molecular weight markers (in kilodaltons) are shown to the sides. Each lane has been cut into two halves and the strips reacted with different primary antibodies. In the left-hand panel the result with a patient's serum at 1/100 is shown beside that with serum from a sheep with Steblay nephritis at 1/200. The human serum recognizes one major 'monomer' band in the 25–30 kD region. The sheep serum recognizes the same band, but also picks out bands at a lower molecular weight (probably human α1 and α2 chains). In the right-hand panel a patient's serum is compared with monoclonal antibody P1[90]. Each picks out one band in the 'monomer' region and three in the 'dimer' region at 50–60 kD. There are minor differences in relative intensity but the bands identified are identical. The overall complexity of these digests is shown in the silver-stained two-dimensional gel in Figure 5.

of disulphide bonds also destroys the antigenicity of the molecule. Collagenase-solubilized GBM is used as the ligand in the standard immunoassays for anti-GBM antibodies, and for immunoblotting (Figure 3).

From these digests it has been shown that the antigen is attached to, or a part of, the major C-terminal non-collagenous domain (NC1 domain) of type IV collagen (Figure 4)[92]. Type IV collagen makes up the structural skeleton of all basement membranes by cross-linking at its N-terminal and C-terminal ends. The globular NC1 domains at the C-terminus are a feature of procollagens, and are cleaved from the procollagen during fibril formation in most interstitial collagens. Each type IV collagen molecule is composed of three chains, most commonly two α1 chains and one α2 (Figure 4). Collagenase destroys the triple-helical, fibrillar part of the molecule, leaving

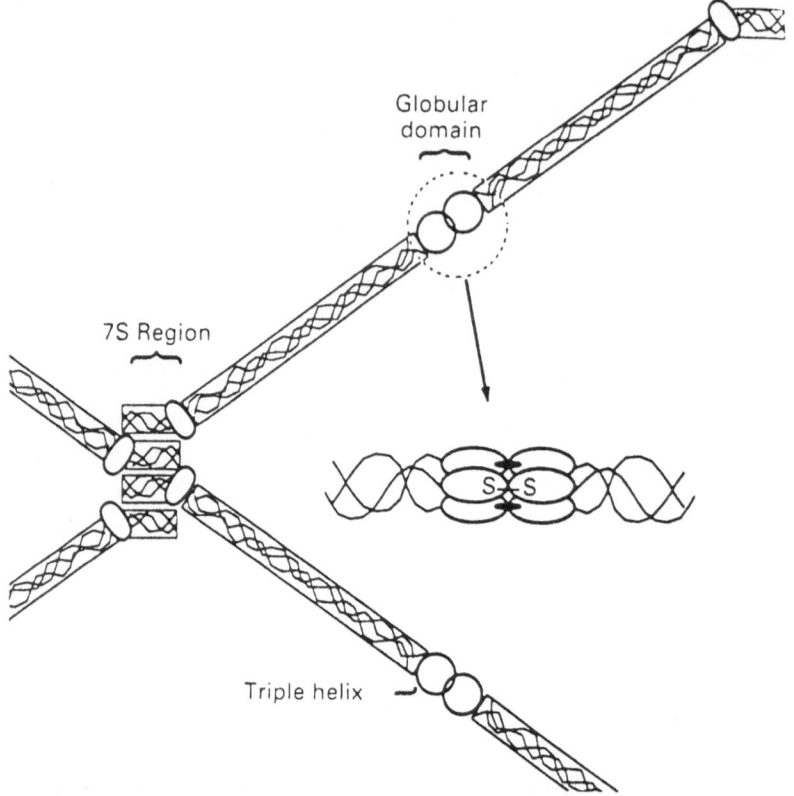

Figure 4 Schematic diagram of a type IV collagen molecule. The majority of the molecule is triple helical, with various 'non-collagenous' interruptions. The largest of the non-collagenous regions is the NC1 domain at the C-terminus, in which each of the three chains making up the molecule are represented (inset). An NC1 domain is covalently (mostly through disulphide bridges) and non-covalently associated with a similar domain from an adjacent molecule. The triple helical regions are destroyed by collagenase to give a digest rich in NC1 domain 'hexamers' (inset). SDS and other dissociating agents separate these hexamers into 'monomers' (25–30 kD), each being the C-terminal end of a single type IV collagen chain, and dimers (50–60 kD), composed of the cross-linked C-terminal domains from chains of two adjacent type IV collagen molecules[92,100,101]. (From *Kidney International*[102], with permission.)

the non-collagenous domains intact and releasing them from the basement membrane network. The α1 and α2 chains have been extensively studied and cloned in both man and the mouse[103,104]. In man their genes lie in a unique arrangement on chromosome 13, head to head and separated by less than 200 base pairs, with common, bidirectional promoter sequences between[105,106]. However, the Goodpasture antigen is only found in some basement membranes, whereas type IV collagen is a major part of all of them.

Evidence from two-dimensional SDS-PAGE and immunoblotting and limited protein sequence data from purified bovine[107,108], sheep[70], and more recently human[109], NC1 domains has suggested that basement membranes

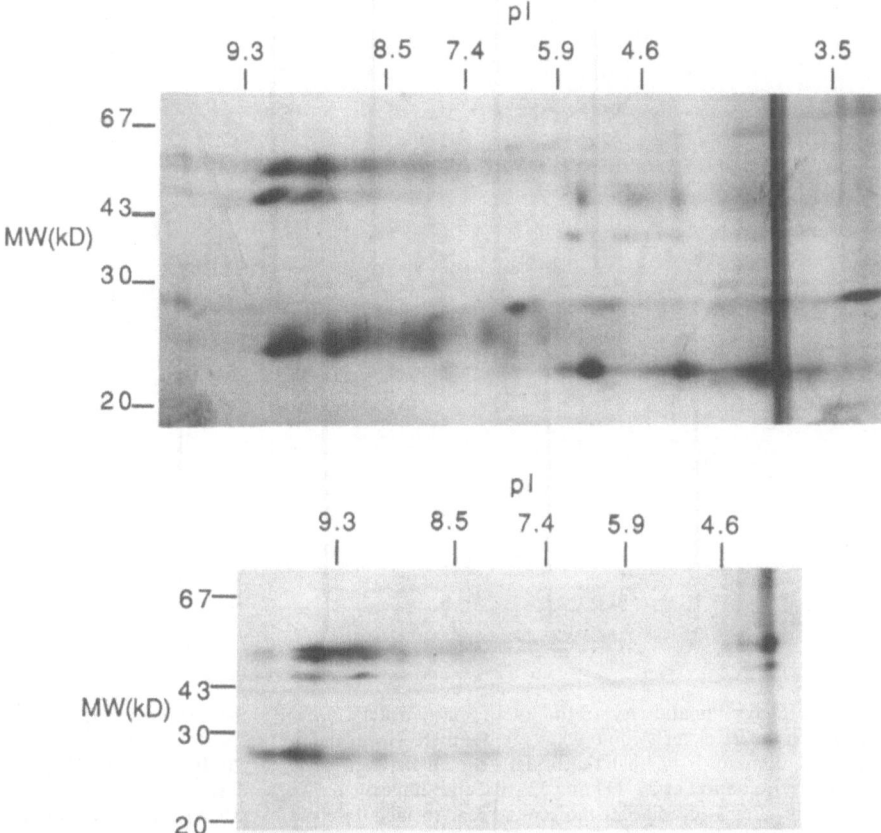

Figure 5 Two-dimensional SDS-PAGE of collagenase-solubilized human GBM: silver-stained gel (upper panel) and immunoblot with patient's serum (lower panel). pI markers are shown along the upper border, and molecular weight markers down the left margin. The vertical line towards the right of the gel and the blot is an artefact from the loading point of the first (isoelectric focusing) stage. Components of interest fall into 'monomer' and 'dimer' groups as described in Figure 4, but each one shows 'charge isoforms', with apparently several isoelectric points. The reason for this phenomenon is not known[110,111]. The antigenic component in immunoblots with patients' serum or the monoclonal antibody P1 (and other monoclonal antibodies believed to recognize the antigen[89]) is highly cationic (positively charged), and the monomer component has a molecular weight of about 28 kD. (Courtesy of C. J. Derry.)

in some tissues contain additional types of type IV collagen chain. Two new chains have been characterized by these techniques, and labelled as α3 and α4 chains. The non-collagenous domain of the α3 chain appears to carry the Goodpasture antigen. It is highly positively charged in comparison with the others (Figure 5), and has more similarities with the α1 chain than with the α2. The α4 chain is more similar to the α2 chain, and it is possible that these 'novel' chains may interact with each other in the same way as do α1 and α2 chains[89,94,108]. Several groups have put considerable effort into attempts

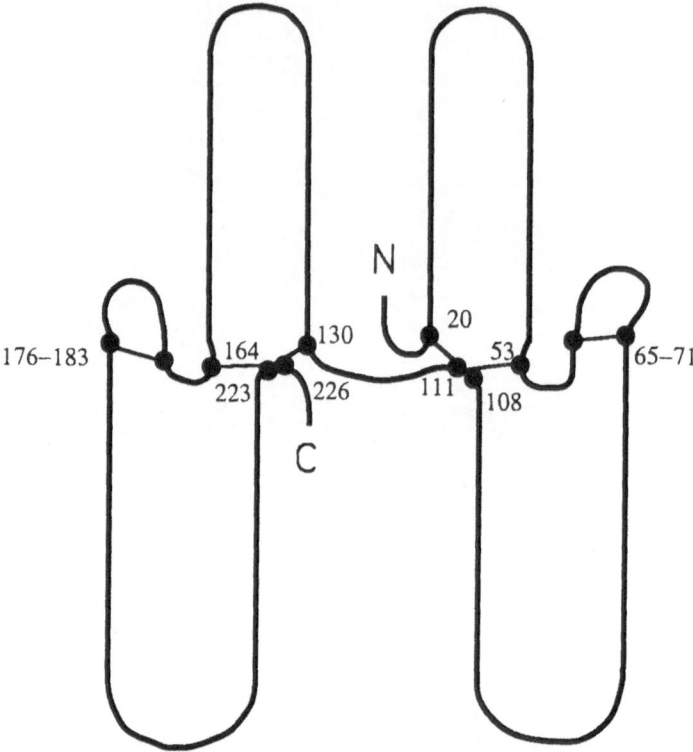

Figure 6 Diagrammatic view of the folding pattern determined by the positions of disulphide bridges in the α1 chain. Amino acids are numbered from the first (most N-terminal) residue of the NC1 domain. Note that the bridges shown between cysteines 20–108 and 53–111 could alternatively connect as 20–111 and 53–108, and similarly in the second pair of loops. Disulphide bridges to chains of adjacent molecules seem to include all four cysteines of this 'disulphide knot'. The NC1 domains of other type IV collagen chains are likely to have an identical folding pattern, as the positions of cysteine residues are highly conserved. (Adapted from Siebold et al.[112])

to define these novel chains at a molecular level, but the full amino acid sequence of the antigenic molecule has yet to emerge. Nevertheless, it is clear from the available data that the new chains are extremely similar to the known chains, which are in any case 63% homologous across the 230 amino acids of the NC1 domain. Each NC1 domain is made up of two similar halves. The positions of the cysteine residues are particularly closely conserved; this is likely to be important for the tertiary structure of the NC1 domain and for its ability to cross-link with adjacent chains, as well as for its antigenicity. The intrachain disulphide bonding pattern for the α1 chain has been solved[112] and is shown in Figure 6. The pattern in the antigenic α3 chain is likely to be identical.

Although there have been suggestions in the past that different antigens were responsible for lung and kidney disease, there can no longer be any doubt that the antigen is the same in the lungs and kidney[8]. It may be differently cross-linked and presented in the lung[113–115], and differences in accessibility to the circulation have been alluded to.

The Goodpasture antigen and Alport's syndrome

Alport's syndrome is an inherited disorder in which a degenerative process affects the glomerular and other basement membranes. Phenotypes vary, but typical cases have renal failure, cochlear degeneration leading to high-tone hearing loss and deafness, and sometimes ocular abnormalities such as lenticonus[116]. Immunohistochemical studies using autoantibodies from patients with Goodpasture's disease or monoclonal antibodies show that the Goodpasture antigen is reduced in amount or absent from the GBM of most of these patients[47,117]. Inheritance of the syndrome is usually X-linked, and males are generally more severely affected than females. Rare cases of autosomal inheritance have also been described[118]. The gene on the X chromosome has been mapped to the Xq22 region by family studies[119,120]. Recently Hostikka *et al.* cloned a new human type IV collagen gene (the $\alpha5$ chain) and localized it to this region of the X chromosome[121]. The new chain is closely similar to the $\alpha1$ chain, especially in the NC1 domain, and less similar to the $\alpha2$ chain. Northern blotting shows it to be expressed in human kidney, and an antibody raised to a peptide deduced from its sequence localized to the glomerular basement membrane. It is curious and fascinating that no evidence for this chain has been found at the protein level. Presumably it is present in even smaller quantities than the $\alpha3$ and $\alpha4$ chains. Assuming that mutations in this gene are responsible for at least some cases of Alport's syndrome, it is not clear how this fits in with observations on the absence of the Goodpasture antigen in the disorder. Perhaps the $\alpha5$ chain is part of a 'novel' network with the $\alpha3$ and $\alpha4$ chains, separate from but adjacent to or interwoven with the $\alpha1$ and $\alpha2$ chains[89,94,108]. An abnormality of one component might then lead to the failure of this whole network, affecting the antigenicity of the $\alpha3$ chain. It will be fascinating to find out.

IMMUNOPATHOGENESIS

Antibodies

Only a few autoantibodies can be shown to be directly involved in the induction or maintenance of the disorder with which they are associated, most emerging only as useful or interesting markers of the disease. Anti-Goodpasture antibodies seem to fall into the small group of directly pathogenic antibodies. It is not clear how much of the tissue damage in the disease is caused by the autoantibodies themselves, and how much is mediated by cellular mechanisms, but it is doubtful whether this is a pathophysiologically relevant question[122]. However, it may be relevant for treatment.

The classic experiments of Lerner, Glassock and Dixon in the 1960s[98] established the pathogenicity of antibodies in Goodpasture's disease. Six to twelve milligrams of ammonium sulphate-precipitated antibodies from patients with Goodpasture's disease were injected into uni-nephrectomized squirrel monkeys. Proteinuria developed with 24 hours, with linear binding of antibody to the GBM and infiltration of neutrophils into the glomeruli. A proliferative nephritis was seen, but no crescent formation. Binding within the kidney was not as extensive as that seen by indirect immunofluorescence, presumably because of differences in accessibility. Similarly, there was no immunoglobulin binding, or other abnormality, in the lungs[98].

The availability of immunoassays for anti-GBM antibodies has revealed an important relationship between the antibody level at presentation and the degree of renal damage[7,18]. As a large part of the renal damage in Goodpasture's disease is irreversible, this level is also related to the renal prognosis. The antibody level shows less relationship to the severity of pulmonary disease[18,45], probably because antibodies do not reach the alveolar basement membrane under normal circumstances.

Finally, in passive immunization experiments the injection of antibodies to GBM components can lead to tissue damage[123-125]. The antibodies that predominate in Goodpasture's disease (IgG1) are complement fixing, and would be expected to be pathogenic if they bound to GBM at an adequate rate. The only way this phenomenon can be observed in man is if it happens to occur by chance during pregnancy. One such case has been reported briefly[45]. In a pregnant and ultimately fatally affected woman, the fetus was apparently unaffected by the transplacental transfer of antibodies in the absence of maternal lymphocytes or other mediators that cannot cross the placenta.

The mechanisms by which anti-GBM antibodies cause renal damage have been investigated in animal models. Three major mechanisms of injury have been demonstrated in these model systems; all could coexist in patients:

(1) Neutrophil-mediated damage, with or without complement binding[126-128];
(2) Complement-mediated damage, via the membrane attack complex (MAC)[129];
(3) Macrophage-mediated damage[130,131].

Cell-mediated immunity

It has to be said that there is only indirect evidence for the involvement of T lymphocytes in the mediation of this, or indeed any other form of human nephritis, although what is known of the immunology of other autoimmune disorders suggests that T lymphocyte responses are crucial to the development of disease. Holdsworth and Tipping review cellular immunity in glomerulonephritis in Chapter 6, and demonstrate clearly that the appropriate effector cells are present. In most types of nephritis the antigens involved are unknown, and investigating the underlying T lymphocyte sensitization without that knowledge is an extremely difficult task. It is to be hoped that this will not be the case for very much longer in Goodpasture's disease.

Goodpasture's disease is strongly associated with HLA DR2 and DR4 alleles, which are carried by almost 90% of patients (Chapter 1). The most economical explanation for disease associations with specific HLA Class II molecules is that they reflect the ability of lymphocytes to recognize and attack (or induce attack against) specific antigens that are important in the pathogenesis of autoimmune disorders. This is exciting because it implies that interfering with such specific recognition might abrogate the disease process without the need for a high level of general immunosuppression. Such experiments are now becoming possible in animal models. In murine experimental allergic encephalomyelitis it has been shown that lymphocyte clones reacting against a relatively simple autoantigen, myelin basic protein, or even fragments of it, can transmit the disease in lymphocyte transfer experiments. Attempts to interfere with the disease by administering antibodies that recognize specific 'families' of T cell receptor have shown promising results[132,133].

Several studies confirm the presence of increased numbers of T lymphocytes (both CD4 and CD8) in the glomeruli of patients with crescentic nephritis (Chapter 6), whether of anti-GBM or vasculitic origin. They are accompanied by macrophages but relatively few B cells. The macrophage infiltration is correlated with the number of T cells[134], and in some model systems can be shown to follow the influx of T lymphocytes[135].

Animal models of anti-GBM disease provide further indirect evidence for the role of T cells and, although problems in interpreting these studies are mentioned below, their general messages about how diseases can be mediated are probably valid. In an avian model it has been possible to dissociate the production of antibodies and the presence of disease, so that transfer of B cells from chickens with anti-GBM disease to irradiated recipients leads to anti-GBM antibody production but no renal disease, while transfer of T cells leads to glomerular disease without evidence of anti-GBM antibody production[136]. Experiments demonstrating transfer of disease by antibodies in experimental[137,138] and human[98] nephritis might seem to contradict such experiments. However, the interpretation of such work is not straightforward, as discussed below, and of course the response of B cells to almost all antigens is T cell-dependent.

Animal models

There have been many attempts to model Goodpasture's disease in animals, and several models are now described where immunization with GBM components, or treatment to induce polyclonal B cell stimulation, generates autoantibody production with linear fixation to the GBM. These models are summarized by Druet in Chapter 2. However, in only Steblay nephritis is linear IgG deposition on the GBM shown to be associated with antibody formation to a molecule similar to the human Goodpasture antigen. Many others provide interesting information on possible mechanisms of immunologically mediated damage, but it is not clear whether they provide true insights into human disease.

Before the existence of anti-GBM antibodies had been demonstrated in man, Steblay showed that sheep immunized with a human GBM preparation in complete Freund's adjuvant developed a progressive and ultimately fatal glomerulonephritis characterized by linear deposition of complement-fixing IgG[139,140]. Antibodies eluted from affected sheep kidneys showed linear fixation to GBM and were capable of causing glomerular injury when injected into lambs. Like human anti-GBM antibodies, such antibodies also react with alveolar basement membranes *in vitro*, and with human alveolar and glomerular basement membranes. Immunization with human lung basement membrane, but not the basement membranes of other tissues, has a similar effect[99]. The pattern of antibody fixation in immunohistochemical studies, and on Western blotting of collagenase-solubilized sheep GBM, is identical to that of the antibodies of patients with Goodpasture's disease[141-143]. Two-dimensional SDS-PAGE results imply that the major antibody target is less cationic than that of Goodpasture's disease, but of similar molecular weight[87]. It is possibly the α4 chain, which seems to have identical tissue distribution to the antigenic (α3) chain[77,89]. There is no evidence so far of genetic restriction in this response, but unfortunately knowledge of sheep histocompatibility antigens is at an early stage in comparison to that of mice and men. This fact, and the difficulties of working with large animals, limits the progress that can be made with this otherwise fascinating model.

Other models of experimental autoimmune glomerulonephritis (EAG) have been developed in various species, and some of these have been mentioned in the sections above. Two models in rats show the development of nephritis in animals immunized with GBM prepared from other strains of the same species[144,145]. This response is strain specific, an interesting analogy with the genetic associations of human Goodpasture's disease, although it has not yet been linked with MHC molecules[145]. The target antigen remains unknown. Experiments demonstrating transfer of disease are particularly interesting. In the Brown Norway model, transfer of T cells from animals with EAG appears to produce a 'priming effect' in recipient animals, and the disease can be blocked by cyclosporin (Reynolds *et al.*, unpublished results). Mercuric chloride nephritis (a rather different model, see Chapter 2) in the same strain has also been shown to be transferable by T cells. In apparent contrast, in the model in WKY rats, in which disease is more severe, antibodies extracted from urine have recently been shown to be capable of inducing a similar renal disease in recipient animals[138]. This model therefore joins Goodpasture's disease and Steblay nephritis, in which antibodies have been shown to be capable of exerting pathogenic effects in transfer experiments[98,137]. Interpretation of these experiments is not straightforward though. As has been mentioned above, passive injection of antibodies to various basement membrane components can induce pathological damage, but that is not very surprising if they are bound at an adequate rate, and particularly if they are complement fixing. However, the effects of such injections may be modulated considerably by the presence of endotoxin or cytokines, or other cytokine-inducing substances, that may also be in the antibody preparation used (see below).

It is notable that pulmonary haemorrhage is not a feature of most animal models of anti-GBM disease induced by injection of heterologous antibody, although it may be an occasional or irregular feature[138,145]. In some it can be induced by exposing the lungs to high concentrations of oxygen[146,147], instillation of petrol[148], or 2 weeks of exposure to cigarette smoke (A. J. Rees, unpublished results), supporting the hypothesis that an extra (usually non-immune) insult is required to precipitate lung damage in anti-GBM disease, perhaps by disrupting the endothelial barrier.

Mediators

The severity of tissue damage is not just a product of B cell and T cell immunity but is dependent on a variety of other factors acting to modulate the degree of injury caused. Although the drawbacks of using animal models have been alluded to, work on the classic animal model of anti-GBM disease, nephrotoxic nephritis, has contributed substantially to understanding of the role played by various inflammatory mediators in glomerulonephritis; for example, the potential roles of neutrophils, complement, and macrophages in antibody-mediated injury as outlined above. One stimulus for pursuing these experiments has been the clinical observation in Goodpasture's disease that disease apparently under control may relapse in association with an intercurrent infection[29]. Such infections are usually remote from the lung or kidneys, and often related to vascular access devices. In rabbits, simultaneous infection potentiates the renal injury caused by injected nephrotoxic globulin (raised by immunizing sheep with rabbit GBM)[149]. Endotoxin, or some of the cytokines released in response to it (TNF and IL-1β), have been shown to have a similar effect in rats[150].

CONCLUDING REMARKS

This rare disease is in many ways the best understood of all the human nephritides, and yet there has been only little change in its treatment or outcome in the last 15 years. Nevertheless, we are on the threshold of another major advance in the understanding of the disorder, with the full sequence of the autoantigen likely to emerge soon. It may then be possible to begin to unravel T cell immunity in the disease, a position which has been achieved in very few autoimmune disorders. If that is so, it will be something of an irony that T cell immunity should be studied first in a disorder that has in the past been thought to be the archetypal antibody-mediated nephritis.

References

1. Goodpasture, E. W. (1919). The significance of certain pulmonary lesions in relation to the etiology of influenza. *Am. J. Med. Sci.*, **158**, 863–870
2. Stanton, M. C. and Tange, J. D. (1958). Goodpasture's syndrome (pulmonary haemorrhage associated with glomerulonephritis). *Aust. N. Z. J. Med.*, **7**, 132–144
3. Scheer, R. L. and Grossman, M. A. (1964). Immune aspects of the glomerulonephritis associated with pulmonary hemorrhage. *Ann. Intern. Med.*, **60**, 1009–1021
4. Wieslander, J., Bygren, P. and Heinegard, D. (1983). Antiglomerular basement membrane antibody: antibody specificity in different forms of glomerulonephritis. *Kidney Int.*, **23**, 855–861
5. Fillit, H., Damle, S. P., Gregory, J. D., Volin, C., Poon-King, T. and Zabriskie, J. (1985). Sera from patients with poststreptococcal glomerulonephritis contain antibodies to glomerular heparan sulfate proteoglycan. *J. Exp. Med.*, **161**, 277–289
6. Bygren, P., Cederholm, B., Heinegard, D. and Wieslander, J. (1989). Non-Goodpasture anti-GBM antibodies in patients with glomerulonephritis. *Nephrol. Dial. Transplant.*, **4**, 254–261
7. Savage, C. O. S., Pusey, C. D., Bowman, C., Rees, A. J. and Lockwood, C. M. (1986). Antiglomerular basement membrane antibody mediated disease in the British Isles 1980–1984. *Br. Med. J. (Clin. Res.)*, **292**, 301–304
8. Turner, N. and Rees, A. J. (1991). Anti-Glomerular basement membrane disease. In Cameron, S. J., Davison, A. M., Grunfeld, J.-P., Kerr, D. N. S. and Ritz, E. (eds.), *Oxford*

Textbook of Nephrology. (Oxford: Oxford University Press)
9. Gossain, V. V., Gerstein, A. R. and Janes, A. W. (1972). Goodpasture's syndrome: a familial occurrence. *Am. Rev. Respir. Dis.,* **105**, 621–624.
10. d'Apice, A. J., Kincaid Smith, P., Becker, G. H., Loughhead, M. G., Freeman, J. W. and Sands, J. M. (1978). Goodpasture's syndrome in identical twins. *Ann. Intern. Med.,* **88**, 61–62
11. Simonsen, H., Brun, C., Thomsen, O. F., Larsen, S. and Ladefoged, J. (1982). Goodpasture's syndrome in twins. *Acta Med. Scand.,* **212**, 425–428
12. Almkuist, R. D., Buckalew, V. M. Jr., Hirszel, P., Maher, J. F., James, P. M. and Wilson, C. B. (1981). Recurrence of anti-glomerular basement membrane antibody mediated glomerulonephritis in an isograft. *Clin. Immunol. Immunopathol.,* **18**, 54–60
13. Rees, A. J., Peters, D. K., Compston, D. A. and Batchelor, J. R. (1978). Strong association between HLA-DRW2 and antibody-mediated Goodpasture's syndrome. *Lancet,* **1**, 966–968
14. Rees, A. J., Peters, D. K., Amos, N., Welsh, K. I. and Batchelor, J. R. (1984). The influence of HLA-linked genes on the severity of anti-GBM antibody-mediated nephritis. *Kidney Int.,* **26**, 445–450
15. Rees, A. J., Demaine, A. G. and Welsh, K. I. (1984). Association of immunoglobulin Gm allotypes with antiglomerular basement membrane antibodies and their titer. *Hum. Immunol.,* **10**, 213–220
16. Heale, W. F., Matthiesson, A. M. and Niall, J. F. (1969). Lung haemorrhage and nephritis (Goodpasture's syndrome). *Med. J. Aust.,* **2**, 355–357
17. Donaghy, M. and Rees, A. J. (1983). Cigarette smoking and lung haemorrhage in glomerulonephritis caused by autoantibodies to glomerular basement membrane. *Lancet,* **2**, 1390–1393
18. Simpson, I. J., Doak, P. B., Williams, L. C. *et al.* (1982). Plasma exchange in Goodpasture's syndrome. *Am. J. Nephrol.,* **2**, 301–311
19. Perez, G. O., Bjornsson, S., Ross, A. H., Aamato, J. and Rothfield, N. A mini-epidemic of Goodpasture's syndrome clinical and immunological studies. *Nephron,* **13**, 161–173
20. Williams, P. S., Davenport, A., McDicken, I., Ashby, D. and Bone, J. M. (1988). Increased incidence of anti-glomerular basement membrane antibody (anti-GBM) nephritis in the Mersey region, September 1984–October 1985. *Q. J. Med.,* **68**, 727–733
21. Wilson, C. B., Dixon, F. J., Evans, A. S. and Glassock, R. J. (1973). Antiviral antibody responses in patients with renal diseases. *Clin. Immunol. Immunopathol.,* **2**, 121–132
22. Beirne, G. J. (1972). Goodpasture's syndrome and exposure to solvents. *J. Am. Med. Assoc.,* **222**, 1555
23. Kleinknecht, D., Morel Maroger, L., Callard, P., Adhemar, J. P. and Mahieu, P. (1980). Antiglomerular basement membrane nephritis after solvent exposure. *Arch. Intern. Med.,* **140**, 230–232
24. Daniell, W. E., Couser, W. G. and Rosenstock, L. (1988). Occupational solvent exposure and glomerulonephritis. A case report and review of the literature. *J. Am. Med. Assoc.,* **259**, 2280–2283
25. Bernis, P., Hamels, J., Quoidbach, A., Mahieu, P. and Bouvy, P. (1985). Remission of Goodpasture's syndrome after withdrawal of an unusual toxin. *Clin. Nephrol.,* **23**, 312–317
26. Briggs, W. A., Johnson, J. P., Teichman, S., Yeager, H. C. and Wilson, C. B. (1979). Antiglomerular basement membrane antibody-mediated glomerulonephritis and Goodpasture's syndrome. *Medicine (Baltimore),* **58**, 348–361
27. Rees, A. J., Lockwood, C. M. and Peters, D. K. (1979). Nephritis due to antibodies to GBM. In Kincaid-Smith, P., d'Apice, A. J. F., Atkins, R. C. (eds.). *Progress in Glomerulonephritis,* p. 347. (New York: Wiley)
28. Bailey, R. R., Simpson, I. J., Lynn, K. L., Neale, T. J., Doak, P. B. and McGiven, A. R. (1981). Goodpasture's syndrome with normal renal function. *Clin. Nephrol.,* **15**, 211–215
29. Rees, A. J., Lockwood, C. M. and Peters, D. K. (1977). Enhanced allergic tissue injury in Goodpasture's syndrome by intercurrent bacterial infection. *Br. Med. J.,* **2**, 723–726
30. Johnson, J. P., Whitman, W., Briggs, W. A. and Wilson, C. B. (1978). Plasmapheresis and immunosuppressive agents in antibasement membrane antibody-induced Goodpasture's syndrome. *Am. J. Med.,* **64**, 354–359
31. Haworth, S. J., Savage, C. O. S., Carr, D., Hughes, J. M. B. and Rees, A. J. (1985). Pulmonary haemorrhage complicating Wegener's granulomatosis and microscopic polyarteritis. *Br. Med. J.,* **290**, 1775–1778

32. Relman, A. S., Dvorak, H. F. and Colvin, R. B. (1971). Case records of the Massachusetts General Hospital. Weekly clinicopathological exercises. Case 46-1971. *N. Engl. J. Med.*, **285**, 1187–1196
33. Wahls, T. L., Bonsib, S. M. and Schuster, V. L. (1987). Coexistent Wegener's granulomatosis and anti-glomerular basement membrane disease. *Hum. Pathol.*, **18**, 202–205
34. Kalderon, A. E., Bogaars, H. A. and Diamond, I. (1973). Ultrastructural alterations of the follicular basement membrane in Hashimoto's thyroiditis. *Am. J. Med.*, **55**, 485–491
35. Blake, D. R., Rashid, H., McHugh, M. and Morley, A. R. (1980). A possible association of partial lipodystrophy with anti-GBM nephritis (Goodpasture's syndrome). *Postgrad. Med. J.*, **56**, 137–139
36. Klassen, J., Elwood, C., Grossberg, A. L. *et al.* (1974). Evolution of membranous nephropathy into anti-glomerular-basement-membrane glomerulonephritis. *N. Engl. J. Med.*, **290**, 1340–1344
37. Moorthy, A. V., Zimmerman, S. W., Burkholder, P. M. and Harrington, A. R. (1976). Association of crescentic glomerulonephritis with membranous glomerulonephropathy: a report of three cases. *Clin. Nephrol.*, **6**, 319–325
38. Beirne, G. J., Wagnild, J. P., Zimmerman, S. W., Macken, P. D. and Burkholder, P. M. (1977). Idiopathic crescentic glomerulonephritis. *Medicine (Baltimore)*, **56**, 349–381
39. Richman, A. V., Rifkin, S. I. and McAllister, C. J. (1981). Rapidly progressive glomerulonephritis. Combined antiglomerular basement membrane antibody and immune complex pathogenesis. *Hum. Pathol.*, **12**, 597–604
40. Kurki, P., Helve, T., von Bonsdorff, M. *et al.* (1984). Transformation of membranous glomerulonephritis into crescentic glomerulonephritis with glomerular basement membrane antibodies. Serial determinations of anti-GBM before the transformation. *Nephron*, **38**, 134–137
41. Hume, D. M., Sterling, W. A., Weymouth, R. J., Siebel, H. R., Madge, G. E. and Lee, H. M. (1970). Glomerulonephritis in human renal homotransplants. *Transplant. Proc.*, **2**, 361–412
42. Guerin, V., Rabin, C., Noel, L. H. *et al.* (1990). Anti-glomerular basement membrane disease after lithotripsy. *Lancet*, **1**, 856–857
43. Weber, M., Pullig, O. and Boesken, W. H. (1990). Anti-glomerular basement membrane disease after renal obstruction. *Lancet*, **2**, 512–513
44. Ma, K. W., Golbus, S. M., Kaufman, R., Staley, N., Londer, H. and Brown, D. C. (1978). Glomerulonephritis with Hodgkin's disease and herpes zoster. *Arch. Pathol. Lab. Med.*, **102**, 527–529
45. Wilson, C. B. and Dixon, F. J. (1981). The renal response to immunological injury. In Brenner, B. M. and Rector, F. C. (eds.) *The Kidney*, p. 1237. (Philadelphia, W. B. Saunders)
46. Curtis, J. J., Bhathena, D., Leach, R. P., Galla, J. H., Lucas, B. A. and Luke, R. G. (1976). Goodpasture's syndrome in a patient with the Nail-Patella syndrome. *Am. J. Med.*, **61**, 401–406
47. McCoy, R. C., Johnson, H. K., Stone, W. J. and Wilson, C. B. (1982). Absence of nephritogenic GBM antigen(s) in some patients with hereditary nephritis. *Kidney Int.*, **21**, 642–652
48. Milliner, D. S., Pierides, A. M. and Holley, K. E. (1982). Renal transplantation in Alport's syndrome: anti-glomerular basement membrane glomerulonephritis in the allograft. *Mayo Clin. Proc.*, **57**, 35–43
49. Querin, S., Noel, L. H., Grunfeld, J. P., Droz, D., Mahieu, P. and Berger, J. (1986). Linear glomerular IgG fixation in renal allografts: incidence and significance in Alport's syndrome. *Clin. Nephrol.*, **25**, 134–140
50. Shah, B., First, M. R., Mendoza, N. C., Clyne, D. H., Alexander, J. W. and Weiss, M. A. (1988). Alport's syndrome: risk of glomerulonephritis induced by anti-glomerular-basement-membrane antibody after renal transplantation. *Nephron*, **50**, 34–38
51. Fleming, S. J., Savage, C. O. S., McWilliam, L. J. *et al.* (1988). Anti-glomerular basement membrane antibody-mediated nephritis complicating transplantation in a patient with Alport's syndrome. *Transplantation*, **46**, 857–859
52. Heuvel, L. P. W. J., Schroder, C. H., Savage, C. S. *et al.* (1989). The development of anti-glomerular basement membrane nephritis in two children with Alport's syndrome after renal transplantation: characterisation of the antibody target. *Pediatr. Nephrol.*, **3**, 406–413
53. Rassoul, Z., Al-Khader, A. A., Al-Sulaiman, M., Dhar, J. M. and Coode, P. (1990). Recurrent allograft antiglomerular basement membrane glomerulonephritis in a patient with Alport's syndrome. *Am. J. Nephrol.*, **10**, 73–76

54. Jayne, D. R. W., Marshall, P. D., Jones, S. J. and Lockwood, C. M. (1990). Autoantibodies to GBM and neutrophil cytoplasm in rapidly progressive glomerulonephritis. *Kidney Int.*, **37**, 965–970

55. O'Donoghue, D. J., Short, C. D., Brenchley, P. E. C., Lawler, W. and Ballardie, F. W. (1989). Sequential development of systemic vasculitis with anti-neutrophil cytoplasmic antibodies complicating anti-glomerular basement membrane disease. *Clin. Nephrol.*, **32**, 251–255

56. Sternleib, I., Bennett, B. and Scheinberg, I. H. (1975). D-Penicillamine induced Goodpasture's syndrome in Wilson's disease. *Ann. Intern. Med.*, **82**, 673–676

57. Banfi, G., Imbasciati, E., Guerra, L., Mihatsch, M. J. and Ponticelli, C. (1983). Extracapillary glomerulonephritis with necrotizing vasculitis in D-Penicillamine-treated rheumatoid arthritis. *Nephron*, **33**, 56–60

58. Devogelaer, J. P., Pirson, Y., Vandenbroucke, J. M., Cosyns, J. P., Brichard, S. and Nagant de Deuxchaisnes, C. (1987). D-Penicillamine induced crescentic glomerulonephritis: report and review of the literature. *J. Rheumatol.*, **14**, 1036–1041

59. Wilson, C. B. and Dixon, F. J. (1973). Anti-glomerular basement membrane antibody-induced glomerulonephritis. *Kidney Int.*, **3**, 74–89

60. Walker, R. G., Scheinkestel, C., Becker, G. J., Owen, J. E., Dowling, J. P. and Kincaid Smith, P. (1985). Clinical and morphological aspects of the management of crescentic anti-glomerular basement membrane antibody (anti-GBM) nephritis/Goodpasture's syndrome. *Q. J. Med.*, **54**, 75–89

61. Rees, A. J. and Lockwood, C. M. (1988). Antiglomerular basement membrane antibody-mediated nephritis. In Schrier, R. W. and Gottschalk, C. W. (eds.) *Diseases of the Kidney*, p. 2091. (Boston: Little, Brown)

62. Heptinstall, R. H. (1983). Schonlein-Henoch syndrome; lung haemorrhage and glomerulonephritis. In Heptinstall, R. H. (ed.) *Pathology of the Kidney*, p. 761. (Boston: Little, Brown)

63. Wilson, C. B. and Dixon, F. J. (1974). Diagnosis of immunopathologic renal disease. *Kidney Int.*, **5**, 389–401

64. Agodoa, L. C., Striker, G. E., George, C. R., Glassock, R. and Quadracci, L. J. (1976). The appearance of nonlinear deposits of immunoglobulins in Goodpasture's syndrome. *Am. J. Med.*, **61**, 407–413

65. Bruijn, J. A., Hoedemaeker, P. J. and Fleuren, G. J. (1990). Pathogenesis of anti-basement membrane glomerulopathy and immune-complex glomerulonephritis: dichotomy dissolved. *Lab. Invest.*, **61**, 480–488

66. Wieslander, J., Bygren, P. G. and Heinegard, D. (1981). Anti-basement membrane antibody: immunoenzymatic assay and specificity of antibodies. *Scand. J. Clin. Lab. Invest.*, **41**, 763–772

67. Bowman, C. and Lockwood, C. M. (1985). Clinical application of a radio-immunoassay for auto-antibodies to glomerular basement membrane. *J. Clin. Lab. Immunol.*, **17**, 197–202

68. Wheeler, J., Simpson, J. and Morley, A. R. (1988). Routine and rapid enzyme linked immunosorbent assays for circulating anti-glomerular basement membrane antibodies. *J. Clin. Pathol.*, **41**, 163–170

69. Saxena, R., Isaksson, B., Bygren, P. and Wieslander, J. (1989). A rapid assay for circulating anti-glomerular basement membrane antibodies in Goodpasture syndrome. *J. Immunol. Meth.*, **118**, 73–78

70. Turner, N., Mason, P. J., Rees, A. J. and Pusey, C. D. (1991). Purification of the Goodpasture antigen from sheep kidney discloses the presence of two new type IV collagen chains. *Nephrol. Dial. Transplant.* (Abstr.) (In press)

71. Bowman, C., Ambrus, K. and Lockwood, C. M. (1987). Restriction of human IgG subclass expression in the population of auto-antibodies to glomerular basement membrane. *Clin. Exp. Immunol.*, **69**, 341–349

72. Weber, M., Lohse, A. W., Manns, M., Meyer zum Buschenfelde, K. H. and Kohler, H. (1988). IgG subclass distribution of autoantibodies to glomerular basement membrane in Goodpasture's syndrome compared to other autoantibodies. *Nephron*, **49**, 54–57

73. Noel, L. H., Aucouturier, P., Monteiro, R. C., Preud Homme, J. L. and Lesavre, P. (1988). Glomerular and serum immunoglobulin G subclasses in membranous nephropathy and anti-glomerular basement membrane nephritis. *Clin. Immunol. Immunopathol.*, **46**, 186–194

74. Border, W. A., Baehler, R. W., Bhathena, D. and Glassock, R. J. (1979). IgA antibasement membrane nephritis with pulmonary haemorrhage. *Ann. Intern. Med.*, **91**, 21–25

75. McPhaul, J. J. Jr and Dixon, F. J. (1970). Characterization of human anti-glomerular basement membrane antibodies eluted from glomerulonephritic kidneys. *J. Clin. Invest.*, **49**, 308–317

76. McIntosh, R. M., Copack, P., Chernack, W. B., Griswold, W. R., Weil, R., III (1975). The human choroid plexus and autoimmune nephritis. *Arch. Pathol.*, **99**, 48–50

77. Cashman, S. J., Pusey, C. D. and Evans, D. J. (1988). Extraglomerular distribution of immunoreactive Goodpasture antigen. *J. Pathol.*, **155**, 61–70

78. Jampol, L. M., Lahov, M., Albert, D. M. and Craft, J. (1975). Ocular clinical findings and basement membrane changes in Goodpasture's syndrome. *Am. J. Ophthalmol.*, **79**, 452–463

79. Lockwood, C. M., Rees, A. J., Pearson, T. A., Evans, D. J. and Peters, D. K. (1976). Immunosuppression and plasma-exchange in the treatment of Goodpasture's syndrome. *Lancet*, **1**, 711–715

80. Benoit, F. L., Rulon, D. B., Theil, G. B., Doolan, P. D. and Watten, R. H. (1964). Goodpasture's syndrome. A clinicopathological entity. *Am. J. Med.*, **37**, 424–444

81. Proskey, A. J., Weatherbee, L., Easterling, R. E., Greene, J. A. Jr and Weller, J. M. (1970). Goodpasture's syndrome. A report of five cases and review of the literature. *Am. J. Med.*, **48**, 162–173

82. Johnson, J. P., Moore, J. Jr, Austin, H. A., Balow, J. E., Antonovych, T. T. and Wilson, C. B. (1985). Therapy of anti-glomerular basement membrane antibody disease: analysis of prognostic significance of clinical, pathologic and treatment factors. *Medicine (Baltimore)*, **64**, 219–227

83. Bygren, P., Freiburghaus, C., Lindholm, T., Simonsen, O., Thysell, H. and Wieslander, J. (1985). Goodpasture's syndrome treated with staphylococcal protein A immunoadsorption (letter). *Lancet*, **2**, 1295–1296

84. Flores, J. C., Taube, D., Savage, C. O. S., Cameron, J. S., Lockwood, C. M. and Ogg, C. S. (1986). Clinical and immunological evolution of oligoanuric anti-GBM nephritis treated by haemodialysis. *Lancet*, **1**, 5–8

85. Dahlberg, P. J., Kurtz, S. B., Donadio, J. V. *et al.* (1978). Recurrent Goodpasture's syndrome. *Mayo Clin. Proc.*, **53**, 533–537

86. Foidart, J. B., Pirard, Y., Foidart, J. M., Dubois, C. U. and Mahieu, P. (1980). Anti-type IV procollagen and anti-laminin antibodies in Goodpasture syndrome. *Kidney Int.*, **18**, 126

87. Kleppel, M. M., Michael, A. F. and Fish, A. J. (1986). Antibody specificity of human glomerular basement membrane type IV collagen NC1 subunits. Species variation in subunit composition. *J. Biol. Chem.*, **261**, 16547–16552

88. Wieslander, J., Kataja, M. and Hudson, B. G. (1987). Characterization of the human Goodpasture antigen. *Clin. Exp. Immunol.*, **69**, 332–340

89. Kleppel, M. M., Santi, P. A., Cameron, J. D., Wieslander, J. and Michael, A. F. (1989). Human tissue distribution of novel basement membrane collagen. *Am. J. Pathol.*, **134**, 813–825

90 Pusey, C. D., Dash, A., Kershaw, M. J. *et al.* (1987). A single autoantigen in Goodpasture's syndrome identified by a monoclonal antibody to human glomerular basement membrane. *Lab. Invest.*, **56**, 23–31

91. Abrahamson, D. R. (1987). Structure and development of the glomerular capillary wall and basement membrane. *Am. J. Physiol.*, **253**, F783–F794

92. Hudson, B. G., Wieslander, J., Wisdom, B. J. and Noelken, M. E. (1989). Goodpasture syndrome: molecular architecture and function of basement membrane antigen. *Lab. Invest.*, **61**, 256–269

93. Sisson, S., Dysart, N. K. Jr, Fish, A. J. and Vernier, R. L. (1982). Localization of the Goodpasture antigen by immunoelectron microscopy. *Clin. Immunol. Immunopathol.*, **23**, 414–429

94. Mounier, F., Gros, F., Wieslander, J. *et al.* (1988). Glomerular distribution of M1 and M2 subunits of the globular domain of the basement membrane collagen. An immunohistochemical study. In Gubler, M. C. and Sternberg, M. (eds.) *Progress in Basement Membrane Research. Renal and Related Aspects in Health and Disease*, p. 53. (Paris: John Libbey Eurotext Ltd.)

95. Butkowski, R. J., Wieslander, J., Kleppel, M., Michael, A. F. and Fish, A. J. (1989). Basement membrane collagen in the kidney: Regional localization of novel chains related to collagen IV. *Kidney Int.*, **35**, 1195–1202

96. Martinez-Hernandez, A. and Amenta, P. S. (1983). The basement membrane in pathology. *Lab. Invest.*, **48**, 656–677

97. Timpl, R., Paulsson, M., Dziadek, M. and Fujiwara, S. (1987). Basement membranes. *Meth. Enzymol.*, **145**, 363–391

98. Lerner, R. A., Glassock, R. J. and Dixon, F. J. (1967). The role of anti-glomerular basement membrane antibody in the pathogenesis of human glomerulonephritis. *J. Exp. Med.*, **126**, 989–1004

99. Steblay, R. W. and Rudofsky, U. H. (1983). Experimental autoimmune antiglomerular basement membrane antibody-induced glomerulonephritis. I. The effects of injecting sheep with human, homologous or autologous lung basement membranes and complete Freund's adjuvant. *Clin. Immunol. Immunopathol.*, **27**, 65–80

100. Weber, S., Engel, J., Wiedemann, H., Glanville, R. W. and Timpl, R. (1984). Subunit structure and assembly of the globular domain of basement-membrane collagen type IV. *Eur. J. Biochem.*, **139**, 401–410

101. Wieslander, J., Langeveld, J., Butkowski, R., Jodlowski, M., Noelken, M. and Hudson, B. G. (1985). Physical and immunochemical properties of the globular domain of type IV collagen. Cryptic properties of the Goodpasture antigen. *J. Biol. Chem.*, **260**, 8564–8570

102. Salant, D. J. (1987). Immunopathogenesis of crescentic glomerulonephritis and lung purpura (clinical conference). *Kidney Int.*, **32**, 408–425

103. Muthukumaran, G., Blumberg, B. and Kurkinen, M. (1989). The complete primary structure for the α_1-chain of mouse collagen IV. *J. Biol. Chem.*, **264**, 6310–6317

104. Hostikka, S. L. and Tryggvason, K. (1988). The complete primary structrure of the $\alpha 2$ chain of human type IV collagen and comparison with the $\alpha 1$(IV) chain. *J. Biol. Chem.*, **263**, 19488–19493

105. Soininen, R., Huotari, M., Hostikka, S. L., Prockop, D. J. and Tryggvason, K. (1988). The structural genes for $\alpha 1$ and $\alpha 2$ chains of human type IV collagen are divergently encoded on opposite DNA strands and have an overlapping promoter region. *J. Biol. Chem.*, **263**, 17217–17220

106. Poschl, E., Pollner, R. and Kuhn, K. (1988). The genes for the $\alpha 1$(IV) and $\alpha 2$(IV) chains of human basement membrane collagen type IV are arranged head-to-head and separated by a bidirectional promoter of unique structure. *EMBO J.*, **7**, 2687–2695

107. Butkowski, R. J., Langeveld, J. P. M., Wieslander, J., Hamilton, J. and Hudson, B. G. (1987). Localization of the Goodpasture epitope to a novel chain of basement membrane collagen. *J. Biol. Chem.*, **262**, 7874–7877

108. Saus, J., Wieslander, J., Langeveld, J. P. M., Quinones, S. and Hudson, B. G. (1988). Identification of the Goodpasture antigen as the α 3(IV) chain of collagen IV. *J. Biol. Chem.*, **263**, 13374–13380

109. Butkowski, R. J., Guo-Qui, S., Wieslander, J., Michael, A. F. and Fish, A. J. (1990). Characterization of type IV collagen NC1 monomers and Goodpasture antigen in human renal basement membranes. *J. Lab. Clin. Med.*, **115**, 365–373

110. Langeveld, J. P. M., Wieslander, J., Timoneda, J. *et al.* (1988). Structural hereogeneity of the noncollagenous domain of basement membrane collagen. *J. Biol. Chem.*, **263**, 10481–10488

111. Yoshioka, K., Kleppel, M. and Fish, A. J. (1985). Analysis of nephritogenic antigens in human glomerular basement membrane by two-dimensional gel electrophoresis. *J. Immunol.*, **134**, 3831–3837

112. Siebold, B., Deutzmann, R. and Kuhn, K. (1988). The arrangement of intra- and intermolecular disulfide bonds in the carboxyterminal, non-collagenous aggregation and cross-linking domain of basement-membrane type IV collagen. *Eur. J. Biochem.*, **176**, 617–624

113. Wieslander, J. and Heinegard, D. (1985). The involvement of type IV collagen in Goodpasture's syndrome. *Ann. N.Y. Acad. Sci.*, **460**, 363–374

114. Weber, M., Meyer zum Buschenfelde, K. H. and Kohler, H. (1988). Immunological properties of the human Goodpasture target antigen. *Clin. Exp. Immunol.*, **74**, 289–294

115. Yoshioka, K., Iseki, T., Okada, M., Morimoto, Y., Eryu, N. and Maki, S. (1988). Identification of Goodpasture antigens in human alveolar basement membrane. *Clin. Exp. Immunol.*, **74**, 419–424

116. Atkin, C. L., Gregory, M. C. and Border, W. A. (1988). Alport syndrome. In Schrier, R. W. and Gottschalk, C. W. (eds.). *Diseases of the Kidney*. (Boston: Little, Brown)

117. Savage, C. O. S., Pusey, C. D., Kershaw, M. J. *et al.* (1986). The Goodpasture antigen in Alport's syndrome: studies with a monoclonal antibody. *Kidney Int.*, **30**, 107–112

118. Feingold, F., Bois, E., Chompret, A., Broyer, M., Gubler, M.-C. and Grunfeld, J. P. (1985).

Genetic heterogeneity of Alport syndrome. *Kidney Int.*, **27**, 672–677

119. Flinter, F. A., Cameron, J. S., Chantler, C., Houston, I. and Bobrow, M. (1988). Genetics of classic Alport's syndrome. *Lancet*, **2**, 1005–1007

120. Atkin, C. L., Hasstedt, S. J., Menlove, L. *et al.* (1988). Mapping of Alport syndrome to the long arm of the X chromosome. *Am. J. Hum. Genet.*, **42**, 249–255

121. Hostikka, S. L., Eddy, R. L., Byers, M. G., Hoyhtya, M., Shows, T. B. and Tryggvason, K. (1990). Identification of a distinct type IV collagen alpha chain with restricted kidney distribution and assignment of its gene to the locus of X chromosome-linked Alport syndrome. *Proc. Natl. Acad. Sci. USA*, **87**, 1606–1610

122. Oliveira, D. B. G. and Peters, D. K. (1989). Autoimmunity and the kidney. *Kidney Int.*, **35**, 923–928

123. Yaar, M., Foidart, J. M., Brown, K. S., Rennard, S. I., Martin, G. R. and Liotta, L. (1982). The Goodpasture-like syndrome in mice induced by intravenous injections of anti-type IV collagen and anti-laminin antibody. *Am. J. Pathol.*, **107**, 79–91

124. Feintzeig, I. D., Abrahamson, D. R., Cybulsky, A. V., Dittmer, J. E. and Salant, D. J. (1986). Nephritogenic potential of sheep antibodies against glomerular basement membrane laminin in the rat. *Lab. Invest.*, **54**, 531–542

125. Wick, G., von der Mark, H., Dietrich, H. and Timpl, R. (1986). Globular domain of basement membrane collagen induces autoimmune pulmonary lesions in mice resembling human Goodpasture disease. *Lab. Invest.*, **55**, 308–317

126. Cochrane, C. G., Unanue, E. R. and Dixon, F. J. (1965). A role of polymorphonuclear leucocytes and complement in nephrotoxic nephritis. *J. Exp. Med.*, **122**, 99

127. Thomson, N. M., Naish, P. F., Simpson, I. J. and Peters, D. K. (1976). The role of C3 in the autologous phase of nephrotoxic nephritis. *Clin. Exp. Immunol.*, **24**, 464–473

128. Pilia, P. A., Boackle, R. J., Swain, R. P. and Ainsworth, S. K. (1983). Complement-independent nephrotoxic serum nephritis in Munich Wistar rats. Immunologic and ultrastructural studies. *Lab. Invest.*, **48**, 585–597

129. Groggel, G. C., Salant, D. J., Darby, C., Rennke, H. G. and Couser, W. G. (1985). Role of terminal complement pathway in the heterologous phase of antiglomerular basement membrane nephritis. *Kidney Int.*, **27**, 643–651

130. Schreiner, G. F., Cotran, R. S., Pando, V. and Unanue, E. R. (1978). A mononuclear cell component in experimental immunological glomerulonephritis. *J. Exp. Med.*, **147**, 369

131. Holdsworth, S. R., Neale, T. J. and Wilson, C. B. (1981). Abrogation of macrophage-dependent injury in experimental glomerulonephritis in the rabbit. Use of an antimacrophage serum. *J. Clin. Invest.*, **68**, 686–698

132. Wraith, D. C., McDevitt, H. O., Steinman, L. and Acha-Orbea, H. (1989). T Cell recognition as the target for immune intervention in autoimmune disease. *Cell*, **57**, 709–714

133. Janeway, C. A. (1989). Immunotherapy by peptides? *Nature*, **341**, 482–483

134. Nolasco, F. E. B., Cameron, J. S., Hartley, B., Coelho, A., Hildreth, G. and Reuben, R. (1987). Intraglomerular T cells and monocytes in nephritis: Study with monoclonal antibodies. *Kidney Int.*, **31**, 1160–1166

135. Tipping, P. G., Neale, T. J. and Holdsworth, S. R. (1985). T lymphocyte participation in antibody-induced experimental glomerulonephritis. *Kidney Int.*, **27**, 530–537.

136. Bolton, W. K., Chandra, M., Tyson, T. M., Kirkpatrick, P. R., Sadovnic, M. J. and Sturgill, B. C. (1988). Transfer of experimental glomerulonephritis in chickens by mononuclear cells. *Kidney Int.*, **34**, 598–610

137. Lerner, R. A. and Dixon, F. J. (1966). Transfer of ovine experimental allergic glomerulonephritis (EAG) with serum. *J. Exp. Med.*, **124**, 431

138. Sado, Y., Naito, I. and Okigaki, T. (1989). Transfer of anti-glomerular basement membrane antibody-induced glomerulonephritis in inbred rats with isologous antibodies from the urine of nephritic rats. *J. Pathol.*, **158**, 325–332

139. Steblay, R. W. (1962). Glomerulonephritis induced in sheep by injections of heterologous glomerular basement membrane and Freund's complete adjuvant. *J. Exp. Med.*, **116**, 253–271

140. Steblay, R. W. and Rudofsky, U. H. (1983). Experimental autoimmune glomerulonephritis induced by anti-glomerular basement membrane antibody. II. Effects of injecting heterologous, homologous, or autologous glomerular basement membranes and complete Freund's adjuvant into sheep. *Am. J. Pathol.*, **113**, 125–133

141. Jeraj, K., Michael, A. F. and Fish, A. J. (1982). Immunologic similarities between

Goodpasture's and Steblay's antibodies. *Clin. Immunol. Immunopathol.*, **23**, 408–413

142. Bygren, P., Wieslander, J. and Heinegard, D. (1987). Glomerulonephritis induced in sheep by immunization with human glomerular basement membrane. *Kidney Int.*, **31**, 25–31

143. Evans, D. J., Dash, A. and Lockwood, M. (1984). Role of Goodpasture antigen in Steblay nephritis. *J. Pathol.*, **42**, A17

144. Sado, Y. and Naito, I. (1987). Experimental autoimmune glomerulonephritis in rats by soluble isologous or homologous antigens from glomerular and tubular basement membranes. *Br. J. Exp. Pathol.*, **68**, 695–704

145. Pusey, C. D., Holland, M. J., Cashman, S. J. *et al.* (1991). Autoimmunity to glomerular basement membrane induced by homologous and isologous antigens in Brown Norway rats. *Nephrol. Dial. Transplant.*, (in press)

146. Jennings, L., Roholt, O. A., Pressman, D., Blau, M., Andres, G. A. and Brentjens, J. R. (1981). Experimental anti-alveolar basement membrane antibody-mediated pneumonitis. I. The role of increased permeability of the alveolar capillary wall induced by oxygen. *J. Immunol.*, **127**, 129–134

147. Downie, G. H., Roholt, O. A,., Jennings, L., Blau, M., Brentjens, J. R. and Andres, G. A. (1982). Experimental anti-alveolar basement membrane antibody-mediated pneumonitis. II. Role of endothelial damage and repair, induction of autologous phase, and kinetics of antibody deposition in Lewis rats. *J. Immunol.*, **129**, 2647–2652

148. Yamamoto, T. and Wilson, C. B. (1987). Binding of anti-basement membrane antibody to alveolar basement membrane after intratracheal gasoline instillation in rabbits. *Am. J. Pathol.*, **126**, 497–505

149. Van Zyl Smit, R., Rees, A. J. and Peters, D. K. (1983). Factors affecting severity of injury during nephrotoxic nephritis in rabbits. *Clin. Exp. Immunol.*, **54**, 366–372

150. Tomosugi, N. I., Cashman, S. J., Hay, H. *et al.* (1989). Modulation of antibody-mediated glomerular injury in vivo by bacterial lipopolysaccharide, tumor necrosis factor, and IL-1. *J. Immunol.*, **142**, 3083–3090.

12
Autoimmunity in Systemic Vasculitis

D. R. W. JAYNE and C. M. LOCKWOOD

DEFINITION

The systemic vasculitides are a group of diseases having in common chronic inflammation and necrosis of blood vessels. They differ one from another in the size and site of vessels involved. Ideally classification should be according to mechanisms of pathogenesis, but until recently so little information was available that classification has been according to morphological criteria (Table 1).

The renal lesion of the more common small-vessel vasculitides—Wegener's granulomatosis and microscopic polyarteritis—is most often a focal necrotizing crescentic glomerulonephritis, but focal segmental proliferative or membrano-proliferative glomerulonephritis has been reported. Extraglomerular arteritis may be seen and is more characteristic of polyarteritis nodosa.

BACKGROUND

Until recently, there has been little direct evidence for autoimmune processes in systemic vasculitis. Circumstantial pointers have been the therapeutic responses to cortisone (1950)[1], cyclophosphamide (1979)[2] and plasma exchange (1976)[3], the presence of immune reactants such as circulating immune complexes, and immunoglobulin deposits and T-cell infiltrates in affected tissues[4-6].

Therefore, the discovery of autoantibodies to neutrophil cytoplasmic antigens (ANCA), and their restriction to diseases within the spectrum of systemic vasculitis, has been particularly important. ANCA were first reported in rapidly progressive glomerulonephritis by Davies et al.[7], and were subsequently found in Wegener's granulomatosis[8], microscopic polyarteritis[9] and other vasculitic syndromes[10-14].

Over the last five years, interest has focused on this autoantibody system

Table 1 The major clinical and pathological syndromes within the spectrum of systemic vasculitis, classified by the size of vessel involved and the presence of granulomata

Size of vessel involved	Granulomata absent	Granulomata present
Small	Microscopic polyarteritis	Wegener's granulomatosis
Medium	Polyarteritis nodosa Kawasaki disease	Churg–Strauss angiitis
Large*	Giant-cell arteritis Takayasu's arteritis	

* Note: Both forms of large-vessel vasculitis may show granuloma formation

and its importance in the diagnosis and management of patients with systemic vasculitis. Also, ANCA have been implicated in the pathogenesis of these disorders and are forming the basis of a new serological classification of the vasculitides.

AUTOANTIGENS IN SYSTEMIC VASCULITIS

Leukocytes

Although in his original description, Davies observed antibody binding to fixed neutrophil leukocytes[7], van der Woude found that antibodies also bound to monocytes and could be internally phagocytosed by neutrophils in suspension[8]. Rasmussen has since demonstrated by density gradient centrifugation that the antigen resides in the primary granule fraction[15]. At the First International ANCA Workshop, two patterns of neutrophil fluorescence were recognized, a granular cytoplasmic or classical pattern (CANCA) and a predominantly perinuclear or atypical appearance (PANCA)[16]. This latter pattern overlaps with that reported earlier by Wiik, for granulocyte-specific anti-nuclear antibodies, present in the sera of some patients with rheumatoid arthritis[17]. The standard ANCA assay assesses binding of antibody to normal neutrophils, alcohol-fixed to glass slides, by indirect immunofluorescence[16]; direct immunofluorescence studies of neutrophils from patients with active disease have not shown binding of autoantibody *in vivo*.

The target for CANCA has been shown independently by Goldschmeding, Ludemann and Niles to be a 29 kD protein[18-20], when neutrophil preparations are run under reducing conditions followed by immunoblotting with ANCA-positive sera. Under non-reducing conditions, a 38 kD protein was also seen by Ludemann[19], while Jones found both 40 kD and 29 kD proteins after immunoprecipitation with HL-60 cell extracts, a myeloid precursor cell line which contains the ANCA antigen[21]. Both Ludemann and Niles have shown homology between the N-terminal sequences of their 29 kD proteins with the serine proteinase family[19,20], and study of its enzymic activity by Ludemann has supported an identity with neutrophil serine proteinase 3[19].

Using size separation of a neutrophil extract by high-pressure liquid chromatography, Lockwood found reactivity of sera from patients with Wegener's granulomatosis with fractions of 2 and 12 kD, whereas sera from patients with microscopic polyarteritis reacted with fractions of 100 and 25 kD; the amino acid sequence of the 2 kD fraction showed homology with alkaline phosphatase[22]. However, using an ANCA assay based on a monoclonal antibody raised against the 29 kD protein, Goldschmeding has shown that all CANCA sera recognize a protein bound by this monoclonal[23], while Falk has completely inhibited fluorescence of a CANCA sera by a monoclonal anti-neutrophil serine proteinase 3[24]. As the complete sequence of neutrophil serine proteinase 3 is unknown, it is possible that the epitope on this protein recognized by Wegener's sera has homology with alkaline phosphatase, but in the latter protein this epitope is only available for antibody binding after enzymic digestion or autolysis.

Pooled sputum was studied as a potential source of antigen by Daha, who found that CANCA sera showed reactivity with a 91 kD glycoprotein[25]. Monoclonal antisera made against this glycoprotein also bound to a 91 kD neutrophil antigen after phorbol myristate acetate stimulation, but to a 29 kD neutrophil antigen after SDS extraction[25].

In 1988, Falk and Jenette proposed myeloperoxidase as a target antigen for ANCA and confirmed myeloperoxidase reactivity by ELISA and dot-blotting[26]. The immunofluorescence pattern of the anti-myeloperoxidase sera was perinuclear, and Falk and Jenette demonstrated that migration of basic myeloperoxidase from the primary granules to the nuclear membrane during alcohol fixation produced this artefactual pattern[27]. Other workers have confirmed the correlation of myeloperoxidase reactivity with PANCA inmmunofluorescence[28,29], but it is not the only PANCA antigen, since antibodies to both lactoferrin and elastase can produce similar immuno-fluorescence appearances[29-31].

Glomerular and endothelial cell antigens

In view of the frequent involvement of the kidney in systemic vasculitis, antibodies against glomerular components have been sought. Using cell lines cultured from human kidneys, Abbot found antibodies in sera from patients with Wegener's granulomatosis that bound to glomerular endothelial and epithelial cells, and similar reactivity was found with a monoclonal antibody, W8 (raised against a neutrophil cytoplasmic extract), with anti-myeloperoxidase activity[32]. Immunoglobulins with ANCA activity have also been eluted from the isolated, washed glomeruli of post-mortem kidneys in two cases of crescentic glomerulonephritis associated with circulating ANCA[33].

Antibodies which were lytic for human umbilical vein endothelial cells were found in Kawasaki disease, a childhood systemic vasculitis (1986)[34]; and more recently they have been demonstrated in adult systemic vasculitis[35-37]. Similar antibodies have also been found in other conditions, such as SLE and scleroderma[38,39]. However, in none has the biochemical nature of the autoantigens been determined.

T cell antigens

T lymphocytes can be the predominant infiltrating cell type in biopsies from affected tissue[5]; and circulating T cells from patients with vasculitis have been shown by one group to proliferate in response to a CANCA antigen preparation, in contrast to T cells from healthy controls[40].

IMPORTANCE OF HUMORAL RESPONSES

Occurrence of ANCA

ANCA are present in almost all cases of untreated, active, primary small-vessel systemic vasculitis and are therefore the first specific serological marker for these conditions. Their value as a diagnostic test has been shown in several studies, in which specificities of up to 99% and sensitivities up to 96% have been reported[9,41]. Such a test has particular importance in localized or early disease[42], when diagnostic histology cannot be obtained, and in rapidly progressive glomerulonephritis, where there may be no other features of vasculitic disease. In a large prospective study, ANCA were present in 30% of sera referred from patients with suspected (but not confirmed) renal vasculitis[43]. In localized disease limited to the respiratory tract, without systemic symptoms, an incidence of 60% has been reported[41].

In vasculitis affecting larger vessels, ANCA has been reported in Churg–Strauss angiitis[12,29] and in hepatitis B-associated polyarteritis nodosa[28,44]. Whether or not ANCA are present in non-hepatitis B-associated macroscopic polyarteritis nodosa (Kussmaul–Maier disease) is uncertain. However, in all these conditions it is difficult to exclude the possibility of overlapping features of microscopic polyarteritis and polyarteritis nodosa[45]. Savage found ANCA in 10 out of 11 sera from children with Kawasaki disease, a non-granulomatous vasculitis of small and medium-sized vessels[11].

In a study of six cases of Takayasu's disease with radiologically proven arteritis, none gave typical ANCA immunofluorescence. However, all showed reactivity with a 200 kD neutrophil antigen prepared by gel chromatography, although none could be shown to react with the whole neutrophil extract[14]. This suggested that there might be cryptic cytoplasmic neutrophil antigens, only revealed after chromatography of the parent material. ANCA were not present in a series of 21 patients with giant cell arteritis or polymyalgia rheumatica (unpublished observations).

Relation to disease activity

The incidence of ANCA positivity falls in clinical remission, and individual patients followed sequentially usually show a close relation between ANCA titre and clinical disease activity[41,46]. Thus, ANCA have acquired a role in monitoring disease activity as well as in diagnosis. Monitoring is particularly important in systemic vasculitis, where the frequency of relapse should preclude the indiscriminate withdrawal of treatment[47]. Previously, activity had been monitored by non-specific indices such as ESR and C-reactive protein, which are affected by other variables such as anaemia and infection[48].

Although ANCA may persist during clinical remission, sequential ANCA titres are valuable in the prediction and diagnosis of relapse. Cohen Tervaert followed 35 patients over 16 months and observed 17 clinical relapses, all preceded by a rise in ANCA a mean of 7 weeks earlier[49]. In another study following 20 patients over 12 months, there were 9 relapses, all preceded by an increase in ANCA a mean of 4 weeks earlier, although on three occasions ANCA rose and fell without clinical sequelae[46]. Both reports noted that most relapses occurred following reductions in therapy. In the latter study, ANCA were compared to C-reactive protein and found to relate much more closely to disease activity[46]. Therefore, absolute levels are not of predictive value, but regular ANCA estimations during follow-up and comparison with earlier values are useful.

In a comparison of ANCA and anti-human umbilical vein endothelial cell antibodies, Frampton found an incidence of anti-endothelial cell antibodies of 30% in sera from patients with active, ANCA-positive, vasculitis; and the titres of anti-endothelial cell antibodies reflected disease activity in patients followed sequentially[37]. The titre of anti-endothelial cell antibodies also correlated with von Willebrand factor release, a marker of endothelial cell injury[50]. Cross-inhibition experiments have confirmed that anti-endothelial cell antibodies recognize a different target from ANCA[37], so some more subtle explanation must underlie the correlations between ANCA, anti-endothelial cell levels, and disease activity.

Immunoglobulin class and disease

Although almost always of IgG class, ANCA restricted to IgM have been found in a few patients, when they have been associated with a common clinical presentation of severe pulmonary haemorrhage and nephritis[33]. Interestingly, three cases followed sequentially showed an ANCA class switch from IgM to IgG[33]. IgA ANCA have been found in Henoch–Schonlein purpura[13], but the presence of IgA rheumatoid factor in this condition may produce a false positive IgA ANCA[51].

In a quantitative study of ANCA IgG subclasses in acute sera, ANCA were found in all subclasses, but were relatively over-represented in the IgG3 and under-represented in the IgG2 fractions[52]. In contrast, the distribution of ANCA-positive remission sera showed a reversal of this pattern[52] (Figure 1). As IgG3 has a much shorter half-life than the other subclasses, it is probably the dominant isotype in the acute ANCA response. Other qualitative studies have found restriction of ANCA to IgG1 and IgG4; the differences in results may be accounted for by varying affinities of the subclass monoclonal reagants[53].

The sequence of IgM to IgG and IgG3 to IgG2 follows the sequence of heavy-chain genomic arrangement of $5'-\mu-\delta-g3-g1-\alpha1-g2-g4-\varepsilon-\alpha2$[54]. If there is an association between the order of heavy-chain genes and immune maturation, then these results suggest that ANCA are either the result of an early immune response or that there are defects in heavy-chain switching. The presence of IgG2 in remission sera may also explain the discrepancy between ANCA and clinical remission seen in some patients, as IgG3 and

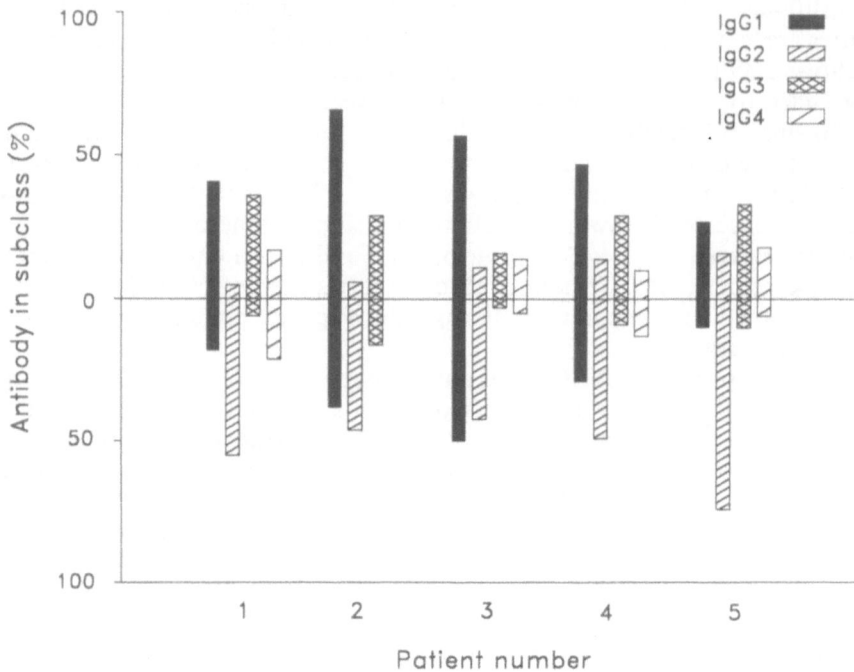

Figure 1 Comparison of ANCA IgG subclass distribution in five patients with persistent ANCA positivity, expressed as the percentage of total ANCA IgG binding between acute disease (above the line) and clinical remission (below the line), a mean of 9 weeks later. IgG1 and IgG3 were the dominant ANCA IgG subclasses associated with acute disease, but in remission maturation of the subclass response was observed with relative reductions in IgG3 and elevations of IgG2.

IgG1 have greater phlogistic potential owing to their ability to fix complement and bind to the macrophage Fc receptor[55]. The maturation of the ANCA response is unusual for an autoantibody and suggests a pathogenetic role for ANCA analogous to that for anti-glomerular basement membrane antibodies.

Classification of vasculitis

Traditionally, the systemic vasculitides have been classified by their clinical and histological features. The presence of the same immunological marker across a range of diseases with vasculitis as their common histological feature argues for the use of systemic vasculitis as a collective term. Of the two ANCA autoantigens defined so far, reactivity to the 29 kD serine proteinase has been correlated with a clinical diagnosis of Wegener's granulomatosis, and that to myeloperoxidase with microscopic polyarteritis and renal-limited vasculitis[23,26,31]. Cases where the clinical diagnosis falls between these two groups have had a mixture of both reactivities[31]. Dual reactivity within the same patient does not seem to be common[29].

Patients with single organ disease and non-diagnostic histology may only be diagnosed when the disease becomes more widespread[56]. The presence of

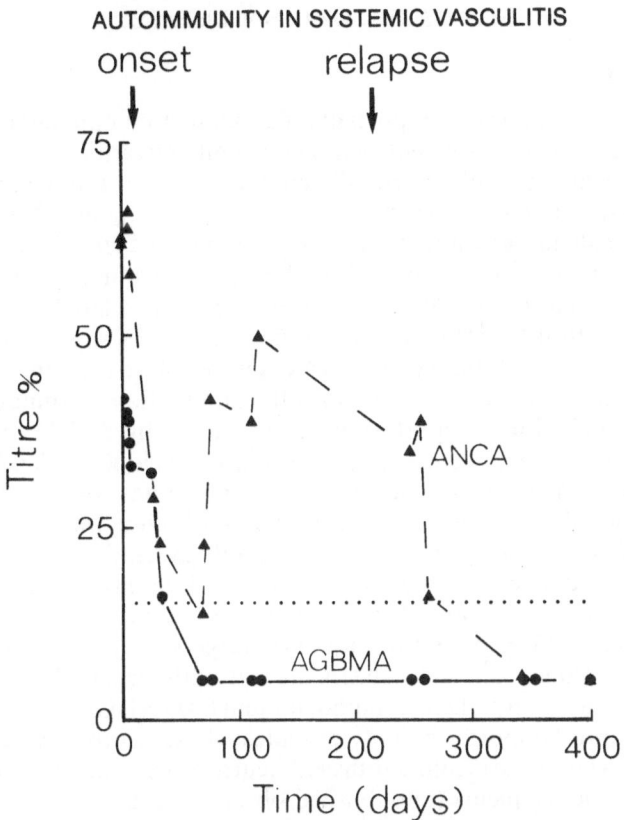

Figure 2 Sequential ANCA and anti-glomerular basement membrane antibody binding (per cent) for a patient with rapidly progressive glomerulonephritis and dual autoantibody positivity. The dotted line represents the upper limit of the normal ranges. Both autoantibody levels fell to the normal range following induction treatment; however, ANCA rose during follow-up and a clinical relapse occurred 8 months after presentation, associated with persistent ANCA positivity and undetectable anti-glomerular basement membrane antibodies.

ANCA during this localized phase validates the inclusion of these patients within the spectrum of systemic vasculitis and simplifies their classification.

A subgroup of anti-glomerular basement membrane disease defined by ANCA positivity accounted for 30% of anti-glomerular basement membrane antibody-positive patients in a study of these markers in rapidly progressive glomerulonephritis[43]. Analysis of their clinical and histological features showed evidence of both vasculitis and anti-glomerular basement membrane disease; in particular, pulmonary haemorrhage was common although few were smokers, and some biopsies showed not only linear IgG immunofluorescence in the glomeruli but also granulomata and extra-glomerular vasculitis[43]. Two features pointed to the clinical importance of this subgroup: first, after treatment with plasma exchange, steroids and cyclophosphamide, three of seven survivors who were initially dialysis dependent recovered satisfactory renal function, an outcome rare for anti-glomerular basement membrane disease but seen in systemic vasculitis[57]; second, two late recurrences of disease activity were seen, both associated with a rise in ANCA and without detectable anti-glomerular basement membrane antibodies[43] (Figure 2).

Pathophysiology

Clearly, the neutrophil is an important inflammatory component in vasculitis and ANCA may play a role either in neutrophil activation or in enhancing the pathological effects of neutrophil activation. $F(ab')_2$ fragments prepared from ANCA-positive IgG exert a specific inhibitory effect on FMLP-induced intracellular calcium flux and calcium inositol-induced entry of calcium into normal human neutrophils, in a dose-dependent manner[58]. This suggests that ANCA bind to a cell surface target closely related to the phosphatidylinositol/DPG pathway and can effect neutrophil signal transduction.

In contrast to this inhibitory effect, ANCA were able to activate neutrophils, as measured by superoxide production, after stimulation by tumour necrosis factor[59]. A preliminary report showed inhibition by ANCA of luminol-dependent chemiluminescence using fluid-phase myeloperoxidase[60], but the effect of ANCA on the enzymic activity of proteinase 3 has not been determined.

A cytolytic effect of anti-endothelial cell antibodies was shown first in Kawasaki disease and more recently in adult systemic vasculitis[34,35]. A pathogenetic sequence of excess monocyte cytokine production activating endothelial cells, which are then lysed by AECA has been proposed by Leung[61]. As ANCA also bind to monocyte targets, they may have a role in initiating this sequence[8]. That ANCA are not pathogenetic in isolation can be inferred from a study where immunoglobulin from ANCA-positive patients was infused into baboons (the only primates whose neutrophils contain the CANCA antigen). Apart from a transient neutropenia, there was no evidence of disease in the recipients (unpublished observations).

TREATMENT AND THE B CELL RESPONSE

Current therapy

The current treatment of vasculitis has evolved empirically, but using ANCA assays it can now be monitored by its effect on the abnormal B cell response. Induction therapy consists of steroids and cyclophosphamide, for example prednisolone 60 mg/day and cyclophosphamide 3 mg/kg/day. The prednisolone is reduced over 6 weeks to maintenance levels of 10 mg/day, and in addition some centres switch cyclophosphamide to azathioprine to avoid cumulative toxicity. Because plasma exchange has been an effective treatment in anti-glomerular basement membrane disease[62], which has many similarities to systemic vasculitis, it has been used in addition to steroids and cyclophosphamide in the presence of pulmonary and renal disease[57].

If ANCA contribute to pathogenesis, then it would be logical to remove them as quickly as possible by plasma exchange, meanwhile suppressing their further synthesis with cyclophosphamide. In a controlled study of the additional benefit of plasma exchange compared to steroids and cyclophosphamide alone, in patients with rapidly progressive glomerulonephritis, Pusey showed a convincing effect of plasma exchange in the group with most advanced renal failure[57].

In a study of plasma exchange as sole therapy for ANCA-positive vasculitis, clinical remission was induced in all four patients treated, but ANCA returned in three of the four between 2 weeks and 3 months later; in two this was associated with minor, self-limiting relapse and in the third with a more major relapse (unpublished observations).

Regulation of the humoral response

Possible mechanisms for the physiological control of B cell autoreactivity are T cell suppression, either active or as a result of T cell deletion or energy, and idiotypic/anti-idiotypic (id/anti-id) interactions. Anti-idiotypic antibodies reactive with ANCA have been demonstrated in pooled normal human immunoglobulin (IVIG), and in ANCA-negative sera from patients who have recovered from vasculitis[63]. The anti-idiotypic antibodies inhibited the binding of ANCA to their target in a dose-dependent manner, and were therefore presumed to interact with the antigen binding site of ANCA.

In post-recovery sera, anti-idiotypic activity has been found in the IgG and IgM fractions; interestingly, latent ANCA activity was produced from ANCA-negative sera by removing the IgM fraction (unpublished observations). A dynamic relationship between idiotypes on ANCA and anti-idiotypic antibodies appears to exist, with disease expression occurring when there is excess ANCA and remission when ANCA is controlled. The presence of anti-idiotypes on normal immunoglobulin suggests that they have a role in the physiological prevention of autoimmune vasculitis, and that a breakdown in this mechanism is associated with disease activation.

Post-recovery immunoglobulin from one patient was able to inhibit the binding of ANCA in acute sera from other patients, so at least some of the idiotypes on ANCA are 'public', which has important implications for the use of pooled immunoglobulin or monoclonal anti-idiotypic antibodies in the treatment of vasculitis[63]. Preliminary results using high-dose IVIG in systemic vasculitis have shown that clinical remission has been successfully induced in 3/3 cases accompanied by marked reduction in ANCA levels (unpublished observations).

IMPORTANCE OF THE T CELL RESPONSE

Evidence for T cell autoreactivity in vasculitis

Study of autoreactive T cells is limited by technical problems and ignorance of the T cell autoantigens. Apart from the report by Daha[25], there is no direct evidence for T cell autoreactivity in systemic vasculitis. Indirect evidence has been obtained from immunohistological studies of the respiratory tract in Wegener's granulomatosis[5], and of the kidney in rapidly progressive glomerulonephritis[4], both of which found T lymphocytes to be a major component of the cellular infiltrate, with an altered subset ratio to that found in the serum. Also, T lymphocytes are present in the prominent perivascular cellular infiltrate in the cutaneous vasculitides[64], and a similar pattern may be seen in systemic vasculitis[65].

T cell therapy

While cyclophosphamide affects B and T cells and other inflammatory components, cyclosporin A specifically blocks T cell IL-2 gene activation and IL-2 synthesis[66]. Isolated reports have shown that cyclosporin A can induce remission in systemic vasculitis[67,68], but further study is required before any conclusions can be reached.

T cell therapy using monoclonal antibodies has an established place in oncology and graft rejection, and offers the opportunity in autoimmunity to target treatment more precisely than current therapy. In one case, a combination of Campath 1H (anti-B-cell, T-cell and monocyte) and an anti-CD4 monoclonal induced lasting remission in a patient with systemic vasculitis refractory to conventional treatment[69]. It has been found in experimental transplantation that anti-CD4 can induce tolerance to foreign antigens[70]; it would be exciting if this effect could be reproduced with respect to self-antigens in man.

AETIOLOGY OF SYSTEMIC VASCULITIS

Genetic mechanisms

Associations of a particular autoimmune disease with major histocompatibility complex (MHC) antigens imply an important T cell contribution, as T cells only see antigen in the context of MHC; and such MHC restriction suggests that only a small number of epitopes are acting as self-antigens. Strong associations occur in anti-glomerular basement membrane disease[71] and membranous nephropathy[72], but the reported MHC associations of systemic vasculitis using serological markers are weak—namely, HLA-B8 and DR4 with Wegener's granulomatosis[73,74] and HLA-Bw22 with Kawasaki disease[75]. These results may be explained by the heterogeneity of autoimmune responses within the systemic vasculitides, and closer associations may be found by looking at B cell autoantigens and at the other Class II loci.

Infection

In the absence of a particular infective agent, several factors have lead to a hypothesis for the pathogenesis of systemic vasculitis initiated by infection: a seasonal variation in incidence[24], frequent prodrome of influenzal symptoms[24], association of relapse with intercurrent infection[76], and the therapeutic response to the antibiotic combination of sulphamethoxazole and trimethoprim[77]. The release of potential neutrophil self-antigens in a genetically susceptible patient would then drive a pathogenic immune response[78]. Both cutaneous and systemic vasculitis occur in cystic fibrosis, where there is both chronic infection and also immunosuppression characterized by depressed T cell responses to environmental antigens and hypergammaglobulinaemia. These cases are not associated with a particular infective agent, but are possibly the result of prolonged immune stimulation[79].

In Davies' original report on ANCA, an association between arbovirus infection and rapidly progressive glomerulonephritis was observed[7], and retroviruses have been implicated in Kawasaki disease[80]. In another study, incorporation of Epstein–Barr virus DNA into the host genome of a patient with a Kawasaki-like disease was demonstrated[81]. However, no confirmatory evidence for the role of any of these agents has been forthcoming.

If infection was operating as a non-specific immune stimulus, then no particular microbial agent would need to be implicated; however, evidence of infection is not invariable, and the induction of systemic vasculitis by drugs such as hydralazine[82] and penicillamine[83] suggest that the autoreactive immune response is not necessarily antigen driven. Both these drugs are polyclonal B cell activators and a polyclonal autoantibody response occurs in vasculitis; in addition to ANCA, anti-glomerular basement membrane and anti-endothelial cell antibodies, rheumatoid factors, and the anti-nuclear antibodies anti-Ro and anti-La, have been reported, and hypergammaglobulinaemia is common.

SUMMARY

An autoimmune component in the aetiology of systemic vasculitides has been established by the discovery of ANCA and other autoantibodies in these conditions. Investigation of these humoral responses has produced valuable specific serological assays for diagnosis and follow-up, and a new classification of systemic vasculitis based on serological reactivity is emerging.

The pathogenetic role for ANCA is unclear; they may cause pathophysiological effects through influences on neutrophil function but they require other factors, possibly autoreactive T-cells or anti-endothelial cell antibodies, to induce inflammation. The interplay between infection and pathogenesis is also complex and is at present unresolved. However, it is likely that, in common with other autoimmune diseases, both genetic susceptibility and environmental triggers will feature in the eventual explanation.

Current treatment is limited by toxicity, generalized immunosuppression and limited efficacy, and several promising new approaches, such as high-dose immunoglobulin and monoclonal antibody therapy, are currently under investigation.

References

1. Moore, P. M., Beard, E. E., Thoburn, T. W. and Williams, H. L. (1951). Idiopathic (lethal) granuloma of the midline facial tissues treated with cortisone: report of a case. *Laryngoscope*, **61**, 320–331
2. Fauci, A. S., Katz, P., Haynes, B. F. and Wolff, S. M. (1979). Cyclophosphamide therapy of severe systemic necrotizing vasculitis. *N. Engl. J. Med.*, **301**, 235–238
3. Lockwood, C. M., Pinching, A. J., Sweny, P., Rees, A. J. and Peters, D. K. (1977). Plasma exchange and immunosuppression in the treatment of fulminating immune-complex nephritis. *Lancet*, **1**, 63–67
4. Nolasco, F., Cameron, J. S., Hartley, B., Coelho, A., Hildreth, G. and Reuben, R. (1987). Intraglomerular T cells and monocytes in nephritis: Study with monoclonal antibodies. *Kidney Int.*, **31**, 1160–1166

5. Rasmussen, N., Petersen, J., Ralfkiaer, E., Avnstrom, S. and Wiik, A. (1988). Spontaneous and induced immunoglobulin synthesis and anti-neutrophil cytoplasm antibodies in Wegener's granulomatosis: relation to leucocyte subpopulations in blood and active lesions. *Rheumatol. Int.*, **8**, 153–158

6. Howell, S. B. and Epstein, W. V. (1976). Circulating immunoglobulin complexes in Wegener's granulomatosis. *Am. J. Med.*, **60**, 259–268

7. Davies, D. J., Moran, J. E., Niall, J. F. and Ryan, G. B. (1982). Segmental necrotizing glomerulonephritis with antineutrophil antibody: possible arbovirus aetiology. *Br. Med. J.*, **285**, 606–609

8. Van der Woude, F. J., Rasmussen, N., Lobatto, S. *et al.* (1985). Autoantibodies against neutrophils and monocytes; tool for diagnosis and marker of disease activity in Wegener's granulomatosis. *Lancet*, **1**, 425–429

9. Savage, C. O. S., Winearls, C. G., Jones, S., Marshall, P. D. and Lockwood, C. M. (1987). Prospective study of radioimmunoassay for antibodies against neutrophil cytoplasm in diagnosis of systemic vasculitis. *Lancet*, **1**, 1389–1393

10. Walters, M. D. S., Savage, C. O. S., Dillon, M. J., Lockwood, C. M. and Barratt, T. M. (1988). Antineutrophil cytoplasm antibody in crescentic glomerulonephritis. *Arch. Dis. Child.*, **63**, 814–817

11. Savage, C. O. S., Tizard, J., Jayne, D. R. W., Lockwood, C. M. and Dillon, M. J. (1989). Antineutrophil cytoplasm antibodies in Kawasaki disease. *Arch. Dis. Child.*, **64**, 360–363

12. Wathen, C. W. and Harrison, D. J. (1987). Circulating anti-neutrophil antibodies in systemic vasculitis. *Lancet*, **1**, 1037 (Letter)

13. Van der Wall Bake, A. W. L., Lobatto, S., Jonges, L., Daha, M. R. and Van Es, L. A. (1987). IgA antibodies directed against cytoplasmic antigens of polymorphonuclear leucocytes in patients with Henoch–Schonlein purpura. *Adv. Exp. Med. Biol.*, **216B**, 1593–1598

14. Lai, K. N., Jayne, D. R. W., Brownlee, A. and Lockwood, C. M. (1990). The specificity of anti-neutrophil cytoplasm autoantibodies in systemic vasculitides. *Clin. Exp. Immunol.*, **82**, 233–237

15. Rasmussen, N., Borregaard, N. and Wiik, A. (1987). Anti-neutrophil-cytoplasm antibodies are not directed against alkaline phosphatase. *Lancet*, **1**, 1488 (Letter)

16. Rasmussen, N., Wiik, A., Hoier-Madsen, M., Borregaard, N. and Van Der Woude, F. (1988). Anti-neutrophil cytoplasm antibodies. *Lancet*, **1**, 706–707

17. Wiik, A., Jensen, E. and Friis, J. (1974). Granulocyte-specific antinuclear factors in synovial fluids and sera from patients with rheumatoid arthritis. *Ann. Rheum. Dis.*, **33**, 515–519

18. Goldschmeding, R., Van der Schoot, C. E., ten Bokkel Huinink, D. *et al.* (1989). Wegener's granulomatosis autoantibodies identify a novel diisopropylflurophosphate-binding protein in the lysosomes of normal human neutrophils. *J. Clin. Invest.*, **84**, 1577–1587

19. Ludemann, J., Utecht, B. and Gross, W. L. (1990). Anti-neutrophil cytoplasm antibodies in Wegener's granulomatosis recognise an elastinolytic enzyme. *J. Exp. Med.*, **171**, 357–362

20. Niles, J. L., McCluskey, R. T., Ahmed, M. F. and Arnaout, M. A. (1989). Wegener's granulomatosis autoantigen is a novel neutrophil serine proteinase. *Blood*, **74**, 1888–1893

21. Jones, S. J. and Lockwood, C. M. (1990). Characterisation of autoantigens in systemic vasculitis. *Kidney Int.*, **37**, 441 (Abstract)

22. Lockwood, C. M., Bates, D., Jones, S. J., Whitaker, K. B., Moss, D. W. and Savage, C. O. S. (1987). Association of alkaline phosphatase with an autoantigen recognised by circulating anti-neutrophil antibodies in systemic vasculitis. *Lancet*, **1**, 716–720

23. Gans, R. O. B., Goldschmeding, R., Donker, A. J. M. *et al.* (1989). Neutrophil cytoplasmic autoantibodies and Wegener's granulomatosis. *Lancet*, **1**, 269–270 (Letter)

24. Falk, R. (1990). Clinicopathologic correlates of anto-myeloperoxidase antibodies. In Panayi, G. S. (ed.) *Recent Advances in Systemic Vasculitis. J. R. Soc. Med.*, **83**, 404–410

25. Daha, M. R., Kramps, J. A., Schrama, E., Van Es, L. A. and Van der Woude, F. J. (1990). Isolation from purulent sputum of an antigen reactive with antibodies in Wegener's serum. In *Proceedings of the 2nd International ANCA Workshop. Neth. J. Med.*, **36**, 117–120

26. Falk, R. J. and Jennette, J. C. (1988). Anti-neutrophil cytoplasmic autoantibodies with specificity for myeloperoxidase in patients with systemic vasculitis and idiopathic necrotizing and crescentic glomerulonephritis. *N. Engl. J. Med.*, **318**, 1651–1657

27. Jennette, J. C., Charles, L. A., Lauritzen, S. L. and Falk, R. J. (1989). The effects of fixation on the neutrophil staining patterns produced by autoantibodies specific for primary granule

constituents. In *Proceedings of the 2nd International ANCA Workshop. Neth. J. Med.*, **36**, 121–125
28. Daha, M. R. and Falk, R. J. (1990). Anti-myeloperoxidase antibodies and clinical associations. In *Proceedings of the 2nd International ANCA Workshop. Neth. J. Med.*, **36**, 152–153
29. Cohen Tervaert, J. W., Goldschmeding, R., Elema, J. D. *et al.* (1990). Autoantibodies to myeloperoxidase are associated with different forms of vasculitis. *Arthritis Rheum.*, **33**, 1264–1272
30. Thompson, R. A. and Lee, S. S. (1989). Anti-neutrophil cytoplasmic antobidies. *Lancet*, **1**, 670-671 (Letter)
31. Noel, L.-H., Chen, N., Nusbaum, P., Lesavre, P. and Grunfeld, J. P. (1990). Characterisation of antineutrophil cytoplasm antibodies (ANCA) in different forms of vasculitis and rapidly progressive glomerulonephritis. *Kidney Int.*, **37**, 444
32. Abbott, F., Jones, S. J., Lockwood, C. M. and Rees, A. J. (1989). Autoantibodies to glomerular antigens in patients with Wegener's granulomatosis. *Nephrol. Dial. Transplant.*, **4**, 1–8
33. Jayne, D. R. W., Jones, S. J., Severn, A., Shaunak, S., Murphy, J. and Lockwood, C. M. (1989). Severe pulmonary haemorrhage and systemic vasculitis in association with circulating anti-neutrophil cytoplasm antibodies of IgM class only. *Clin. Nephrol.*, **32**, 101–106
34. Leung, D. Y. M., Collins, T., Lapierre, L. A., Geha, R. S. and Pober, J. S. (1986). IgM antibodies in the acute phase of Kawasaki syndrome lyse cultured vascular endothelial cells stimulated with gamma interferon. *J. Clin. Invest.*, **77**, 1428–1435
35. Brasile, L., Kremer, J. M., Clarke, J. L. and Cerilli, J. (1989). Identification of an autoantibody to vascular endothelial cell-specific antigens in patients with systemic vasculitis. *Am. J. Med.*, **87**, 74–80
36. Bagueley, E. and Hughes, G. R. V. Lytic IgG anti-endothelial cell antibodies in vasculitis. *Lancet*, **2**, 907 (Letter)
37. Frampton, G., Jayne, D. R. W., Lockwood, C. M. and Cameron, J. S. (1990). Antibodies to endothelial cells and neutrophil cytoplasm in systemic vasculitis. *Clin. Exp. Immunol.*, **82**, 227–232
38. Heurkens, A. H. M., Hiemstra, P. S., Lafeber, G. J. M., Daha, M. R. and Breedveld. (1989). Anti-endothelial cell antibodies in patients with rheumatoid arthritis complicated by vasculitis. *Clin. Exp. Immunol.*, **78**, 7–12
39. Cines, D. B., Ltss, A. P., Reeber, M. and DeHoritias, R. J. (1984). Presence of complement fixing anti-endothelial cell antibodies in systemic lupus erythematosus. *J. Clin. Invest.*, **73**, 611–625
40. van der Woude, F. J., van Es, L. A. and Daha, M. R. (1990). The role of the CANCA antigen in the pathogenesis of Wegener's granulomatosis. *Neth. J. Med.*, **36**, 169–171
41. Nolle, B., Specks, U., Ludemann, J., Rohrbach, M. S., Deremee, R. A. and Gross, W. L. (1989). Anticytoplasmic autoantibodies: their immunodiagnostic value in Wegener granulomatosis. *Ann. Intern. Med.*, **111**, 28–40
42. Hoare, T. J., Jayne, D. R. W., Rhys Evans, P., Croft, C. B. and Howard, D. J. (1989). Wegeners granulomatosis, subglottic stenosis and antineutrophil cytoplasm autoantibodies. *J. Laryngol. Otol.*, **103**, 1187–1191
43. Jayne, D. R. W., Marshall, P. D., Jones, S. J. and Lockwood, C. M. (1990). Autoantibodies to GBM and neutrophil cytoplasm in rapidly progressive glomerulonephritis. *Kidney Int.*, **37**, 965–970
44. O'Donoghue, D. J., Nusbaum, P., Halbwachs-Mecarelli, L., Lesaure, P., Noel, L.-H. and Guillevin, L. (1991). Anti-neutrophil cytoplasm antibodies associated with polyarteritis nodosa, Churg-Strauss syndrome and HIV infection. *Am. J. Kidney Dis.*, (Abstr.) (in press)
45. Heptinstall, R. H. (1983). Polyarteritis (periarteritis) nodosa, other forms of vasculitis, and rheumatoid arthritis. In Heptinstall, R. H. (ed.) *Pathology of the Kidney*, pp. 793–838. (Boston/Toronto: Little Brown)
46. Jayne, D. R. W., Heaton, A., Evans, D. B. and Lockwood, C. M. (1990). Sequential anti-neutrophil cytoplasm antibody titres in the management of systemic vasculitis. *Nephrol. Dial. Transplant.*, **5**, 309–310 (Abstract)
47. Bradley, J. D., Brandt, K. D. and Katz, B. P. (1989). Infectious complications of cyclophosphamide treatment for vasculitis. *Arthritis Rheum.*, **32**, 45–53
48. Hind, C. R. K., Winnearls, C. G. and Pepys, M. B. (1985). Correlation of disease activity in systemic vasculitis with serum C-reactive protein measurement. A prospective study of thirty-eight patients. *Eur. J. Clin. Invest.*, **15**, 89–94
49. Cohen Tervaert, J. W., van Der Woude, F., Fauci, A. S. *et al.* (1989). Association between active Wegener's granulomatosis and anticytoplasmic antibodies. *Arch. Intern. Med.*, **149**, 2461–2465

50. Brown, Z., Neild, G. H., Willoughby, J. J., Somia, N. V. and Cameron, J. S. (1986). Increased factor VIII as an index of vascular injury in cyclosporin nephrotoxicity. *Transplantation*, **42**, 150–154

51. Brouwer, E., Cohen Tevaert, J. W., Horst, G., Huitema, M. G., van der Giessen, M., Limburg, P. C. and Kallenberg, C. G. M. (1991). Predominance of IgG1 and IgG4 subclasses of anti-neutrophil cytoplasmic autoantibodies (ANCA) in patients with Wegener's granulomatosis and related disorders. *Clin. Exp. Immunol.*, **83**, 379–386

52. Jayne, D. R. W., Weetman, A. P. and Lockwood, C. M. (1988). The IgG subclass distribution of anti-neutrophil cytoplasm autoantibodies in systemic vasculitis. *Nephrol. Dial. Transplant.*, **4**, 387 (Abstract)

53. Weetman, A. P. and Cohen, S. B. (1986). The IgG subclass distribution of thyroid autoantibodies. *Immunol. Lett.*, **13**, 335–341

54. Flanagan, J. G. and Rabbits, T. H. (1982). Arrangement of human immunoglobulin heavy chain constant region genes implies evolutionary duplication of a segment containing gamma, eta and alpha genes. *Nature*, **300**, 709–713

55. Waldmann, H. (1989). Manipulation of T-cell responses with monoclonal antibodies. *Annu. Rev. Immunol.*, **7**, 407–444

56. Waxman, J. and Bose, W. J. (1986). Laryngeal manifestations of Wegener's granulomatosis: case reports and review of the literature. *J. Rheumatol.*, **13**, 408–411

57. Pusey, C. D. and Lockwood, C. M. (1984). Plasma exchange for glomerular disease. In Robinson, R. R. (ed.) *Nephrology*, pp. 1474–1485. (New York: Springer)

58. Lai, K. N. and Lockwood, C. M. (1991). Effect of anti-neutrophil cytoplasm autoantibodies on signal transduction in human neutrophils and HL-60 cells. *Kidney Int.*, **37**, 442 (Abstract)

59. Falk, R. J., Terrell, R., Huneycutt-Calder, L. and Jennette, J. C. (1989). Anti-neutrophil cytoplasmic autoantibodies (ANCA) stimulate neutrophil activation in vivo. *Kidney Int.*, **35**, 346 (Abstract)

60. Lee, S. S., Adu, D. and Thompson, R. A. (1990). Anti-myeloperoxidase antibodies in systemic vasculitis. *Clin. Exp. Immunol.*, **79**, 41–46

61. Leung, D. Y. M., Kurt-Jones, E., Newburger, J. W., Cotran, R. S., Burns, J. C. and Pober, J. S. (1989). Endothelial cell activation and high interleukin-1 secretion in the pathogenesis of acute Kawasaki disease. *Lancet*, **1**, 1298–1302

62. Lockwood, C. M., Rees, A. J., Pearson, T. A., Evans, D. J. and Peters, D. K. (1976). Immunosuppression and plasma exchange in the treatment of Goodpasture's syndrome. *Lancet*, **1**, 711–715

63. Jayne, D. R. W., Rossi, F., Kazatchkine, M. D. and Lockwood, C. M. (1989). Anti-idiotypes against autoantibodies to neutrophil cytoplasmic antigens are present in pooled human immunoglobulin and post-recovery sera. In *7th International Congress of Immunology*, p. 273 (Abstract)

64. Soter, R. A. and Austen, K. F. (1980). Pathogenetic mechanisms in the necrotizing vasculitides. *Clin. Rheum. Dis.*, **6**, 233

65. McCluskey, R. T. and Fienberg, R. (1983). Vasculitis in primary vasculitides, granulomatoses and connective tissue diseases. *Hum. Pathol.*, **14**, 305

66. Strom, T. B. and Kelley, V. E. (1989). Towards more selective therapies to block undesired immune responses. *Kidney Int.*, **35**, 1026–1033

67. Borleffs, J. C. C., Derksoen, R. H. W. M. and Hene, R. J. (1987). Wegener's granulomatosis and cyclosporine. *Ann. Rheum. Dis.*, **46**, 175–177

68. Gremmel, F., Druml, W., Schmidt, P. and Graninger, W. (1988). Cyclosporin in Wegener's granulomatosis. *Ann. Intern. Med.*, **108**, 491

69. Mathieson, P. W., Lockwood, C. M., Grant, J. W. and Waldmann, H. (1990). Induction of remission in systemic vasculitis with monoclonal antibody Campath 1H. *Br. J. Dermatol.*, (In press)

70. Qin, S., Cobbold, S. P., Tighe, H., Benjamin, R. and Waldmann, H. (1987). CD4 Mab pairs for immunosuppression and tolerance induction. *Eur. J. Immunol.*, **17**, 1559

71. Rees, A. J., Peters, D. K., Compston, D. A. S. and Batchelor, J. R. (1978). Strong association between HLA DRw2 and antibody mediated Goodpasture's syndrome. *Lancet*, **1**, 966–968

72. Klouda, P. T., Manos, J., Acheson, E. J. *et al.* (1979). Strong association between idiopathic membranous nephropathy and HLA-DRw3. *Lancet*, **2**, 770–771

73. Katz, P. (1979). Association of Wegeners granulomatosis and HLA B-8. *Clin. Immunol.*

Immunopathol., **14**, 268–272

74. Elkon, K. B., Sutherland, D. C. and Rees, A. J. (1983). HLA antigen frequencies in systemic vasculitis: increase in HLA DR4 in Wegener's granulomatosis. *Arthritis Rheum.*, **26**, 102–104

75. Kato, S., Kimura, M., Tsuji, K. *et al.* (1978). HLA antigens in Kawasaki disease. *Paediatrics*, **61**, 252–255

76. Pinching, A. J., Lockwood, C. M., Pussell, B. A. and Peters, D. K. (1983). Wegeners granulomatosis: presentation, pathology and prognosis. *Q. J. Med.*, **53**, 435–460

77. Deremee, R. A. (1989). The treatment of Wegener's granulomatosis with trimethoprim/sulfamethoxazole: illusion or vision? *Arthritis Rheum.*, **31**, 1068–1073

78. Van der Woude, F. J., Daha, M. R. and Van Es, L. A. (1989). The current status of neutrophil cytoplasmic antibodies. *Clin. Exp. Immunol.*, **78**, 143–148

79. Finnegan, M. J., Hinchcliffe, J., Russell-Jones, D. *et al.* (1989). Vasculitis in cystic fibrosis. *Q. J. Med.*, **22**, 609–622

80. Shulman, S. T. and Rowley, A. H. (1986). Does Kawasaki disease have a retroviral aetiology? *Lancet*, **2**, 545–546

81. Kikuta, H., Taguchi, Y., Tomisawa, K. *et al.* (1988). Epstein-Barr virus genome positive T lymphocytes in a boy with chronic active EBV infection associated with a Kawasaki-like disease. *Nature*, **333**, 455 (Letter)

82. Mason, P. D. and Lockwood, C. M. (1986). Rapidly progressive nephritis in patients taking hydralazine. *J. Clin. Lab. Immunol.*, **20**, 151–153

83. Banfi, G., Imbasciati, E. and Guerra, L. (1983). Extracapillary glomerulonephritis with necrotizing vasculitis in D-penicillamine treated rheumatoid arthritis. *Nephron*, **33**, 56

13
Immunopathogenic Mechanisms of Interstitial Nephritis

C. M. MEYERS and C. J. KELLY

Primary tubulointerstitial nephritis causes a significant proportion of both acute and chronic renal disease[1]. Advances in our knowledge of clinico-pathological correlates, moreover, have also established a prognostic importance for the tubulointerstitium in other primary types of renal disease[2]. Studies evaluating renal function in primary glomerular disease, for example, have demonstrated the importance of tubulointerstitial damage in determining the ultimate prognosis[2,3]. In some settings, indices of tubulointerstitial damage display a better correlation with glomerular filtration rate than do indices of glomerular damage[4,5]. Such findings have stimulated a growing interest in understanding mechanisms of injury to the tubulointerstitium.

It is generally accepted that acute inflammatory interstitial nephritis represents an early and reversible stage of renal injury. Chronic interstitial nephritis, with its attendant tubular atrophy and fibrosis, reflects irreversible damage. Although acute and chronic interstitial nephritis are traditionally classified as having distinct aetiologies, there is most likely considerable overlap. Acute interstitial nephritis can progress to a lesion with a chronic histological appearance and progressive renal insufficiency. What is typically regarded as chronic interstitial nephritis may evolve out of a clinically silent acute inflammatory stage. While most research has been directed towards understanding pathogenic mechanisms underlying acute inflammation, there is a growing enthusiasm for studying mechanisms of fibrogenesis.

Despite the varied inciting factors of acute and chronic interstitial nephritis, the histology of the lesions is quite similar. Mononuclear cell infiltration and occasionally giant-cell formation are typically seen in acute interstitial nephritis, with variable degrees of immunoglobulin and complement deposition in the interstitium[1]. Chronic interstitial nephritis may also display a mononuclear cell infiltrate, in addition to the characteristic interstitial fibrosis and tubular atrophy. Such findings suggest that immune mechanisms are important either

271

Table 1 Nephritogenic immune response to tubulointerstitial antigens

Afferent mechanisms	Regulatory mechanisms	Effector mechanisms

1. Tissue expression of antigen	1. Regulatory T cells	*Antigen specific*
		1. Antigen-specific T cells
		  (a) Cytotoxicity
		  (b) Delayed-type hypersensitivity

2. Antigen processing and presentation	2. Anti-idiotypic antibodies	2. Antibodies
		  (a) Deposition of circulating immune complexes
		  (b) *In situ* formation of immune complexes

3. Antigen recognition by helper T cells bearing heterodimeric T cell antigen receptors		*Antigen non-specific* 1. Macrophages, natural killer cells 2. Complement

in initiating the interstitial damage or in amplifying primary interstitial injury from non-immune causes. Most knowledge regarding the role of both humoral and cell-mediated immune phenomena in interstitial nephritis has been obtained from studies performed in experimental models of autoimmune interstitial nephritis. In this review, we describe a general approach to understanding immune-mediated parenchymal tissue damage, and use this approach as a framework for discussing our current understanding of the immunopathogenesis of several distinct phenotypic forms of interstitial nephritis.

MINIMAL REQUIREMENTS FOR ORGAN-SPECIFIC AUTOIMMUNITY

An immunological response targeted to parenchymal tissue antigens, such as those expressed in the tubulointerstitium, represents a complex interaction of multiple cell types and biochemical mediators whose function can be analysed at several levels. Attention has traditionally been focused on the effector mechanisms of autoimmune tissue damage, the antibodies, antigen-specific T cells, T cell products and other humoral components (such as complement) which effect tissue damage. Such an analysis, however, largely ignores host genetic and environmental factors which underlie the expression and development of these effector mechanisms. A more comprehensive approach to understanding determinants of susceptibility to an autoimmune disease utilizes the current understanding of requirements for expression of an immune response, and applies these principles to the unique environment of the tubulointerstitium.

The requirements for the generation of a T cell-dependent immune response to a parenchymal antigen (be it a native or planted antigen) can be divided into three broad categories, which encompass phases of classically described immune responses (Table 1). Since the B cell response to parenchymal tissue antigens is probably T cell-dependent, this approach is also applicable to developing antibody responses. The requirements for immune responsiveness include those events required for antigen presentation, those events which potentially regulate the development or expression of an induced immune response, and those events which serve as effector mechanisms of the immune response[6].

Implicit in the notion of antigen presentation is organ expression of the target antigen. It is now clear that renal target antigens of autoimmune responses can be polymorphic in their expression[7,8]. Such polymorphism may apply to the entire protein or be restricted to immunogenic epitopes of that protein. In addition to target antigen expression as an initial requirement for a susceptible phenotype, the target antigen must also be immunologically visible to circulating lymphocytes. Such visibility requires that the antigen should not be sequestered in an immunologically privileged site. Sequestration may be an important mechanism for maintaining tolerance to many tissue-specific antigens, which only become exposed to circulating immune cells following non-immune tissue damage. Visibility also requires that the target epitope of the antigen be non-covalently associated with major histocompatibility complex (MHC) antigens, primarily MHC Class II antigens, for presentation to CD4+ helper T cells[9].

The nature of the cells in parenchymal tissues which present antigens to T cells is currently an active area of investigation. Several organ-specific cells such as astrocytes[10], islet cells[11], and renal tubular cells[12-14], may express small amounts of MHC Class II antigens on their surface and, in some instances, function as antigen-presenting cells[10,12-16]. MHC Class II expression on many of these cells is inducible with gamma-interferon, which can be produced by infiltrating T cells and macrophages. This raises the possibility that antigen presentation by organ-specific cells may be important in amplifying an autoimmune response. MHC Class II antigen expression by parenchymal tissue cells also raises the possibility that structurally aberrant forms of MHC Class II may render immunogenic those parenchymal antigens previously recognized as self by the T cell repertoire. An alternative hypothesis is that the glycoprotein targets of autoimmune diseases are processed by traditional antigen-presenting cells, either as they traffic through the organ or as they encounter soluble antigen in a peripheral lymphoid organ.

The final major requirement for antigen presentation to helper T cells is the presence in the T cell repertoire of lymphocytes bearing heterodimeric T cell receptors which can recognize the target antigen. Thymic deletion of T cells recognizing self antigens is a classically proposed mechanism for explaining self-tolerance, which has gained recent experimental support. There is, for example, a T cell receptor $V\beta$ gene segment which preferentially recognizes murine Class II I-E MHC antigens[17]. T cells expressing this variable region, $V\beta 17a$, are deleted during thymic maturation in mice expressing the I-E gene product on cell surfaces[18]. $V\beta 17a$-bearing T cells mature and are found in the peripheral lymphoid organs of mice who do not express the I-E region gene product[18]. Whether this elegantly delineated mechanism for tolerance to self I-E antigens is applicable to parenchymal tissue antigens as well has not been determined.

Regulatory events which modulate the quantitative and qualitative expression of an induced autoimmune response may function either during the development of that immune response or after the immune response is fully formed. Such regulatory responses may be mediated by T cells[19] or anti-idiotypic antibodies[20], and have been demonstrated in several experimental models of tubulointerstitial disease to be important in determining host susceptibility.

The final phase in which the nature of the immune response can be analysed is the efferent or effector phase. This phase encompasses those mediators which result in tissue destruction. In the nephritogenic immune response these consist of antigen-specific T cells, non-specific immune effector cells (macrophages, natural killer cells), immune complexes, and tissue-specific antibodies, as well as other humoral mediators. In the following sections we will examine models of immune complex tubulointerstitial nephritis, anti-tubular basement membrane (TBM) disease mediating interstitial nephritis, and purely T cell-mediated interstitial nephritis, with particular regard to those factors determining susceptibility to disease.

IMMUNE MECHANISMS IN PHENOTYPICALLY DISTINCT FORMS OF TUBULOINTERSTITIAL NEPHRITIS

Immune complex-mediated tubulointerstitial nephritis

Immune complexes can be deposited in the tubulointerstitium both in primary tubulointerstitial disease and in diseases which also cause immune complex deposition in the glomerulus. Immune complex disease has been much more thoroughly evaluated in the context of glomerular disease. The precise role of immune complex deposition in the induction of tubulointerstitial injury is unclear. In both experimental models and human disease, the presence of discontinuous granular immune deposits along the TBM does not correlate well with either the degree of interstitial injury or the level of renal function[3,21]. Isolated tubulointerstitial nephritis following immune complex deposition is quite rare. Experimental models studying immune complex deposition in the interstitium have been developed primarily in rabbits, using homologous renal antigen in adjuvant[22], and in rats, using Tamm–Horsfall protein[21]. Rats[21,23] or mice[24] iummunized with Tamm–Horsfall protein develop immune complex deposits at the base of tubular cells in the thick ascending limb. In animals made proteinuric, anti-Tamm–Horsfall antibody will bind the luminal surfaces of these cells[25]. In some cases such immune deposits are associated with mononuclear cell infiltration[26]. It is unclear whether such immune deposits damage cells of the thick ascending limb or alter their function. There are other models in which antibodies to tubular cell antigens can be shown to induce tubular cell damage. Antibodies to Fx1A, for example, can induce tubular epithelial cell lysis in the absence of complement[27,28]. There may well be other settings, however, in which immune complexes activate complement and lead to inflammatory cell infiltrates. It has also been suggested that the location of immune deposits may influence the degree of interstitial damage[29]. Formation of deposits on the tubular side of the basement membrane appears to incite less of an inflammatory response[29].

Interstitial immune complex disease occurs in other models of chronic glomerular inflammation, for example serum sickness[29-31], Heymann nephritis[27,32], immune complex glomerulonephritis[33], and virally induced glomerulonephritis[34]. In these models, the presence of the tubulointerstitial deposits does not correlate well with the degree of renal insufficiency, and the mechanism of inflammation is unexplained.

Interstitial immune complex disease has been reported in humans, but generally not as an isolated finding, although an idiopathic form of this disease has been reported[30,35]. Approximately 50% of patients with systemic lupus erythematosus (SLE), in published studies, have tubulointerstitial deposits apparent on biopsy in association with glomerular inflammation[3,36,37]. Just as in experimental models, the degree of renal insufficiency correlates best with the degree of interstitial inflammation irrespective of immune complex deposition[3]. Other diseases associated with tubulointerstitial deposition include Sjögren's syndrome[38], and isolated cases of proliferative glomerulonephritis[39], essential mixed cryoglobulinaemia[29], and cutaneous vasculitis[40].

Anti-TBM antibody-associated interstitial nephritis

Target antigen expression and susceptibility to disease

Anti-TBM disease producing interstitial nephritis is an autoimmune disease in humans, with a well-studied experimental counterpart in rodents. In humans, linear deposition of IgG along the TBM associated with mononuclear cell infiltration of the interstitium has been identified in drug-induced tubulointerstitial nephritis (primarily as a complication of methicillin therapy[41], but other drugs have been implicated[42]), as a complication of anti-glomerular basement membrane (GBM) disease[43], in SLE[44], following renal transplantation[45,46], and as a primary or idiopathic disease[47,48]. Our understanding of the immunopathogenesis of human anti-TBM disease is scanty. It appears that the target antigen of human anti-TBM disease is highly homologous to the purified rabbit antigen used to induce experimental anti-TBM disease[49-51]. This antigen has been purified from human renal tubular basement membranes by several laboratories using different techniques[49,50]. If collagenase-solubilized human renal tubular antigen is used as a starting preparation, the target antigen recognized by human anti-TBM, but not anti-GBM, antibodies, migrates as a 48 kD protein under reducing conditions on SDS-polyacrylamide gels[49]. Solubilization of human renal tubular antigens with 6 M guanidine results in the purification of a 58 kD protein which is reactive with human anti-TBM sera[50]. It is most likely that this variability in molecular weight, as determined by SDS-PAGE, relates to the technique of isolation. Some of the size discrepancy may also represent polymorphic antigen expression of this glycoprotein antigen. Polymorphic forms of the antigen may also exist without significant M_r differences. Such polymorphisms may well underlie the observation that anti-TBM antibodies are seen periodically in recipients of renal allografts[45,46,52]. The renal allograft may express a tubular antigen which was not present on the host's native kidney, or an isoform of a common antigen to which the host is not tolerant.

Experimental anti-TBM disease is induced by immunization of susceptible strains of guinea pigs, rats, or mice with heterologous renal tubular antigen (RTA) in complete Freund's adjuvant[53-56]. The time course of the disease varies among the different species. Mononuclear cell infiltration within the tubulointerstitium can be demonstrated in immunized guinea pigs and rats 2–3 weeks following immunization, whereas such lesions take 6–8 weeks to develop in susceptible mouse strains. Circulating and deposited anti-TBM antibodies can be demonstrated, however, in all species by 1–2 weeks following immunization. By immunofluorescence, these appear as linear deposition of IgG along the proximal tubular basement membrane. The mononuclear cell infiltrate is composed of a heterogenous population of T cells, B cells, plasma cells, natural killer cells, and macrophages[57,58]. This active inflammatory lesion is eventually replaced by progressive derangement of the tubular architecture and interstitial fibrosis. The latter histological findings are accompanied by evidence of progressive and irreversible renal insufficiency.

The determinants of susceptibility to murine anti-TBM disease have been extensively studied. The glycoprotein target antigen of anti-TBM disease was originally purified from a collagenase-solubilized preparation of rabbit renal tubular antigens by immunoaffinity chromatography[51]. The antibody coupled to this resin was a monoclonal antibody which stained the proximal tubules of Brown Norway (BN) rat kidneys but not kidneys from the Lewis rat strain. It had been known for some time that the target antigen of this disease was not expressed, or was not immunologically visible, in the kidneys of Lewis rats[55]. This monoclonal antibody identifies a 48 kD glycoprotein in rabbit renal tubular basement membranes. This antigen has been called 3M-I[51] and it displays conserved antigenicity across several mammalian species, although there is some molecular-weight variation (rabbit and human, 48 kD; rat, 42 kD; mouse, 30 kD). Immunization with purified 3M-1 results in typical anti-TBM-associated interstitial nephritis[51], whereas immunization with collagenase-solubilized renal tubular antigens depleted of 3M-1 does not result in either antibody deposition or interstitial inflammation. By immunoelectron microscopy, 3M-1 can be localized to the most lateral aspect of the tubular basement membrane in proximal tubular cells[51]. The basis for non-expression of this antigen in the Lewis rat strain is an active area of investigation; it may be controlled at a transcriptional or translational level. Recently, a murine proximal tubular epithelial cell line (MCT) which synthesizes the 3M-1 antigen has been established in long-term culture[14]. mRNA from this cell line was used to construct a cDNA library, which has been screened with polyclonal antisera to 3M-1. The majority of the cDNA encoding murine 3M-1 has been sequenced[59]. The open reading frames of this cDNA sequence have been used to construct several synthetic peptides, which might be expected, on the basis of their hydrophilicity and alpha-helical configuration, to be immunogenic peptides. One of these peptides is recognized by both CD4+ (helper) and CD8+ (effector) 3M-1-reactive T cell lines, as well as by a monoclonal anti-3M-1 antibody[59]. These findings raise the possibility that expression of the 3M-1 glycoprotein, as defined by immunofluorescence, may reflect the presence or absence of a very small region of the entire glycoprotein.

In induced anti-TBM disease, antigen presentation to T cells probably occurs largely in the peripheral lymphoid organs, since both T and B cells reactive with RTA can be isolated from draining lymph nodes and spleen within 7 days following immunization[60]. However, in considering how the education of T cells occurs in a spontaneous disease, one must consider the possibility that renal cells actually present target antigens, such as 3M-1, to circulating T cells. Recent studies support the notion that renal tubular epithelial cells can act as antigen-presenting cells under defined circumstances. Studies performed using the MCT cells have shown that antigen presentation by tubular epithelium conforms to models derived from studies with conventional antigen-presenting cells[15,58]. T cell recognition of 3M-1 synthesized by the MCT cells is dependent on both antigen and MHC Class II expression, and utilizes CD4 associative recognition determinants. Such local antigen presentation by parenchymal tissue cells may become even more important in the chronic phase of autoimmune injury, when infiltrating inflammatory cells can potentially augment MHC Class II expression through the release of gamma-interferon[61].

Thymic deletion does not appear to be a relevant mechanism for determining non-susceptibility to anti-TBM disease in either the B or T cell compartment. All strains of inbred rodents that have been examined thus far are able to mount anti-TBM responses following immunization, regardless of whether they develop interstitial nephritis[7,54]. The situation with RTA-reactive T cells is more complicated. The expression of RTA-reactive T cells from strains of rats susceptible and non-susceptible to anti-TBM disease has been evaluated[62]. These two strains (BN and Lewis) differ in that Lewis rats, as mentioned previously, do not express the 3M-1 antigen in the renal tubule. One might therefore expect that animals expressing the target antigen (BN) would have deleted 3M-1-reactive T cells from their repertoire. If one examines peripheral lymphocytes from BN and Lewis rats immunized with BN RTA, there is a distinct difference in T cell reactivity. Draining lymph node cells from Lewis rats demonstrate delayed-type hypersensitivity (DTH) reactivity to BN RTA in acute adoptive transfer assays, whereas similarly prepared lymphocytes from BN rats do not demonstrate such reactivity[62]. The absence of this reactivity, however, is not due to thymic deletion but rather to the presence of RTA-specific suppressor cells in the BN rat. This can be confirmed by demonstrating suppression of the Lewis DTH response by lymphocytes from genetically compatible, RTA-immunized, 3M-1-expressing rats[62]. One can also show that BN lymphocytes depleted of suppressor cells demonstrate DTH reactivity to 3M-1, and that BN rats treated with low-dose cyclophosphamide (a manoeuvre which eliminates suppressor cells) are susceptible to disease[62]. These studies suggest that thymic deletion may not be the only mechanism by which tolerance to parenchymal self antigens is maintained; there may also be an important role for regulatory T cells.

Events modulating the expression of the induced anti-3M-1 immune response

There is clearly an important role for regulatory T cells in the differentiation of 3M-1-specific T cells in mice susceptible and non-susceptible to anti-TBM disease. Susceptibility to anti-TBM disease in mice is an autosomally dominant trait which maps to the MHC Class I H-2K^{s,d} locus[54]. In susceptible strains of mice, the 3M-1-specific effector T cells found within the interstitial infiltrate (as well as in peripheral lymphoid organs) are CD8+, CD4− T cells genetically restricted by MHC Class I antigens. These T cells also bear idiotypes cross-reactive with those found on antibodies eluted from nephritic kidneys[63]. This 3M-1-reactive CD8 + subpopulation demonstrates cytotoxicity towards monolayers of renal tubular epithelial cells[54], and induces interstitial nephritis within 7 days following subcapsular transfer to naive syngeneic mice[60,63]. The CD8+ subpopulation is also reactive in DTH responses to 3M-1 following adoptive transfer to syngeneic mice[63]. The cytotoxic T cells and the DTH-reactive T cells probably represent distinct CD8+ clonal subpopulations, both which are antigen-specific.

Although non-susceptible mice mount an anti-TBM antibody response which is indistinguishable from that of susceptible mice (see below), they do not develop interstitial infiltrates. This absence of interstitial infiltrates, however, does not represent an absence of 3M-1-specific T cells[63]. Non-susceptible strains of mice do develop 3M-1-specific T cells, but the phenotype of these effector cells is CD4+, CD8−. Studies have established that both CD8+ and CD4+ T cell subpopulations are present in peripheral lymph nodes following immunization with RTA/CFA in both susceptible and non-susceptible strains of mice[63]. The critical determinant of non-susceptibility is the selective maturation of CD4+ effector cells. Conversely, the critical determinant of susceptibility is the selective maturation of CD8+ effector cells. Both CD4+ and CD8+ 3M-1-specific T cells recognize tubular antigen and mediate DTH responses in the skin following the antigen challenge. CD4+ T cells, however, do not infiltrate and destroy the renal tubulointerstitium following transfer into syngeneic mice. These CD4+ T cells are MHC Class II restricted (I-A), and do not express the cross-reactive idiotype[63]. In large part, their lack of nephritogenicity may relate to the low basal levels of MHC Class II antigen expression by the renal tubular epithelium. Recent studies have shown that if such MHC Class II expression is first augmented by injections of gamma-interferon, then the CD4+ T cells are capable of mediating an inflammatory interstitial lesion[64].

Given the observation that both CD4+ and CD8+ 3M-1-specific T cells initially differentiate in both susceptible and non-susceptible strains of mice, one must explain the preferential selection of each phenotype in different strains. This selection process itself appears to be mediated by 3M-1-specific regulatory T cells, whose expression differs in susceptible and non-susceptible strains[65]. Both susceptible and non-susceptible strains express a 3M-1-specific CD8+ suppressor T cell whose function is to suppress the potentially self-injurious CD8+ effector cells. This suppression allows, in non-susceptible mice, for the preferential development of CD4+ effector cells[65]. In susceptible mice, however, these suppressor cells are counteracted by another regulatory T cell subpopulation, the Vicia Villosa lectin-adherent contrasuppressor cells, which negate suppressor cell function and allow for preferential maturation of CD8 + T cells[66]. Therefore, differential regulation of T cell differentiation appears to be a critical factor in determining susceptibility to this disease.

There are multiple means by which the expression of CD8 + T cells and the inflammatory interstitial lesion can be inhibited. These immunosuppressive regimens include both antigen-non-specific and antigen-specific modalities. The non-specific immunosuppressive modalities which are effective in experimental anti-TBM disease include cyclophosphamide[67], cyclosporin[68], prostaglandin E_1 [69], and protein-caloric restriction[70]. PGE_1 inhibits an early step in the differentiation of CD8 + effector cells. This inhibition can be overcome by recombitant IL-1[69]. Antigen-specific immunosuppression has been achieved by a variety of techniques, including immunization with large amounts of tubular antigen in incomplete Freund's adjuvant[71], injection of tubular antigen-reactive T lymphoblasts which bear a cross-reactive idiotype[20], anti-idiotypic antisera[72], and induced suppressor T cell networks[19,73]. Suppressor T cells can be induced in susceptible mice following intravenous injection of splenocytes to which tubular antigens have been chemically coupled with 1-ethyl-3-(3-dimethylaminopropyl)-carbodiimide[73]. Such antigen presentation induces two types of suppressor T cells which are phenotypically and functionally distinct[73]. Suppressor inducer cells bear the CD4 + phenotype and express a cross-reactive idiotype[73]. These cells inhibit an early stage in the differentiation of the CD8 + nephritogenic effector cells, and also function to induce a population of CD8 + suppressor effector lymphocytes[19,73]. Suppression by the CD4 + suppressor cells is mediated by an antigen-binding soluble protein factor[74] that bears variable-region gene products of the T cell receptor. Suppression by this soluble protein requires prostaglandin synthesis as well as new mRNA and protein synthesis[75]. The CD8 + suppressor cells acutely inhibit the function of fully formed nephritogenic effector cells through a non-cytotoxic mechanism. This suppression is also mediated by a soluble, cell-derived protein. These suppressor effector cells down-regulate anti-TBM disease even if transferred to an animal following disease onset[76]. Thus, they represent a potentially important therapeutic strategy in autoimmune disease.

Effector mechanisms in anti-TBM disease

If B and T cells of the appropriate antigenic specificity have been allowed to differentiate and contact their target antigen within the tubulointerstitium, what then are the mechanisms by which these immune products cause tissue injury? A number of studies have suggested that the deposition of anti-TBM antibodies alone is insufficient to cause interstitial nephritis[7,54,69,71]. Antibody titres, expression of the cross-reactive idiotype, and epitopic specificity of the anti-TBM antibody response do not distinguish antibody responses in susceptible and non-susceptible strains of mice[77]. Moreover, a variety of immunosuppressive modalities have been described which selectively inhibit the 3M-1-specific T cell response but not the antibody response, with effective suppression of interstitial inflammation. Although, in some species, serum from immune animals is capable of transferring interstitial nephritis, this does not necessarily mean that the damage is due to antibody deposition alone. Transferred antibody may induce antigen-specific T cells which are then capable of causing interstitial inflammation. Antibody deposition may, however, have other important effects on the target tubuloepithelium. Recent studies have shown that anti-TBM antibodies are capable of inhibiting Class II expression by murine proximal tubular epithelial cells in culture, implying that anti-TBM antibodies may further serve to protect the host from autoimmunity by suppressing already low levels of MHC Class II antigen[64]. Antibodies to tubular cell antigens may also alter other tubular cell functions, such as ion transport, without causing overt cell injury.

Activation of complement has also been implicated in the anti-TBM immune response, as complement components are frequently identified along the TBM by immunofluorescence[78]. Complement depletion is protective in certain species immunized to produce anti-TBM disease[78]. It has also been demonstrated that anti-TBM antibodies can act as an informational bridge between the humoral and cellular immune response via antibody-dependent cell-mediated cytotoxicity[79].

The underlying mechanisms of CD8 + T cell injury are active areas of investigation. It seems likely that CD8 + DTH-reactive T cells produce a local hypersensitivity response within the kidney, with influx of macrophages and other antigen-non-specific inflammatory cells. Macrophages elaborate a number of secretory products, such as collagenases, elastases, and lysozymes, which are capable of tissue damage[80]. Cytotoxic T cells may also play a role in the tubular cell destruction and resultant tubular atrophy seen in this disease. Recent investigations into the mechanisms of cytotoxicity by T cells have established a role for serine proteases[81], which can form pores in cell membranes much like the activated membrane attack complex of the complement cascade[81]. Cytotoxicity provides a direct explanation for tubular drop-out. There may also be more subtle mechanisms by which cytotoxic cells injure epithelium expressing the target antigen. At low effector:target ratios, for example, these CD8 + T cells may release cytokines which affect basement membrane synthesis, alter tubular cell function, or stimulate the proliferation of interstitial fibroblasts[82].

T cell-mediated tubulointerstitial nephritis

Many cases of human tubulointerstitial nephritis display mononuclear cell infiltrates without specific antibody deposition. Such findings suggest that the interstitial injury is predominantly accounted for by cell-mediated mechanisms of interstitial injury. Evidence for cell-mediated immunity in human interstitial nephritis is derived primarily from analysis of mononuclear infiltrates within the tubulointerstitium. Phenotypic evaluation of these cells by several investigators has exhibited a predominance of T cells and macrophages, with fewer B cells and mature plasma cells[36,83,84]. Both CD4 + and CD8 + T cell subsets have been identified in these infiltrates. The predominant subset expressed, however, has varied between study groups and the underlying aetiology of the interstitial nephritis, be it drug-induced or infection-related. The predominant T cell population may also be related to specific therapy prior to biopsy, or to the particular stage of disease at the time of biopsy[36]. In addition to T cell-specific determinants, expression of MHC Class II antigens has been noted, suggesting activation of infiltrating cells[85]. More extensive characterization of functional properties of the infiltrating T cells, as well as target renal tubular antigens, has been problematic in humans. Investigators have noted Tamm–Horsfall protein deposition within interstitial infiltrates in several tubulointerstitial diseases, including medullary cystic disease, chronic obstructive pyelonephritis, hydronephrosis, and chronic idiopathic tubulointerstitial nephritis[86]. Whether this protein represents a target antigen for infiltrating T cells is unclear.

Many drugs, as well as bacterial and viral infections, have been associated with interstitial nephritis in humans[36,87]. In addition to analysis of the infiltrating mononuclear cells by immunofluorescence, cell-mediated immunity has been implicated by the findings of both *in vivo* (DTH) and *in vitro* (lymphoblast transformation) evidence of hypersensitivity to specific inciting antigens[87,88]. It has been postulated that chemical or infection-related disease may represent an immune response directed against altered endogenous antigens. Alternatively, interstitial injury caused by either drugs or infectious agents may expose antigens previously 'sequestered' from the immune system. These may be antigens to which the host is not tolerant. Exploration of this hypothesis in either drug- or infection-induced disease, however, has been hampered by the lack of an experimental model.

Cell-mediated immunity is clearly important in human allograft rejection. Allograft rejection appears to be dependent on MHC determinants on the host's native organs, as well as on donor-passenger lymphoctyes contained within the allograft. T cells derived from rejected allografts in animal models or human transplants demonstrate donor-specific cytotoxicity[89,90]. In some cases this cytotoxicity has been shown to be directed against specific MHC Class I determinants of the allograft donor. There may also be other, non-MHC, renal allograft antigens to which the host mounts an immune response. Since MHC Class II expression can be increased in the kidney in any setting associated with inflammatory cell infiltrates[91], it is possible that some aspects of allograft rejection are 'autoimmune'. As it is largely unknown whether non-MHC, kidney-specific antigens are polymorphic in the human, one can only speculate as to how many of these antigens may be able to stimulate an immune response following engraftment.

Experimental models of cell-mediated interstitial nephritis

There are several rodent models of primarily cell-mediated interstitial nephritis. Initial studies demonstrated interstitial inflammation without antibody deposition after challenge with intrarenal aggregated antigen[92], and (in Lewis rats) following immunization with syngeneic renal tissue in complete Freund's adjuvant[93]. The Lewis rat, a strain which does not express the relevant antigen of anti-TBM disease, can develop interstitial nephritis following immunization with homologous renal basement membranes derived from a strain which does express the 3M-1 antigen (the BN rat). The natural history of the disease is characterized by focal mononuclear cell infiltrates during the second week, with progressive cortical involvement[94]. By the fourth week following immunization, infiltrates begin to abate, with evidence, however, of tubular destruction and some peritubular fibrosis. Biochemical abnormalities consist of an elevated creatinine 14 days after immunization which improves towards control values by day 28. Proteinuria and glycosuria are not apparent during this time[53,94].

Although the Lewis rat mounts a significant antibody response following immunization with homologous renal antigen, significant TBM or GBM IgG fixation is not found in diseased kidneys. Areas of inflammation consist of mononuclear cells which express MHC Class II determinants[53]. A large portion of these infiltrating cells also express T cell-specific determinants. Activated T cells, therefore, constitute a significant percentage of cells in this inflammatory lesion. Not unexpectively, disease cannot be transferred with immune serum, but intravenous transfer of B cell-depleted spleen cells from immunized Lewis rats induces disease in naive recipients within 7 days. The histology of transferred disease is identical to that of active disease, although the interstitial lesions occur more readily in the former[53]. The specific target renal tubular antigen of this disease has not been isolated. Indeed, it is interesting that preliminary studies have noted that lymph node cells from immunized Lewis rats demonstrate significant proliferative responses *in vitro* to the immunogenic renal tubular antigens derived from animals which express the anti-TBM disease target antigen, but only minimal proliferation to autologous Lewis rat renal basement membrane antigen[53]. An alteration in endogenous renal tubular antigen may, perhaps, be instrumental in cell-mediated disease induction. There are other studies which have not demonstrated this lesion in Lewis rats after immunization with BN antigen, but the immunization regimen and adjuvant used were different[62].

Another model of cell-mediated disease has been studied extensively in mice. kdkd mice, a mutant subline of the CBA/Ca strain, develop a spontaneous and progressive tubulointerstitial nephritis[95]. Transmission of this disease follows an autosomal recessive pattern with high penetrance[95]. The animals appear normal at birth, but disease develops predictably at 8 weeks of age. Histologically the lesions begin with peritubular mononuclear cell infiltrates and tubular dilatation in the cortex. The progressive nature of the disease is evident, however, with eventual tubular drop-out and interstitial fibrosis. Death usually occurs by 20–28 weeks of life from uraemia[95,96].

Humoral immunity does not appear to contribute significantly to the immunopathogenesis of this disease, as no renal-specific antibodies in serum or kidney have been isolated from diseased animals[96]. Cell-mediated immunity has been implicated not only by the presence of mononuclear cell infiltrates but also by the demonstration of disease transfer through radiation bone-marrow chimaeras and by protection from disease following thymectomy[96]. The specific target renal tubular antigen in this disease is distinct from the 3M-1 glycoprotein of anti-TBM disease, and appears to be a 56 kD glycoprotein (C. Kelly, unpublished observations). Tubular antigen-reactive immune cells have been isolated from peripheral lymph nodes and kidneys of diseased kdkd mice[97]. The predominant effector T cell population in these isolates are CD8 + T cells which are MHC Class I restricted (H-2K^k)[97]. This CD8 + population from nephritic kdkd mice not only mediates DTH responses to CBA/Ca renal tubular antigen, but also produces typical infiltrating lesions in the tubulointerstitium following subcapsular transfer of cells[97].

The immune regulation of this spontaneous nephritogenic response remains an area of continued investigation. As suppressor T cells in anti-TBM disease have clearly been implicated in abrogating expression of disease, similar studies of suppression have been conducted in kdkd mice. T cell preparations from the non-disease prone CBA/Ca strain suppress the tubulointerstitial nephritis in kdkd mice[98]. Interestingly, however, T cells with identical suppressor function have been isolated from kdkd mice. Therefore, disease induction is not simply a result of deletion of suppressor cells from the T cell repertoire in kdkd mice. Further characterization of T cell subpopulations in nephritic animals has revealed the presence of antigen-specific contrasuppressor T cells, which function to inhibit the antigen-specific T suppressor cells and therefore allow the expression of the nephritogenic effector cells[98]. The absence of disease in CBA/Ca mice, therefore, is not due to a lack of tubular antigen-reactive effector cells, as the presence of such cells can be demonstrated either by deleting the suppressor cells in CBA/Ca mice or by admixing contrasuppressor cells from kdkd mice to CBA/Ca splenocytes[98]. Protection from disease in these mice is due to the predominant expression of antigen-specific suppressor cells and the relative absence of contrasuppression, which, on the balance, maintain tolerance to this self antigen. These findings, as discussed earlier in the section on anti-TBM disease, argue strongly against a thymic deletion model as the sole means for maintaining tolerance to parenchymal self antigens. They do not rule out, however, the possibility that thymic deletion may eliminate the majority of self-reactive cells, with the remaining cells being kept under control by the actions of regulatory T cells.

References

1. Cotran, R. S., Rubin, R. H. and Tolkoff-Rubin, N. E. (1986). *Tubulointerstitial Diseases*. In Brenner, B. M. and Rector, F. C. (eds.) *The Kidney*, pp. 1143–1173. (Philadelphia: W. B. Saunders)
2. Sloper, J. C., de Wardener, H. and Woodrow, D. F. (1980). Relationship between renal structure and function derived from renal biopsies. In Leaf, A., Giebisch, G., Bolis, L., Gorini, S. (eds.) *Renal Pathophysiology*, pp. 109–120. (New York: Raven Press)
3. Park, M. H., D'Agati, V., Appel, G. B. and Pirani, C. L. (1986). Tubulointerstitial disease in lupus nephritis: Relationship to immune deposits, interstitial inflammation, glomerular changes, renal function, and prognosis. *Nephron*, **44**, 309–319
4. Risdon, R. A., Sloper, J. C. and de Wardener, H. E. (1968). Relationship between renal function and histological changes found in renal biopsy specimens from patients with persistent glomerular nephritis. *Lancet*, **1**, 363–366
5. Rosenbaum, J. L. (1974). Evaluation of clearance studies in lupus nephritis. *Clin. Nephrol.*, **2**, 47–51
6. Neilson, E. G. and Zakheim, B. (1983). T cell regulation, anti-idiotypic immunity, and the nephritogenic immune response. *Kidney Int.*, **24**, 289–302
7. Neilson, E. G., Gasser, D. L., McCafferty, E., Zakheim, B. and Phillips, S. M. (1983). Polymorphism of genes involved in anti-tubular basement membrane disease in rats. *Immunogenetics*, **17**, 55–65
8. Kleppel, M. M., Kashtan, C. E., Butkowski, R. J., Fish, A. J. and Michael, A. F. (1987). Alport familial nephritis. Absence of 28 kilodalton non-collagenous monomers of type IV

collagen in glomerular basement membrane. *J. Clin. Invest.*, **80**, 263–266

9. Dialynas, D. P., Wilde, D. B., Marrack, P., Pierres, A., Wall, K. A., Havran, W., Otten, G., Loken, M. R., Pierres, M., Kappler, J. and Fitch, F. W. (1983). Characterization of the murine antigenic determinant, designated L3T4a, recognized by monoclonal antibody GK1.5; expression of L3T4a by functional T cell clones appears to correlate primarily with Class II MHC antigen-reactivity. *Immunol. Rev.*, **74**, 29–56

10. Fierz, W., Endler, B., Reske, K., Wekerle, H. and Fontano, A. (1985). Astrocytes as antigen-presenting cells. I. Induction of Ia antigen expression on astrocytes by T cells via immune interferon and its effects on antigen presentation. *J. Immunol.*, **134**, 3785–3793

11. Steiniger, B., Klempnauer, J. and Wonigeit, K. (1985). Altered distribution of class I and class II MHC antigens during acute pancreas allograft rejection in the rat. *Transplantation*, **40**, 234–239

12. Mayrhofer, G. and Schon-Hegrad, M. A. (1983). Ia antigens in rat kidney, with special reference to their expression in tubular epithelium. *J. Exp. Med.*, **157**, 2097–2109

13. Halloran, P. F., Wadgymar, A. and Autenried, P. (1986). The regulation of expression of major histocompatibility complex products. *Transplantation*, **41**, 413–420

14. Haverty, T. P., Kelly, C. J., Hines, W. H., Amenta, P. S., Watanabe, M., Harper, R. A., Kefalides, N. A. and Neilson, E. G. (1988). Characterization of a renal tubular epithelial cell line which secretes the autologous target antigen of autoimmune experimental interstitial nephritis. *J. Cell Biol.*, **107**, 1359–1368

15. Hines, H. W., Haverty, T. P., Elias, J. A., Neilson, E. G. and Kelly, C. J. (1989). T cell recognition of epithelial self. *Autoimmunity*, **5**, 37–47

16. Wuthrich, R. P., Glimcher, L. H. and Kelley, V. E. (1989). Antigen presenting capacity of MHC class II positive proximal tubular cells in MRL/lpr mice with lupus nephritis. *Kidney Int.*, **35**, 366a

17. Kappler, J. W., Wade, T., White, J., Kushnir, E., Blackman, M., Bill, J., Roehm, N. and Marrack, P. (1987). A T cell receptor Vβ segment that imparts reactivity to a class II major histocompatibility complex product. *Cell*, **49**, 263–271

18. Kappler, J. W., Roehm, N. and Marrack, P. (1987). T cell tolerance by clonal elimination in the thymus. *Cell*, **49**, 273–280

19. Kelly, C. J., Clayman, M. D., Hines, W. H. and Neilson, E. G. (1987). Therapeutic immune regulation in experimental interstitial nephritis with suppressor T cells and their soluble factors. *Ciba Foundation Symposia*, **129**, 73–87

20. Neilson, E. G. and Phillips, S. M. (1982). Suppression of interstitial nephritis by auto-anti-idiotypic immunity. *J. Exp. Med.*, **155**, 179–189

21. Hoyer, J. H. (1980). Tubulointerstitial immune complex nephritis in rats immunized with Tamm–Horsfall protein. *Kidney Int.*, **17**, 284–292

22. Klassen, J., Milgrom, F. M. and McCluskey, R. T. (1977). Studies of the antigens involved in immunologic renal tubular lesions in rabbits. *Am. J. Pathol.*, **88**, 135–141

23. Seiler, M. W. and Hoyer, J. R. (1981). Ultrastructural studies of tubulointerstitial immune complex nephritis in rats immunized with Tamm–Horsfall protein. *Lab. Invest.*, **45**, 321–327

24. Fasth, A., Hoyer, J. R. and Seiler, M. W. (1982). Renal tubular immune complex formation in mice immunized with Tamm–Horsfall protein. *Am. J. Pathol.*, **125**, 555–562

25. Ishidate, T., Hoyer, J. R. and Seiler, M. W. (1983). Influence of altered glomerular permeability on renal tubular immune complex formation and clearance. *Lab. Invest.*, **49**, 582–588

26. Friedman, J., Hoyer, J. R. and Seiler, M. W. (1982). Formation and clearance of tubulointerstitial immune complexes in kidneys of rats immunized with heterologous antisera to Tamm–Horsfall protein. *Kidney Int.*, **21**, 575–582

27. Noble, B., Mendrick, D. L., Brentjens, J. R. and Andres, G. A. (1981). Antibody-mediated injury to proximal tubules in the rat kidney induced by passive transfer of homologous anti-brush border serum. *Clin. Immunol. Immunopathol.*, **19**, 289–301

28. Noble, B., Andres, G. A. and Brentjens, J. R. (1983). Passively transferred anti-brush border antibodies induce injury of proximal tubules in the absence of complement. *Clin. Exp. Immunol.*, **56**, 281–288

29. McCluskey, R. T. (1983). Immunologically mediated tubulointerstitial nephritis. *Contemp. Issues Nephrol.*, **10**, 121–149

30. Andres, G. A. and McCluskey, R. T. (1975). Tubular and interstitial renal disease due to immunologic mechanisms. *Kidney Int.*, **13**, 271–289

31. Brentjens, J., O'Connell, D. W. and Pawlowski, I. B. (1974). Extra-glomerular lesions associated with deposition of circulating antigen–antibody complexes in kidneys of rabbits with chronic serum sickness. *Clin. Immunol. Immunopathol.*, **3**, 112–126
32. Allison, M. E., Wilson, C. B. and Gottchalk, C. W. (1974). Pathophysiology of experimental glomerulonephritis in rats. *J. Clin. Invest.*, **53**, 1402–1423
33. Couser, W. G. (1985). Mechanism of glomerular injury in immune-complex disease. *Kidney Int.*, **28**, 569–583
34. Smith, R. D. and Wehner, R. W. (1980). Acute cytomegalovirus glomerulonephritis: An experimental model. *Lab. Invest.*, **43**, 278–286
35. Spital, A., Panner, B. J. and Sterns, R. H. (1987). Primary acute idiopathic tubulointerstitial nephritis: Report of two cases and review of the literature. *Am. J. Kidney Dis.*, **9**, 710–718
36. Cameron, J. S. (1989). Immunologically mediated interstitial nephritis: Primary and secondary. *Adv. Nephrol.*, **18**, 207–248
37. Magil, A. B. and Tyler, M. (1984). Tubulointerstitial disease in lupus nephritis: A morphometric study. *Histopathology*, **8**, 81–87
38. Winer, R. L., Cohen, A. H., Sawhney, A. S. and Gorman, J. T. (1977). Sjogren's Syndrome with immune-complex tubulointerstitial renal disease. *Clin. Immunol. Immunopathol.*, **8**, 494–503
39. Lehman, D. H. and Dixon, F. J. (1975). Extra-glomerular immunoglobulin deposits in human nephritis. *Am. J. Med.*, **58**, 765–796
40. Nojimi, Y., Terai, C., Takehara, K., Yamanda, A. and Takaku, F. (1986). Tubulointerstitial immune complex nephritis in a patient with cutaneous vasculitis. *Clin. Nephrol.*, **25**, 48–51
41. Border, W. A., Lehman, D. H., Egan, J. D., Sass, H. J., Glode, J. E. and Wilson, C. B. (1974). Anti-tubular basement membrane antibodies in methicillin-associated interstitial nephritis. *N. Engl. J. Med.*, **291**, 381–384
42. Hyman, L. R., Ballow, M. and Knieser, M. R. (1978). Diphenylhydantoin interstitial nephritis. Roles of cellular and humoral immunologic injury. *J. Pediatr.*, **92**, 915–920
43. Andres, G., Brentjens, J., Kohli, R., Antone, S., Beliah, T., Montes, M., Mookeigie, B. K., Prezyna, A., Sepulveda, M., Venuto, R. and Elwood, C. (1978). Histology of human tubulointerstitial nephritis associated with antibodies to renal basement membranes. *Kidney Int.*, **13**, 480–491
44. Makker, S. P. (1980). Tubular basement membrane antibody-induced interstitial nephritis in systemic lupus erythematosus. *Am. J. Med.*, **79**, 949–952
45. Klassen, J., Kano, K., Milgrom, F., Menno, A. B., Anthone, S., Anthone, K., Sepulveda, M., Elwood, C. M. and Andres, G. A. (1973). Tubular lesions produced by autoantibodies in tubular basement membrane in human allografts. *Int. Arch. Allergy Appl. Immunol.*, **45**, 675–689
46. Roteller, C., Noel, L. H., Droz, D., Kreis, H. and Berger, J. (1986). Role of antibodies against tubular basement membranes in human renal transplantation. *Am. J. Kidney Dis.*, **7**, 157–161
47. Graber, M. L., Logan, M. G. and Connor, D. G. (1978). Idiopathic acute interstitial nephritis. *West. J. Med.*, **129**, 72–76
48. Cattran, D. C. (1980). Circulating anti-tubular basement membrane antibody in a variety of human renal diseases. *Nephron*, **26**, 13–19
49. Clayman, M. D., Michaud, L., Brentjens, J., Andres, G. A., Kefalides, N. A. and Neilson, E. G. (1986). Isolation of the target antigen in human anti-tubular basement membrane nephritis. *J. Clin. Invest.*, **77**, 1143–1147
50. Fliger, F. D., Wieslander, J., Brentjens, J. R., Andres, G. A. and Butkowski, R. J. (1987). Identification of a target antigen in human anti-tubular basement membrane nephritis. *Kidney Int.*, **31**, 800–807
51. Clayman, M., Martinez-Hernandez, A., Michaud, L., Alper, R., Mann, R., Kefalides, N. A. and Neilson, E. G. (1985). Isolation and characterization of the nephritogenic antigen producing anti-tubular basement membrane disease. *J. Exp. Med.*, **161**, 290–305
52. Wilson, C. B., Lehman, D. H., McCoy, R. C. *et al.* (1974). Antitubular basement membrane antibody after renal transplantation. *Transplantation*, **18**, 447–431
53. Bannister, K. M., Ulich, T. R. and Wilson, C. B. (1988). Immunological mechanisms in experimental models of tubulointerstitial nephritis. In Davison, A. M. (ed.) *Nephrology*, pp. 618–635. (London: Ballière Tindall)
54. Neilson, E. G. and Phillips, S. M. (1982). Murine Interstitial Nephritis. I. Analysis of disease susceptibility and its relationship to pleomorphic gene products defining both immune-response genes and a restrictive requirement for cytotoxic T cells at H-2K. *J. Exp. Med.*, **155**, 1075–1085

55. Lehman, D. H., Wilson, C. B. and Dixon, F. J. (1974). Interstitial nephritis in rats immunized with heterologous tubular basement membrane. *Kidney Int.*, **5**, 187–195
56. Neilson, E. G. and Phillips, S. M. (1979). Cell-mediated immunity in interstitial nephritis. I. T lymphocyte systems in nephritic guinea pigs: the natural history and diversity of the immune response. *J. Immunol.*, **123**, 2373–2378
57. Mampaso, F. M. and Wilson, C. B. (1983). Characterization of inflammatory cells in autoimmune tubulointerstitial nephritis in rats. *Kidney Int.*, **23**, 448–457
58. Zakheim, B., McCafferty, E., Phillips, S. M., Clayman, M. D. and Neilson, E. G. (1984). Murine interstitial nephritis. II. The adoptive transfer of disease with immune T lymphocytes produces a phenotypically complex interstitial lesion. *J. Immunol.*, **133**, 324
59. Neilson, E. G., Sun, M. J., Emery, J., Kelly, C. J., Haverty, T., Clayman, M. and Cooke, N. (1991). Molecular characterization of a major nephritogenic domain in the autoantigen of anti-tubular basement membrane disease. *Proc. Natl. Acad. Sci. USA*, **88**, 2006–2010
60. Mann, R., Zakheim, B., Clayman, M., McCafferty, E., Michaud, L. and Neilson, E. (1985). Murine interstitial nephritis. IV. Long-term cultured L3T4$^+$ T cell lines transfer delayed expression of disease as I-A-restricted inducers of the effector T cell repertoire. *J. Immunol.*, **135**, 286–293
61. Wadgymar, A., Urmson, J., Baumal, R. and Halloran, P. F. (1984). Changes in Ia expression in mouse kidney during acute graft-vs-host disease. *J. Immunol.*, **132**, 1826–1832
62. Kelly, C. J., Silvers, W. K. and Neilson, E. G. (1985). Tolerance to parenchymal self. Regulatory role of major histocompatibility complex-restricted OX8$^+$ suppresor T cells specific for autologous renal tubular antigen in experimental interstitial nephritis. *J. Exp. Med.*, **162**, 1892–1903
63. Neilson, E. G., McCafferty, E., Mann, R., Michaud, L. and Clayman, M. (1985). Murine interstitial nephritis. III. The selection of phenotypic (Lyt and L3T4) and idiotypic (RE-Id) T cell preferences by genes in Igh-1 and H-2K characterizes the cell-mediated potential for disease expression: Susceptible mice provide a unique effector T cell repertoire in response to tubular antigen. *J. Immunol.*, **134**, 2375–2382
64. Haverty, T. P., Watanabe, M., Neilson, E. G., and Kelly, C. J. (1989). Protective modulation of class II MHC gene expression in tubular epithelium by target antigen-specific antibodies. *J. Immunol.*, **143**, 1133–1141
65. Mann, R., Kelly, C. J., Hines, W. H., Clayman, M., Blanchard, N., Sun, M. J. and Neilson, E. G. (1987). Effector T cell differentiation in experimental interstitial nephritis. I. The development and modulation of effector lymphocyte maturation by I-J$^+$ regulatory T cells. *J. Immunol.*, **136**, 4200–4208
66. Kelly, C. J., Mok, H. and Neilson, E. G. (1988). The selection of effector T cell phenotype by contrasuppression modulates susceptibility to autoimmune injury. *J. Immunol.*, **141**, 3022–3028
67. Agus, D., Mann, R., Clayman, M. D., Kelly, C. J., Michaud, L. and Neilson, E. G. (1986). The effects of daily cyclophosphamide administration on the development and extent of primary experimental interstitial nephritis in rats. *Kidney Int.*, **29**, 635–640
68. Shih, W., Hines, W. H. and Neilson, E. G. (1988). Effects of cyclosporin A on the development of immune-mediated interstitial nephritis. *Kidney Int.*, **33**, 1113–1118
69. Kelly, C. J., Zurier, R. B., Krakauer, K. A., Blanchard, N. and Neilson, E. G. (1987). PGE-1 inhibits effector T cell induction and histologic disease in experimental murine interstitial nephritis. *J. Clin. Invest.*, **79**, 782–789
70. Agus, D., Mann, R., Cohn, D., Michaud, L., Kelly, C. J., Clayman, M. and Neilson, E. G. (1985). Inhibitory role of dietary protein restriction on the development and expression of immune mediated anti-tubular basement membrane induced tubulointerstitial nephritis in rats. *J. Clin. Invest.*, **76**, 930–936
71. Kelly, C. J., Clayman, M. D. and Neilson, E. G. (1986). Immunoregulation in experimental interstitial nephritis: Immunization with renal tubular antigen in incomplete Freund's adjuvant induces major histocompatibility complex-restricted, OX8$^+$ suppressor T cells which are antigen-specific and inhibit the expression of disease. *J. Immunol.*, **136**, 903–907
72. Clayman, M. D., Sun, M. J., Michaud, L., Brill-Dashoff, J., Riblet, R. and Neilson, E. G. (1988). Clonotypic heterogeneity in experimental interstitial nephritis. Restricted specificity of the anti-tubular basement membrane B cell repertoire is associated with a disease-modifying cross-reactive idiotype. *J. Exp. Med.*, **167**, 1296–1312

73. Neilson, E. G., McCafferty, E., Mann, R., Michaud, L. and Clayman, M. (1985). Tubular antigen-derivatized cells induce a disease protective, antigen-specific, and idiotype-specific suppressor T cell network restricted by I-J and Igh-V in mice with experimental interstitial nephritis. *J. Exp. Med.*, **162**, 215–230

74. Neilson, E. G., Kelly, C. J., Clayman, M. D., Hines, W. H., Haverty, T., Sun, M. J. and Blanchard, N. (1987). Murine interstitial nephritis VII. Suppression of renal injury following treatment with soluble suppressor factor TsF₁. *J. Immunol.*, **139**, 1518–1535

75. Kelly, C. J. and Neilson, E. G. (1989). Recognition of murine suppressor-inducer T cells and inhibition of their function by anti-2H4 antibodies. *Kidney Int.*, **35**, 352a

76. Mann, R. and Neilson, E. G. (1986). Murine intestitial nephritis V. The auto-induction of antigen-specific Lyt-2⁺ suppressor T cells diminishes the expression of interstitial nephritis in mice with antitubular basement membrane disease. *J. Immunol.*, **136**, 908–912

77. Clayman, M., Michaud, L. and Neilson, E. G. (1987). Murine interstitial nephritis VI. Characterization of the B cell response in anti-tubular basement membrane disease. *J. Immunol.*, **139**, 2242–2249

78. Rudofsky, V. H., McMaster, P., Ma, W. and Pollara, B. (1974). Experimental autoimmune renal cortical tubulointerstitial disease in guinea pigs lacking the fourth component of complement (C4). *J. Immunol.*, **112**, 1387–1393

79. Neilson, E. G. and Phillips, S. M. (1981). Cell-mediated interstitial nephritis IV. Anti-tubular basement membrane antibodies can function in antibody-dependent cellular cytotoxicity reactions: Observations on a nephritogenic effector mechanism acting as an informational bridge between the humoral and cellular immune response. *J. Immunol.*, **126**, 1990–1993

80. Nathan, C. (1987). Secretory products of macrophages. *J. Clin. Invest.*, **79**, 319–326

81. Young, J. D.-E. and Cohn, Z. A. (1987). Cellular and humoral mechanisms of cytotoxicity: structural and functional analogies. *Adv. Immunol.*, **41**, 269–330

82. Neilson, E. G., Jimenez, S. A. and Phillips, S. M. (1980). Cell-mediated interstitial nephritis III. T lymphocyte mediated fibroblast proliferation and collagen synthesis: An immune mechanism for renal fibrogenesis. *J. Immunol.*, **125**, 1708–1714

83. Bender, W. L., Whelton, A., Beschorner, W. E., Darwish, M., Hall-Craggs, M. and Solez, K. (1984). Interstitial nephritis, proteinuria and renal failure caused by nonsteroidal anti-inflammatory drugs. Immunologic characteristics of the inflammatory infiltrate. *Am. J. Med.*, **76**, 1006–1012

84. Brunati, C., Brando, B., Confalonieri, R., Belli, L. S., Lavagni, M. G. and Minetti, L. (1986). Immunophenotyping of mononuclear cell infiltrates associated with renal disease. *Clin. Nephrol.*, **26**, 15–20

85. Husby, G., Tung, K. S. and Williams, R. C. (1981). Characterization of renal tissue lymphocytes in patients with interstitial nephritis. *Am. J. Med.*, **70**, 31–38

86. Zager, R. A., Cotran, R. S. and Hoyer, J. R. (1978). Pathologic localization of Tamm-Horsfall protein in interstitial deposits in renal disease. *Lab. Invest.*, **38**, 52–57

87. Appel, G. B. and Kunis, C. L. (1983). Acute tubulointerstitial nephritis. *Contemp. Issues Nephrol.*, **10**, 151–185

88. McLeish, K. R., Senitzer, D. and Gohara, A. F. (1979). Acute interstitial nephritis in a patient with aspirin hypersensitivity. *Clin. Immunol. Immunopathol.*, **14**, 64–69

89. Lafferty, K. J., Prowse, S. J. and Simeonovic, C. J. (1983). Immunobiology of tissue transplantation: A return to the passenger leukocyte concept. *Annu. Rev. Immunol.*, **1**, 143–173

90. Mayer, T. G., Fuller, A. A., Fuller, T. C., Lazarovits, A. I., Boyle, L. A. and Kurnick, J. T. (1985). Characterization of in vivo activated allospecific T lymphocytes propagated from human renal alograft biopsies undergoing rejection. *J. Immunol.*, **134**, 258–264

91. Halloran, P. F., Jephthah-Ochola, J., Urmson, J. and Farkas, S. (1985). Systemic immunologic stimuli increase class I and class II antigen expression in mouse kidney. *J. Immunol.*, **135**, 1053–1060

92. Van Zwieten, M. J., Leber, P. D., Bhan, A. K. and McCluskey, R. T. (1977). Experimental cell-mediated interstitial nephritis induced with exogenous antigens. *J. Immunol.*, **118**, 589–593

93. Sugisaki, T., Yoshida, T., McCluskey, R. T., Andres, G. A. and Klassen, J. (1980). Autoimmune cell-mediated tubulointerstitial nephritis induced in Lewis rats by renal antigens. *Clin. Immunol. Immunopathol.*, **15**, 33–43

94. Bannister, K. M., Ulich, T. R. and Wilson, C. B. (1987). Induction, characterization and cell transfer of autoimmune tubulointerstitial nephritis in the Lewis rat. *Kidney Int.*, **32**, 642–651

95. Lyon, M. F. and Hulse, E. V. (1971). An inherited kidney disease of mice resembling human nephronophthis. *J. Med. Genet.*, **8**, 41–48
96. Neilson, E. G., McCafferty, E., Feldman, A., Clayman, M., Zakheim, B. and Korngold, R. (1984). Spontaneous interstitial nephritis in kdkd mice I. An experimental model of autoimmune renal disease. *J. Immunol.*, **133**, 2560–2565
97. Kelly, C. J., Korngold, R., Mann, R., Clayman, M., Haverty, T. and Neilson, E. G. (1986). Spontaneous interstitial nephritis in kdkd mice II. Characterization of a tubular antigen-specific, H-2K-restricted Lyt-2$^+$ effector T cell that mediates destructive tubulointerstitial injury. *J. Immunol.*, **136**, 526–531
98. Kelly, C. J. and Neilson, E. G. (1987). Contrasuppression in autoimmunity. Abnormal contrasuppresion promotes the expression of nephritogenic effector T cells and histologic interstitial nephritis in kdkd mice. *J. Exp. Med.*, **165**, 107–123

Index

aetiological fraction (EF), HLA antigens and
        disease   9–10
aggregates, Ig-containing   188–90
    kinetics and clearances   189–90
alkylating agents, MCN   174
allergens, proteinuria in MCN   169
Alport's syndrome, Goodpasture antigen   243
alveolar epithelial injury, IgA complexes   191
ANCA
    disease activity relationships   258–9
    Goodpasture's disease   232–3
    IgG/IgM, systemic vasculitis   259–60
    myeloperoxidase sensitivity   257
    systemic vasculitis   255–63, 265
    types   256–7
anti-GBM antibodies, measurement,
        Goodpasture's disease   235
anti-GBM disease   1, 2–4, 10, 29–31, 229–47
    ANCA positivity   261
    HLA-DR/DQ association   10–11
    nomenclature   229–30
    passive homologous   105
anti-Goodpasture antibodies   243–4
anti-idiotypic antibodies, ANCA binding
        inhibition   263
anti-laminin antibodies   36, 37
anti-mesangial cell antibodies   195
anti-TBM disease
    effector mechanisms   279–80
    target antigen   275–7
antibody-dependent cell-mediated
        cytotoxicity   98, 113
antigen processing   1
antigens, platelet-activated, growth factor
        release   142–3
antiplatelet therapy   146, 203
arachidonic acid metabolism,
        intrarenal   124–5
arboviruses, RPGN   265
Arthus reaction   81
aspirin, low-dose, renal cyclooxygenase
        effects   144
atopy, in MCN   171–2
autoantibodies

IgA nephropathy   194–5
immune reactant synergism   196–7, 198
nephrotoxicity   195–6
autoantigens, and viruses   197, 199
autoimmune glomerulonephritis
    allogeneic reaction-induced   34–5
    bacterial products-induced   33
    drug-induced   35–8
    parasite-induced   33
    and polyclonal activation   32–8
autoimmunity
    glomerular-specific   29–32
    IgA nephropathy   193–9
    mechanisms   194
    organ-specific   272–4
azathioprine   174, 262

B cells
    autoreactive, Heymann nephritis   31, 32
    function, MCN   170–1
    glomerulonephritis   102
    polyclonal activation   33, 36

C3 nephritic factor (NeF)   215
    action mechanisms   217
    atypical factors   219–20
    clinical associations   220
    detection methods   217–19
    historical aspects   215–17
    and local complement activation   223–3
    pathogenetic mechanisms in
            MPGN   221–3
    stabilization assay   219
C4 nephritic factor (C4 Nef)   220
C5b-9 complex   83, 87–90
    as cell function mediator   84–5
    formation   83–4
    glomerular cell stimulation   85, 87
    glomerular reaction mediation   90–1
calcium, intracellular, vasodilator prostaglandin
        release   128–9
CD4+ (helper/inducer) lymphocytes, HLA Class
        II binding   7
CD4+ (helper/inducer) T cells,
        glomerulonephritis   102

CD8 + (suppressor/cytotoxic) T cells   102
  natural killer activity   98–9, 102–3, 113–14
cell-mediated immunity   30–1
  definition/classification   97–9
  demonstration criteria   99–100
  effectors cells   100–4
  glomerulonephritis   97–116, 142
  Goodpasture's disease   244–5
  human glomerulonephritis   114–16
  interstitial nephritis   280–3
  patterns   98–9, 111–14
  T cells/macrophages, crescent formation   114
chlorambucil, MCN   174
Churg–Strauss angiitis   258
CNS lupus, immune complexes   64–5
coeliac disease   187, 190
collagen synthesis, podocyte, C5b-9
    effects   85, 87
collagen type IV   239–40
  novel chains   241–2
competence factors   131
complement
  abnormalities, infections in MCN   172
  activation
    anti-TBM disease   280
    C5b-9 complex formation   83–4
    IgA nephropathy   192
    inflammation mediators   81, 82
  deficiency, SLE   19–20
  and immune complexes   65–7
  leukocytes and glomerulonephritis   81, 82
  and MCN   164, 166
  nucleated cell interaction   84
complotypes   7
coronary arteritis, immune complexes,
    SLE   64
crescentic glomerulonephritis   18
  anti-GBM-mediated   29
cryoglobulinaemia, essential mixed   275
cyclooxygenase pathway inhibition, impaired
    renal function   129
cyclophosphamide   236
  IgA nephropathy   203
  MCN   169, 174
  systemic vasculitis   262, 264
cyclosporin A   109
  IL-2 inhibition   264
  MCN   175
cystic fibrosis   264
cytokines   125–7
  epithelial cells response   104
  in experimental nephritis   141–3
  glomerular cell interaction   129–32
  and human disease   148–9
  renal damage initiation   141
  see also growth factors

D-penicillamine, autoimmunity induction   38,
    233
delayed type hypersensitivity   98
  fibrin role   112
  glomerulonephritis   111–12

dermatitis herpatiformis   187
diabetes, HLA association   11
dietary antigens, IgA nephropathy   187–8
dipeptidyl-peptidase IV, Heymann nephropathy   52
direct cellular cytotoxicity   98–9
DNA amplification technique   5

eicosanoids   124–5
  in experimental glomerulonephritis   133–4
  and glomerular cells   128–9
  polyunsaturated fatty acid
      relationships   139–40
  release by C5b-9   85, 90
  urinary, glomerular disease   143–5
eicosapentanoic acid (EPA)   139, 148
ELAM-1   126
encephalomyelitis, autoimmune, experimental
      (EAE), T cell receptor genes   4
endothelial cells
  antigens, systemic vasculitis   257
  glomerular, cytokine/growth factor
      effects   132–3
  glomerulonephritis   103–4
endotoxin, macrophage activation   109
environmental antigens, hypersensitivity   187–8,
      195–6
epithelial cells
  glomerular, cytokine/growth factor effects
      132–3
  glomerulonephritis   103
Epstein–Barr virus, Kawasaki-like disease   265
erythrocyte CR1
  immune complex transport/
      clearance   68–9, 190, 223
  loss in disease states   70, 71
  NeF effects   223
essential fatty acids, deficiency
  macrophage /inflammatory response effects
      138–9
  SLE   138

fatty acids, dietary manipulation, and renal
      disease   138–41, 147–8
fibrin
  and delayed type hypersensitivity   112
  deposition, crescentic glomerulonephritis
      107
fish oils, renal disease effects   139–41, 147–8
focal glomerulosclerosis   161–2
  lymphokine/circulating factor effects   166–8
focal proliferative glomerulonephritis, anti-GBM
      antibodies   30
GALT, immunoglobulins   199–200
giant cells, interstitial nephritis   271
gliadian, serum IgA binding   187
glomerular basement membrane
  charge, lymphokine/circulating factor effects
      166–8, 176
  Goodpasture antigen studies   238–42
  monocyte TNF and IL-1 synthesis   130
glomerular cells
  antigens, systemic vasculitis   257
  tissue culture studies   127–8

glomerular injury
  immune reactant mechanisms   190–1
  serum antibody mechanisms   187
glomerulonephritis
  C5b-9 complex   83, 87–90
  cell-mediated immunity   97–116, 142
  complement deposits   81
  HLA association   8
  immune negative   115
  macrophage accumulation timing   104–5
  and MHC   2–4
  severity, HLA allele effects   21–2
  virus-induced   275
  see also various types
glomerulosclerosis
  C5b-9 association   87
  fish oil effects   139–40
  thromboxane inhibition effects   136
glucocorticosteroids, MCN   174
gluten, dietary, IgA immune complexes   187, 190
Gm allotypes, SLE   21
gold, autoimmunity induction   38
Goodpasture antigen   229, 237–43
  Alport's syndrome   243
  distribution/localization   235, 237
  nature   238–42
  non-collagenous domain   241–2
Goodpasture's disease   230
  animal models   245–6
  autoantibodies   243–4
  cell-mediated immunity   244–5
  clinical/laboratory features   234–5
  disease associations   232–3
  environmental aspects   231–2
  genetic factors/susceptibility   230, 231, 233
  HLA associations   231, 233
  immunopathogenesis   243–7
  incidence   230–1
  mediators   247
  resolution   236–7
  treatment   230, 236
Goodpasture's syndrome   10, 229, 234
gp330   48–52
graft-versus-host reaction (GVHR)   30
granulomata, cell-mediated immune
      response   105
growth factors   125
  cell cycle functions   131
  cell surface receptor interaction   142–3
  glomerular cell interaction   129–32

haematuria
  IgA nephropathy   193
  and IgA secretion   200
Henoch–Schönlein nephritis   202–3
  steroid-responsive   203–4
Henoch–Schönlein purpura   185, 193, 194,
      202–3
  anti-mesangial cell antibodies   195, 196
  rheumatoid factors   195
  serological abnormalities   202
hepatic dysfunction, IgA nephropathy   201–2

5-HETE   128
12-HETE   128, 136
Heymann nephritis   4, 12, 31–2, 45–6, 275
  complement fractions and proteinuria   88
  immune deposit formation   50–2
  immune deposit origins   46–7
  microvillar protein role   52
  nephritogenic antigen   47–50
  passive/active   46
HLA antigens
  disease association strength   8–10
  disease and racial groups   8
  HLA Class I genes, loci   5
  HLA Class II β chain genes   6
  HLA Class II genes, loci   5
  HLA Class II pseudogenes   5
  HLA Class III region   7
  HLA-A2, structure   6
HLA-DR
  anti-GBM disease association   10–11
  idiopathic membranous nephropathy
      association   12–14
  TNF secretion effects   21
HLA-DR7
  atopy and MCN   171
  minimal-change nephropathy   164
Hodgkin's disease, Goodpasture's disease   233
humoral immunity, interstitial nephritis   282
humoral responses, systemic vasculitis   258–62
hydrocarbons, Goodpasture's disease   232
hypercoagulability, anti-cardiolipin
      antibodies   64
hypocomplementaemia, systemic, MPGN   222

ICAM-1   126
IgA, glomerular deposit generation   191–2
IgA complexes, alveolar epithelial injury   191
IgA immune response, induction   186–8
IgA nephropathy   183–202
  anti-mesangial cell antibodies   195, 196
  autoimmunity   193–9
  complement activation   192
  environmental antigen hypersensitivity   187–8
  experimental   191–3
  hepatic dysfunction   201–2
  HSP vasculitis   202, 203
  Ig-containing aggregates   188–90
  IgA/IgG kappa:lambda ratios   187
  immune complexes, mucosal surface   185–6
  immunoregulation   200–1
  mucosal immunity   184–6
  polyclonal B cell activation   194
  rheumatoid factors   195
  treatment   203–4
  urinary abnormalities and immune reactants
      192–3
  virus infections   194, 199
IgA nephropathy, mesangial   14–16
  complement-derived mediators   83
  D-penicillamine   38
  familial incidence   14
  HLA association   14–16, 22

HLA and race 8
IgA-IgM mesangial proliferative
    nephropathy 191
IgG, GBM linear binding, RPGN 234
IgG anti-mesangial cell antibodies,
    nephritis 196–7, 198
immune complexes
    and aggregates 188
    C1q binding 60
    and complement 65–7
    composition/size, SLE 60–1
    cross-linking 51
    formation 191–2
    Heymann nephritis 46–7
    inflammatory damage mechanisms 63–4
    MCN 172
    mucosal surface-derived 185–6
    red cell CR1 binding 68
    renal localization 61–4
    SLE severity 60
    soluble clearance 67–72
    subendothelial/mesangial 63
    subepithelial 61, 63
    transport defects and NeF 223
immune responses
    efferent/effector phase 274
    T cell-mediated, parenchymal antigen 272–3
immunization, antigen-specific immune
    response 186
immunoglobulins, immunoadsorption 236
immunoregulation 199–200
infections, and MCN onset 172–3
interleukin-1 (IL-1) 91, 107, 125, 126
    experimental nephritis 141–3
    mesangial cell effects 107, 132
    synthesis, C5b-9 85, 86, 90
interstitial nephritis 271–283
    anti-TBM antibody-associated 275–9
    drug therapy-related 275
    immune complex-mediated 274–5
    T cell-mediated 280–3
    target antigen expression 275–7

Kawasaki disease 258, 264, 265
Kussmaul–Meier disease 258

lactate dehydrogenase (LDH) virus, SLE
    development inhibition 21
leukocyte antigens, systemic vasculitis 256–7
leukotrienes
    efferent glomerular arteriolar resistance
        137
    glomerular injury 128, 134
    nephrotoxic serum nephritis 136–7
levamisole, MCN 175
lipoxygenase products, inhibition, and glomerular
    injury 136–7
lung disease, immune complexes, SLE 64
lupus erythematosus, systemic see systemic lupus
    erythematosus (SLE)
lupus nephritis
    interleukin-1/TNF 107

murine 38–9
    polyunsaturated fatty acid effects 139
lymphocytes
    blastogenesis inhibitor 168
    transformation by mitogens 169
    see also B cells; T cells
lymphokines 125
lymphoma, Goodpasture's disease 233
lymphomas, and MCN 173

3M-1 antigen 276–9
    immune response modulation 278–9
macrophage procoagulant inducing factor 112
macrophages
    binding to GBM 129–30
    cell-mediated immune
        glomerulonephritis 100–1
    depletion/repletion, glomerular injury 105,
        107
    glomerular
        activation regulation 108–9
        effector function/activation status 107–8
        glomerulonephritis mediation 104–9
        mesangial cell interaction 130
Masugi (nephrotoxic) nephritis 191, 193
membrane attack complex (MAC), and
        complement activation 192
membranoproliferative glomerulonephritis
        (MPGN)
    historical aspects 215–17
    types 221
membranous nephropathy
    experimental 45
    familial, HLA association 12
    HLA associations 164
        RR/EF differences 9–10
    HLA and race 8
    lymphokine/circulating factor effects
        166–8
membranous nephropathy, idiopathic
        (IMN) 11–14, 22
mercuric chloride
    autoimmunity induction 35–8
    B cell polyclonal activation 36
mesangial cells
    glomerulonephritis 103
    proliferation, PDGF effects 131
    TNF and growth response 132
methicillin, interstitial nephritis association 275
MHC
    antigen bearing T cell receptor binding 2
    extended haplotypes 7–8
    human 3, 4–10
    structure 165
migration–inhibition factor, lymphocyte
        release 115
minimal-change nephropathy (MCN) 115
    aetiology/pathogenesis 175–6
    associated diseases 172–4
    atopy 171–2
    B cell function 170–1
    definition 161–2

drug-induced 173-4
familial history 162
genetics 162-6
histology 162
HLA associations 16-17, 18, 161, 162-6
HLA and race 8
HLA-B8/B12 and severity 22
humoral response 170-1
immune complexes 172
immunogenetics 161, 162-6
lymphokine/circulating factor effects 166-8
MHC Class III associations 164, 166
monocyte/lymphocyte relationships 170
patients' lymphocyte function 168-71
T-suppressor cell function 169
treatment 174-5
mitogens 125
monocytes, cell-mediated immune
glomerulonephritis 100-1
monokines 125
mononuclear cells, interstitial nephritis 271
MT DR antigens 13
mucosal immunity, IgA nephropathy 184-6
myeloproliferative nephritis, C3-nephritic factor-
positive 89-90

natural killer activity, cytotoxic T cells 98-9,
102-3, 113-14
nephritic factors (NeFs) see C3 nephritic factor
(NeF); C4 nephritic factor
nephritis
autoimmunity 1
immunogenetics 1-22
progression and NeF 224
nephrotic syndrome
eicosanoid effects 133
indomethacin and dextran clearance 145
proteinuria, thromboxane role 146-7
TNF levels 148-9
neutrophil cytoplasm, autoantibodies to see
ANCA
neutrophils, role in glomerulonephritis 81-2
NSAIDs
IgA nephropathy 203
MCN association 173-4
urinary prostaglandins 144

organ-specific autoimmunity 272-4

parenchymal antigens, interstitial nephritis 273
penicillamine
autoimmunity induction 38
Goodpasture's disease 233
pericarditis, SLE, immune complexes 64
phospholipase A_2, translocation/release, TNF
and IL-1 132
plasma exchange 203, 236
systemic vasculitis 262-3
platelet-activating factor 127
platelet-derived growth factor (PDGF) 127
platelets
activated, growth factor release 142
in experimental glomerulonephritis 133
glomerulosclerosis 145-6

polyarteritis, microscopic (MPA) 18, 19, 232,
255, 260
polyarteritis nodosa, hepatitis B-associated
258
polycoclonal B cell activation (PCBA) 194
polymerase chain reaction (PCR) 5
polymers, IgA-containing, nephritis 188
polymorphonuclear leukocytes (PMN),
GBM 130
polyunsaturated fatty acids, renal disease
effects 139-41
post-streptococcal glomerulonephritis
(PSGN) 17-18
prednisolone 236, 262
preventive fraction (PF), HLA antigens and
disease 9-10
primary nephropathies, secretory component
absence 185-6
procoagulant activity 111-112
progression factors 131
prostacyclin (PGI$_2$) 127, 128-9
prostaglandin E_2 126, 128-9, 134
seminal fluid 144
synthesis, IL-1/TNF effects 129
prostaglandin $F_{2\alpha}$ 128
prostaglandins, renal failure protective effects
137-8
proteinuria
cyclooxygenase inhibitors 145
IgA nephropathy 193
lymphokine/circulating factor effects
166-8, 176
thromboxanes 135

rapidly progressive glomerulonephritis
(RPGN) 18-19, 229-47
ANCA/anti-GBM antibody binding 261
HLA-DR association 19
T cell autoreactivity 263
reactive oxygen species 113
relative risk (RR), HLA antigens and
disease 8-10
renal allografts, NeF and MPGN 224
renal failure, dialysis-dependent 236
renal homeostasis, vasodilator/vasoconstrictor
balance 144
renal insufficiency, tubulointerstitial fibrosis
276
renal transplantation, postoperative
Goodpasture's disease 237
renal tubular antigen 276-7
renal tubular epithelial cells, antigen-presenting
cells 277
restriction fragment length polymorphism (RFLP)
analysis, MHC genes 5
reticuloendothelial saturation, immune
complexes 67
rheumatoid arthritis, anti-nuclear antibodies 256
rheumatoid factors 195, 196-7, 198

scarlatina, nephritis 1
scleroderma 257

serum sickness 1, 46, 184–5, 275
Shalhoub's hypothesis, MCN 167, 175
Sjögren's syndrome 275
skin, immune complexes, SLE 64
smoking, lung haemorrhage 232
spleen, hypofunction, nephrotic syndrome 172
Steblay nephritis 245–6
steroid-resistant nephrotic syndrome
    (SRNS) 174
steroid-responsive nephrotic syndrome (SRNS),
    HLA associations 163–4, 166
systemic lupus erythematosus (SLE) 19–21, 59,
    257
  AIgG clearance 67–8
  circulating immune complexes,
      measurement 59–61
  essential fatty acid deficiency effects 138
  HLA-DR association 20
  immune complexes
    clearance mechanisms 65–73
    tissue injury 61–5
  interstitial nephritis 275
  low erythrocyte CR1 70, 71, 72
  neutrophil/lymphocyte CR1 loss 72
  prostaglandin effects 138
  red cell defective adherence 68–9
  urinary thromboxane levels 145, 146
  see also lupus nephritis
systemic vasculitis
  aetiology 264–5
  anti-Goodpasture antibodies 232–3
  autoantigens 256–8
  B cell responses 262–3
  classification 260–1
  definition 255
  genetic mechanisms 264
  HLA associations 264
  humoral responses 258–62, 263
  infection association 264–5
  morphological classification 255, 256
  pathophysiology 262
  T cell response 263–4
  treatment 262–3

T cell antigens, systemic vasculitis 258
T cells
  autoreactive, Heymann nephritis 31, 32
  cell-mediated immune glomerulonephritis
      101–2

glomerulonephritis initiation/mediation
    109–11
  receptor genes 4
Takayasu's disease 258
tetanus immunization, polymeric/monomeric IgA
    antibodies 186
thromboxane A$_2$ (TXA$_2$), vasoconstriction
    135
thromboxane B$_2$ (TXB$_2$) 128
thromboxane receptors, blockade 147
thromboxane synthase inhibition
  endoperoxide accumulation 147
  GFR effects 135–6
  nephropathy progression effects 135–6
thromboxanes
  in experimental glomerulonephritis 133–4
  and glomerular damage 145, 146–7
  inhibition, experimental nephritis 134–6
thymectomy, autoimmune nephritis 31, 32
tissue factor 112
tonsillectomy, in IgA nephropathy 203
tonsils, abnormalities, IgA-positive plasma
    cells 185
trimolecular complex (MHC/antigen/T cell
    receptors) 2
tubulointerstitial nephritis see interstitial nephritis
tumour necrosis factor (TNF) 107, 113, 125,
    126–7
  experimental nephritis 141–3
  mesangial cell effects 132
  SLE 20

vascular permeability, lymphokine/circulating
    factor effects 166–8
vasculitis 275
  renal-limited, anti-myeloperoxidase
      ANCA 260
  small vessel 18, 19
  see also systemic vasculitis
vasoconstrictors, vasodilator prostaglandin
    release 128
viruses, and autoantigens 197, 199

Wegener's granulomatosis 18, 19, 232, 255
  ANCA 260
  HLA associations 264
  respiratory T cell autoreactivity 263